SOUTHERN MISSIONARY COLLEGE
Division of Nursing Library Southern Missionary College
Division Of Nursing, Library
711 Lake Estelle Drive
Orlando, Florida 32803

Fundamentals of patient-centered nursing

2013
DF

ILLUSTRATED

Fundamentals of patient-centered nursing

RUTH V. MATHENEY, R.N., Ed.D.
Professor and Chairman, Department of Nursing,
Nassau Community College, Garden City, N. Y.

BREDA T. NOLAN, R.N., M.A.
Assistant Professor, Department of Nursing,
Nassau Community College, Garden City, N. Y.

ALICE M. EHRHART, R.N., M.A.
Assistant Professor, Department of Nursing,
Bronx Community College of the City University
of New York, Bronx, N. Y.

GERALD J. GRIFFIN, R.N., M.A.
Associate Professor and Head, Department of Nursing,
Bronx Community College of the City University
of New York, Bronx, N. Y.

JOANNE KING GRIFFIN, R.N., M.A.
Lecturer in Nursing Science, Department of Nursing,
Bronx Community College of the City University
of New York, Bronx, N. Y.

WY
100
F981

4039

The C. V. Mosby Company SAINT LOUIS 1964

SOUTHERN MISSIONARY COLLEGE
Division of Nursing Library

Copyright © 1964 by

The C. V. Mosby Company

All rights reserved

Printed in the United States of America

Library of Congress Catalog Card Number 64-10798

Distributed in Great Britain by Henry Kimpton, London

Preface

T̶his book is designed for beginning students in nursing and is based upon fundamental concepts that are applicable to all clinical areas in nursing. As such, it provides the basis upon which the unique aspects of each of the major clinical areas (medicine, surgery, obstetrics, pediatrics, and psychiatry) can be built. Because of the approach used, the book necessarily draws something from each of the clinical areas, and the material from each is included here because it applies to every other area. The fundamentals of nursing fall into four broad areas: (1) the basic needs of patients for physical hygiene and comfort, safely provided, (2) the general patterns of physical or overt health problems that patients may face, (3) the psychological need for a recognition of the patient as a person with his own uniqueness, and (4) the rehabilitative needs of patients with life modifications so common in long-term illness. All four aspects are presented on a fundamental level.

Certain assumptions underlie the use of this book. One important assumption is that even a fundamental or first course in nursing does not exist in a vacuum but rests upon knowledge acquired in the areas of the social, biological, and physical sciences. Therefore, the science knowledge from these fields is not repeated in detail. Certain key concepts from social and biological sciences are identified and repeated for emphasis, but, in general, a basic knowledge of human biology, sociology, and psychology is assumed. Students either may have had the courses or may be taking them concurrently. In addition, no attempt has been made to duplicate, to any great extent, content material from traditional text areas such as nutrition and diet therapy or pharmacology. Texts on these subjects may be used in conjunction with this book.

Very basic concepts are presented in the early units and are referred to in later chapters. It is hoped that references to such material will be taken seriously, for going back to review in the light of increasing knowledge and increasing experience should build depth in such concepts.

The emphasis here is upon fundamental concepts, not upon procedures and techniques. The teaching of details, particularly of procedures, is best done in the actual setting, consistent with the particular procedure used there as an illustration of the application of scientific principles.

Throughout the book, the interrelationships of systems, the physical-emotional-cultural interrelationship within the individual, and the unity of man have been stressed. Nursing care is for people, and each person is unique. Therefore, each nursing care plan is unique and must be designed for the specific patient with recognition of all the factors that affect his total behavior.

Since this is a fundamentals text, development of observational skills is stressed throughout.

The bibliography is a selected rather than a comprehensive one. Recent and pertinent material has been indicated, and, in addition, primary sources of material have been identified.

Appreciation must first be expressed to the many students in nursing who have taught us not only how to teach but how to enjoy teaching. We are grateful to colleagues at Nassau Community College, Bronx Community College, and Queens College of the City of New York who have participated in the development of the approach to fundamentals of nursing presented here. Our appreciation is also extended to the members of the staff of the Meadowbrook Hospital, Long Island, N. Y., who were so pleasantly cooperative in providing space, equipment, and personnel for pictures. In particular, Miss Edith M. Augustson, Associate Director of Nursing Education at Meadowbrook Hospital, was extremely helpful. To Miss Evelyn P. Straus, photographer, supporter, and encourager, we are all grateful for the hours of work that went into getting illustrations ready. To Mrs. Estelle Rancer who labored faithfully and diligently (and with an accurate eye for grammar and spelling) on the manuscript, our thanks!

Ruth V. Matheney
Breda T. Nolan
Alice M. Ehrhart
Gerald J. Griffin
Joanne King Griffin

Contents

8   *Contents*

Overt nursing problems

Rehabilitation problems

Appendix, 325

Glossary, 332

Fundamentals of patient-centered nursing

Health problems and nursing

Chapter 1

Health problems and health teams

Nursing constitutes one of the occupational groups involved in providing health services to society. Health is the concern of many, and the provision of health services has become a major business.

What is health? The Constitution of the World Health Organization states that "health is a state of complete physical, mental and social well-being and not just the absence of disease or infirmity." It further states that "the enjoyment of the highest attainable standard of health is one of the fundamental rights of every human being without distinction of race, religion, political belief, economic or social condition" and that "the health of all peoples is fundamental to the attainment of peace and security and is dependent upon the fullest co-operation of individuals and States."

Looking at the multitude of factors that influence health on a broad, world-wide scale, they tend to fall into three major categories: social, economic, and cultural. Yet, even these cannot be wholly separated. Their interrelatedness and interdependency becomes self-evident.

The effect of social and economic conditions on health has long been recognized. In the presence of disease there is loss of wages, coupled with the concurrent cost of medical care and the loss of earning capacity. All of these combine to produce a very real and direct economic loss. By the same token, social and economic factors act to influence the occurrence of disease. For example, they:

1. Determine the character of home environment
2. Determine character of food and nutrition
3. May determine unhygienic industrial conditions
4. May make it impossible for necessary care and attention to home and family
5. Determine availability of qualified medical care and treatment and the possibility of following such advice
6. Determine character of personal hygiene
7. Determine amount of healthful recreation
8. Determine degree of community education*

---

*Bolduan, Charles F.: Public health and hygiene, Philadelphia, 1929, W. B. Saunders Co., pp. 37-39.

SOUTHERN MISSIONARY COLLEGE
Division of Nursing Library

That "health is wealth" is a truth expressed in varying forms in nearly every language of the world.

"Without health—in the fullest meaning of the word—man cannot produce according to his needs. He cannot raise his standard of life. He is condemned forever to be the slave of his environment.

"Given health his labor can reap the full reward of its merits. He can grow more, make more and eat better. He can achieve and maintain a state of complete well-being."[*]

The influence of culture on the health of individuals or groups is equally as revealing. Jacques May describes Northern Vietnam where the terrain is such that the people live either in the very fertile delta region where rice is grown or in the less fertile hill region with forest cover where lumber is abundant. These two regions account for only two cultural, but important, differences.

In the delta, houses are built on the ground with stables on one side of the house and the kitchen on the other. Meals are brought into the house after being cooked.

In the hill region, houses are built on stilts rising eight to ten feet above ground. Animals are kept under the houses, and cooking is done in the living rooms which are usually filled with smoke. There is a very fierce malaria vector found in this hill region. However, the mosquitoes seldom fly above nine to ten feet and so encounter only the animals under the houses. In addition the fumes and smoke within the houses play a role in driving away any mosquitoes who find themselves up there.

In the delta region, there is no such malaria vector. However, there is economic pressure from overpopulation of this fertile area. People from the delta, seeking relocation in the hills where space is abundant, take their delta culture with them. They build their houses on the ground, keep their animals outside, and keep their houses free of smoke by cooking outdoors.

As a result, the mosquito becomes an active transmitter of malaria. The people of the delta have become discouraged from participating in relocation plans, believing there are "evil spirits" in the hills that do not like delta people.

May further describes a small Chinese village in which one-half of the inhabitants were nearly decimated by a hookworm infestation. The other half of the village had no such health problem. In exploring the local cultures, the following was revealed:

1. Almost all the patients were rice growers who spent their working hours knee deep in mud, which explained the penetration of the hookworm larvae through the skin.
2. The healthy people bought their rice and had nothing to do

_____

[*]Chisholm, Brock: WHO Newsletter, vol. VI, no. 3, March 1953, p. 3.

with its cultivation. Further, they were engaged in silkworm farming and spent their working hours on ladders tending mulberry trees.*

It becomes apparent very quickly that social, economic, and cultural conditions affect health. This is not, however, a one-way street. The relationship is a reciprocal one, each influencing the other.

CHANGING WORLD—CHANGING HEALTH PROBLEMS

We are living in an era of profound changes. Technological and scientific advances have, in a large measure, enabled man to understand and to control his environment.

The diseases that killed our great-grandfathers, often while they were still young, are decreasing in importance almost everywhere. Yet, this intensive technical and scientific progress, which continues to transform the lives of people everywhere, subjects man to new stresses. Dr. H. von Zile Hyde has described these changes as having three basic forms: chemical, physical, and social.†

Chemical changes

Synthetic organic chemicals and radiation wastes are a major characteristic of our era. These chemicals are finding their way increasingly into our water supply, the food we eat, the medications we take, and the air we breathe.

Thousands of industrial plants discharge their chemical wastes into our rivers and streams. Population wastes, such as detergents, and agricultural poisons, like fertilizers, find their way into our water supply.

Chemicals are added to food to modify its color, taste, texture, appearance, stability, and nutritive value. Insecticides are used in the cultivation of fruits and vegetables. The ever increasing practice of self-medication adds to man's intake of inorganic chemicals. Many of these chemicals are not always adequately tested for their effect on man.

Gases are discharged into the air each day by motor vehicles and industry. Air pollution results from virtually the same causes as water pollution. In some areas, this is further compounded because of geography and weather conditions. The "smog" in Southern California and in England is a case in point. The continued testing of atomic weapons by the great national powers has caused widespread concern. The potential health hazard in the presence of a continuing increase in "radioactive fall-out" is of almost incomprehensible magnitude.

---

*May, Jacques: The ecology of human disease, Annals of the New York Academy of Sciences 84:789, 1960-1961.
†Hyde, H. von Zile: A glance back and a look forward—ten years of public health progress, Office of Public Information, Pan-American Sanitary Bureau, Regional Office of WHO, 1958.

Physical changes

This is an age of ever-increasing speed—the age of the superhighway and the jet-propelled plane. As greater speeds are attained in vehicles operating in the air, on the highway, and on the sea, new hazards are created in our environment. In many countries, automobile accidents are emerging as one of the leading causes of death.

Social changes

In the presence of this ever-changing physical environment, our social environment is becoming increasingly more complex. Changes often come suddenly, with little time for adjustment. The abrupt introduction of mechanization and automation sweeps custom and tradition aside by its assault.

This rapid progress brings stress in its wake, the effects of which cannot be ignored. The number of persons with mental disease in some of the highly industrialized countries give stark evidence of the toll of this intense social strain.

CURRENT HEALTH PROBLEMS

While this changing world has produced new problems, it has eliminated many of the old ones. In the presence of technical and scientific progress, what has evolved as current major health problems?

Table 1. *Expectation of life at birth* (Industrial policyholders,†*
Metropolitan Life Insurance Company, 1879-1894 to 1962)

Calendar year	Expectation in years	Calendar year	Expectation in years	Calendar year	Expectation in years
1962	70.9	1946‡	65.6	1930	57.4
1961	70.8	1945‡	64.9	1929	55.8
1960	70.5	1944‡	64.4	1928	55.9
1959	70.4	1943‡	63.9	1927	56.4
1958	70.1	1942‡	64.3	1926	55.0
1957	70.0	1941	63.4	1925	55.5
1956	70.2	1940	62.9	1924	55.6
1955	70.0	1939	62.5	1923	54.5
1954‡	69.8	1938	61.9	1922	55.0
1953‡	68.9	1937	60.7	1921	55.1
1952‡	68.5	1936	60.3	1919–20	51.1
1951‡	68.4	1935	60.2	1911–12	46.6
1950‡	68.3	1934	59.5	1909	46.3
1949	67.7	1933	59.2	1879–94	34.0
1948	67.2	1932	58.8		
1947	66.5	1931	57.9		

Gain, 1962 since 1909, 24.6 years; since 1879-1894, 36.9 years

*Statistical bulletins, 1963; courtesy Metropolitan Life Insurance Co.
†The figures for 1954 and prior years relate to weekly and monthly premium-paying policies; those for 1955-1962 include, in addition, persons with premium-paying ordinary policies for small amounts of insurance.
‡Excludes death from enemy action.

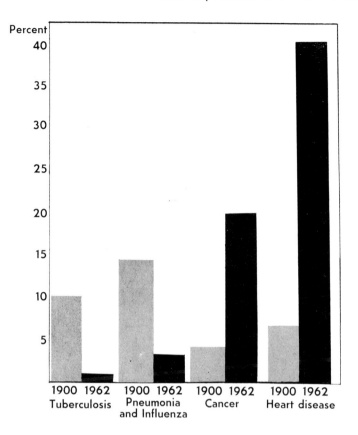

Fig. 1. Change in percentage cause of total deaths—two leading causes 1900-1962.

In the United States, life expectancy has increased from 46.3 years in 1909 to some 70 years in 1962 (Table 1). This accomplishment means larger numbers reach comparatively old age. The chronic and degenerative diseases associated with an older population are becoming more prominent. Heart disease, cancer, and diabetes rank among the top five leading causes of death in the United States.

The stresses in a rapidly changing world have been described earlier. As a greater percent of the total population continues to reach an increased age, mental health will persist as a major health problem.

Communicable diseases have been largely brought under control. This is primarily due to immunization, sanitation, and the advent of new drugs, principally antibiotics. In 1900, tuberculosis and pneumonia ranked first and second as causes of death. Although they cannot be entirely overlooked, they are well down on the list of major health problems. This is generally true of all communicable diseases.

However, one has only to read a newspaper or magazine to realize there is current reemphasis on communicable diseases. In this age of jet travel, once inaccessible corners of the world have become pleasant stopovers on a vacation itinerary. The recent worldwide spread of Asian influenza and the more limited spread of typhoid fever from a ski resort in Switzerland serve to remind us that such diseases can travel thousands of miles a day.

The treatment of communicable diseases and eradication of the causative agents have recently come under closer scrutiny. Prolonged use of antibiotics and insecticides has produced resistance to them. Some malaria vectors have developed resistance to DDT, some bacteria have changed their characteristics so as to survive in the presence of certain antibiotics, and human beings have developed resistance to specific antibiotics after prolonged use. All of these factors serve as reminders that communicable diseases cannot be entirely ignored as health problems.

Some twenty or thirty years ago, accidents ranked seventh as a leading cause of death in the United States. Today they rank third. The majority are accounted for by accidents in the home and on the highway. Increasing speeds and superhighways leave in their wake about 38,000 deaths and 1,400,000 disabling injuries in the United States each year. Industrial accidents continue to decline, largely due to improved working conditions and to intensive safety campaigns.

In taking a broad look at our health situation, we see that life expectancy has been increased to some seventy years, that communicable diseases have been brought under control, and that chronic diseases, accidents, and mental illness evolve as the major health problems. These phenomena, however, are true for the most part only in the Western Hemisphere, and more specifically in the United States. They are equally untrue for more than half the total population of the world.

A look at the worldwide health situation soon reveals a totally different picture. The leading cause of death in the world is malaria. Yet, it is almost nonexistent in the United States. Although pneumonia has tended to level off, it is still among the top ten leading causes of death in many underdeveloped countries. In Europe, venereal disease is the second greatest health problem. It is readily apparent that communicable diseases rank as major international health problems.

The greatest single health problem facing the world at the present time is not a "disease"—but malnutrition. Hundreds of millions of people are starving. In the presence of this problem, the world's population will double within the next forty-one years. This means adding more to our numbers than has been added in the whole period of human existence.* This "population explosion" in the presence of an already existing food problem presents a staggering prospect for the future of the world.

RESOURCES FOR HEALTH—
WORLD, NATIONAL, STATE, AND LOCAL

It is readily apparent that such complex and far-reaching problems cannot be handled by any one organization. As a result, many

---

*Chisholm, Brock: The expanding concept of public health, American Journal of Public Health **50**:88-94, June 1960.

groups are involved in the provision of health facilities. These organizations are of two types: official (nonvoluntary) and nonofficial (voluntary). Official or nonvoluntary agencies are tax supported and operated by federal, state, or local governments. Nonofficial or voluntary agencies are supported by donations, endowments, patients' fees, campaign subscriptions, etc.

World agencies

The most comprehensive, worldwide organization is the World Health Organization. Its Constitution was adopted in 1946 in conformity with the Charter of the United Nations. It has as its objective "the attainment by all peoples of the highest possible level of health."

This organization functions as the coordinator of international health. It provides assistance to government and groups through information and counsel, technical assistance, and, in emergencies, direct aid. It is concerned with the improvement of sanitary conditions and the prevention of infectious and contagious diseases. It also recommends standards for food and drugs, provides statistical services, and promotes improved standards of education in related health fields.

Because of the broad scope of its activities, the World Health Organization functions primarily through committees, commissions, institutions, and other organizations as necessary. It is sponsored by the governments which are members of the United Nations and, as such, is an official agency.

There are also international voluntary organizations concerned with health. The International Red Cross and the Rockefeller Foundation are examples. The International Red Cross is perhaps most widely known for its relief activities associated with war and disaster. The Rockefeller Foundation is primarily concerned with research related to health problems. Most professional organizations also have international branches, such as the International Medical Association and the International Congress of Nurses. These, too, are voluntary organizations concerned with improvement of standards of education and practice as well as exchange of information and research in the interest of advancement of health practices.

National agencies

The Constitution of the United States does not specifically delegate health responsibilities to the Federal Government, but rather to the states. Yet, the government has long been associated with problems of health through the establishment of various agencies, through financial support to state health programs, and through other departments whose functions in some way affect health. The Children's Bureau, the Food and Drug Administration, and the Veterans Administration are examples of such agencies and departments. The United States Public Health Service came into existence in 1798, not as a federal agency originally but as a voluntary relief agency for merchant seamen.

Over the years there has been considerable reorganization until in 1953 the Department of Health, Education, and Welfare was established. This brought many of the existing agencies under one department which is concerned with all matters pertaining to economic security, education, and health. The Secretary of this Department has Cabinet rank.

It is not possible to discuss all the numerous federal agencies concerned with health. A few, however, bear mentioning. The United States Public Health Service is the oldest of the federal agencies concerned with health problems. It provides medical care for merchant seamen through what have come to be known as "marine hospitals." It is responsible for the Quarantine Service, the maintenance of specialized hospitals for the care of alcoholics and narcotic addicts, and the prevention and control of communicable diseases. It is vitally concerned with health education and with research both through its own activities and by financial grants to individuals and groups engaged in research activity. The National Institutes of Health in Bethesda, Maryland, is the research center for the Public Health Service. The Veterans Administration, while concerned with a wide variety of veterans' services, is extensively engaged in the provision of medical and hospital services for veterans. It maintains 169 hospitals and a large number of outpatient treatment centers throughout the United States. As such, it is the largest single medical service program in the world.

There are numerous national voluntary agencies concerned with health. The American Heart Association, the American Cancer Society, the National Tuberculosis Association, and the March of Dimes are examples. These agencies, as their names indicate, are concerned with specific diseases. They engage in research and education and assist in the provision of facilities necessary for the care of persons with these particular health problems. The Rockefeller Foundation, the Ford Foundation, and the Commonwealth Fund, as voluntary agencies, engage in and/or provide large financial grants for research and education in the field of health. The professional organizations, such as the American Medical Association, the American Dental Association, the American Nurses Association and the National League for Nursing are also examples of voluntary agencies.

State agencies

As noted earlier, the Constitution gives the states the power and responsibility for health services. The major agency at the state level is known as a department of health under the direction of a commissioner of health. State departments of health generally provide a wide range of services. They engage in the control of communicable diseases, sanitation, and laboratory services and in the maintenance of hospitals, especially those for the care of the mentally ill. They are concerned with research and with education through their support of medical, dental, and nursing schools. A state department of health is an official agency supported by state and/or federal funds.

Voluntary agencies at the state level are generally branches of the national voluntary agencies.

Local agencies

The local agency is known as a county or city department of health and is also headed by a commissioner of health. These agencies are engaged in services similar to the state agencies, but their activities are generally local in scope. A department of health on a local level is an official agency supported by local and/or state funds. There are other official agencies whose activities are concerned with community health. The fire and police departments are readily recognized as such agencies at the local level.

Voluntary agencies on the local level are usually smaller functioning units of the national and state voluntary agencies.

Although there are basically four levels (world, national, state, and local) of health agencies, their activities are not confined to a specific level. They work cooperatively with each other and with related agencies in the interest of improved health for all people.

THE HEALTH TEAM

Many occupational groups are involved in the provision of health services to society. The groups make up what is known as the health team. Basic to an understanding of the health team is the recognition that the patient is the most important member of the team. It is his health problems that are the focus of all health activities. Yet many concerned with health services make their contributions to society as a whole rather than directly to the individual patient. For this reason, consideration of the team will be on three levels: the over-all health team, the professional health team, and the nursing team.

Over-all health team

The general fields of science and technology are basic to all activities related to health. The fields concerned are numerous. It is not possible to list all of them, but to indicate the following few will suffice to show the variety and scope: biology, chemistry, physics, sociology, and mathematics. Those actively engaged in these basic fields may be concerned primarily with study and research or with the application of this knowledge to specific health situations.

Sanitary engineers are concerned with water supplies, sewage disposal, drainage, lighting, heating, ventilation, etc. Veterinarians are concerned with diseases of animals that may affect human beings (bovine tuberculosis, rabies, and others); entomologists, with the study of disease-bearing insects; and mathematicians, with formulas and testing procedures used in the interpretation of numerical data. These are only a few occupational groups whose contributions to society make them indispensable members of the over-all health team.

Professional health team

The professional health team functions in a more circumscribed environment, namely, the home, physician's office, hospital, or other health agencies.

The physician is the leader of the professional health team. Although he is responsible for the patient's total medical care plan, certain responsibilities are delegated to others. The addition of others to the team is determined by the degree and variety of the patient's health problems.

Members of the team are the patient and his family, the physician, graduate nurse, social worker, nutritionist, clergyman, physical therapist, occupational therapist, and members of other allied professional groups. Participation by these members will be more or less active, depending on the patient's response to illness and to therapy.

Nursing team

The nursing team functions in much the same environment as the professional health team. The patient and his family and the graduate nurse are members of both the professional health team and the nursing team. As such, they function as a liaison between the two teams. As previously noted, certain aspects of the total medical care plan are delegated to others. Those responsibilities delegated to the graduate nurse may not be met by the nurse as an individual, but rather by the nursing team.

The nursing team is most easily identified as it is seen on the ward unit of a hospital. Members of the nursing team are the patient and his family, the graduate nurse, the student nurse, the practical nurse, auxiliary personnel, and volunteers. The graduate nurse, as the leader of the nursing team, is responsible for the total nursing care of the patient. However, certain aspects of care may be delegated to other team members. To do this, a sound knowledge of the preparation, experience, and capabilities of each team member is essential. The backgrounds of the team members are as varied as the individual members themselves. There are, however, some broad generalities that apply to the various groups of nursing service personnel.

Variations in patterns of nursing education are discussed later in this chapter. The preparation of auxiliary personnel (hospital aides, orderlies, attendants, and others) varies with each hospital. Most hospitals provide some form of organized, on-the-job training program. In others, however, the training is dependent on orientation by the personnel of the patient care unit. Volunteers usually are not regular members of the unit personnel, but may vary from day to day. They usually come to the hospital through community service organizations, such as Red Cross, B'nai Brith, and American Legion, but may also be individuals who volunteer their time for the benefit of hospitalized patients without associating with any organization. Some may have specific preparation, like the Red Cross nurse's aides, and others may or may not have any preparation or experience. Generally speaking, auxiliary personnel and volunteers can do simple functions based on common knowledge.

The success of any team is dependent on the desire to work with others toward a common goal. The patient and his health problems are the point of departure and focus of all activities of the nursing team. Among the members there must be recognition, acceptance, and understanding of the goal, knowledge of the capabilities and responsibilities of each member, and coordinated planning and evaluation of activities with provision for full two-way communication both vertically and horizontally.

If the personnel is to successfully meet the needs of the individual patient or groups of patients, there must be *teamwork*. Basic to any team activity is the recognition that each member can and does make a valuable contribution although the levels of education, preparation, and experience may be widely varied.

PATTERNS IN BASIC NURSING EDUCATION

Basic nursing education, as contrasted with graduate education, includes the programs that prepare students for the licensing examination for becoming registered nurses. The term "registered nurse" is a legal title, not to be confused with an academic degree or a diploma. A student who graduates from a basic nursing curriculum may receive a diploma, an associate degree, or a baccalaureate degree. A graduate is entitled to use the term "registered nurse" only after passing the current National League for Nursing State Board Test Pool Examination.

In general, all basic nursing curriculums prepare for first level or beginning positions. This means, rather literally, that graduates are prepared for those jobs in nursing for which the only requirement is an RN. Such positions include staff nursing in any of the major clinical areas, private duty nursing, and office nursing. Specialized positions such as teaching, administration, public health, school nurse, clinical specialist, and research require preparation beyond the basic registered nurse program.

At the present time, there are three types of basic nursing curriculums. The oldest, and still the largest in terms of student enrollment, is the diploma school. Such a school is typically three calendar years in length, is controlled by a hospital, and grants a diploma upon the completion of the course of study. In 1960, there were 891 such schools with a total enrollment of 94,812.* Although the number of students in such schools has grown slowly, the number of schools has decreased somewhat. The total percentage of all students who are enrolled in diploma programs has been decreasing slowly but steadily in recent years. In 1960, for the first time in history, the percentage of students enrolled in diploma schools went below 80%. The diploma school of nursing prepares students for first level positions and emphasizes the physical care of sick patients.

The second basic curriculum in nursing in terms of age and enrollment is the baccalaureate program, which may be either four or five years in length. The baccalaureate program, in addition to preparing for beginning practice in nursing, also emphasizes the preparation of the student as a person and a citizen, usually includes preparation for public health nursing, and builds an academic background on which graduate study can be based. Graduates are capable of advancing the first step beyond the beginning lev-

---

*Facts about nursing, American Nurses Association, 1961, p. 81.

els of nursing with experience and without additional academic preparation. In 1960, there were 158 baccalaureate programs with an enrollment of 20,-783 students.* The number of students in baccalaureate program has increased very slowly in recent years.

The third type of basic nursing curriculum is the associate degree program, launched in 1952. A pilot project to demonstrate the ability of the junior or community college to prepare registered nurses was conducted under the direction of Dr. Mildred L. Montag of Teachers College, Columbia University. The ability of the graduates to pass State Board Examinations, obtain licensure, and function adequately in first level nursing positions was clearly demonstrated. Before the completion of the pilot project, the associate degree program began to expand rapidly. Between 1954 and 1960, the enrollment in the associate degree program rose from 359 to 3,254.† The number of such schools was 57 in 1960‡ and 82 in 1963. The associate degree program represents a major break with traditional patterns of nursing education. The prescribed curriculum is completed in two academic or two calendar years and includes an approximately even distribution between nursing and general education. The clinical areas are used much as laboratories are used in other sicence courses, and broad area courses in nursing have replaced the typical fragmented subject matter approach of the traditional curriculum. Pharmacology, diet therapy, pathology, and many other courses have become part of the broad area courses rather than being taught as isolated subjects. Since this program is associated with the community college movement, which is the most rapidly expanding part of higher education in the United States at present, it can be anticipated that the associate degree program in nursing will continue its rapid rate of growth.

---

*Facts about nursing, American Nurses Association, 1961, p. 102.
†Facts about nursing, American Nurses Association, 1961, p. 101.
‡Facts about nursing, American Nurses Association, 1961, p. 81.

BIBLIOGRAPHY

1. Bolduan, Charles F.: Public health and hygiene, Philadelphia, 1929, W. B. Saunders Co., pp. 37-39.
2. Hyde, H. von Zile: A glance back and a look forward, ten years of public health progress, Office of Public Information, Pan-American Sanitary Bureau, Regional Office of WHO, 1958.
3. Lambertson, Eleanor C.: Education for nursing leadership, Philadelphia, 1958, J. B. Lippincott Co.
4. Mustard, Harry S., and Stebbins, E. L.: An introduction to public health, New York, 1959, The Macmillan Co.
5. Wolman, Engabel: The changing physical and biological environment of man, American Journal of Public Health **51**:1631-1637, Nov. 1961.

Chapter 2

Nursing and the problem-solving process

Nursing is an applied science. It draws on the basic biological, physical, and social sciences, and it assumes its own unique configuration through selection of knowledge from these sciences. Although nursing shares knowledge and skills with other disciplines, its content is drawn from this unique configuration.

As in all other sciences, either basic or applied, development and future advances are solidly confined to the use of the scientific method, the method of inquiry or, as we shall use, the problem-solving approach to nursing care. Before going into the problem-solving process, it might be helpful to discuss briefly the thought processes we use to meet ordinary everyday situations.

The type of mental activity we are principally concerned with is generally called reflective thinking. This differs from daydreaming, "woolgathering," reverie, or "brain storming" primarily because it is directed or controlled for the solution of a problem. Dewey gives a wonderful example of this difference:

". . . . let us consider a rudimentary case of thinking, lying between careful examination of evidence and a mere irresponsible stream of fancies. A man is walking on a warm day. The sky was clear the last time he observed it; but presently he notes, while occupied with other things, that the air is cooler. It occurs to him that it is probably going to rain; looking up, he sees a dark cloud between him and the sun, and he then quickens his steps. What, if anything, in such a situation can be called thought? Neither the act of walking nor the noting of the cold is a thought. Walking is one direction of activity; looking and noting are other modes of activity. The likelihood that it will rain is, however, something suggested. The pedestrian feels the cold; first he thinks of clouds, then he looks and perceives them, and then he thinks of something he does not see; a storm. This suggested possibility is the idea, the thought. If it is believed in as a genuine possibility which may occur, it is the kind of thought which falls within the scope of knowledge and which requires reflective consideration.

"Up to a certain point there is the same sort of situation as when one who looks at a cloud is reminded of a human figure and face. Thinking in both of these cases (the cases of belief and of fancy) involves noting or perceiving a fact, followed by something else that is not observed but that is brought to mind, suggested by the thing seen. One thing reminds us, as we say, of the other. Side by side, however, with this factor of agreement in the two cases of suggestion is a factor of marked disagreement. We do not believe in the face suggested by the cloud; we do not consider at all the probability of its being a fact. There is no reflective thought. The danger of rain, on the contrary, presents itself to us as a genuine possibility—a fact of the same nature as the observed coolness. Put differently, we do not regard the cloud as meaning or indicating a face, but merely as suggesting it, while we do consider the coolness may mean rain."*

Informal reflective thinking will perhaps go through several complete acts. Whitney defines them as follows:

"There is first of all (a) a feeling of deficiency or need, then (b) a more or less definite delimitation of the problem situation involved, followed by (c) the acceptance of a tentative conclusion, (d) its critical examination in terms of evidence, and (e) its experimental corroboration or rejection. If it is abandoned as unsatisfactory, another cycle of the thought act is inaugurated, and so on."†

If we take this ordinary reflective thought process as a base, we can proceed to sharpen and define certain aspects and easily reach what is technically called the scientific method, or the problem-solving approach. Taken by themselves, the steps of the problem-solving approach involve ordinary mental activities carried out daily by every person. Taken collectively, they amount to the most dynamic technique devised by man to know and to control our environment.

The development of the problem-solving approach in the pursuit of knowledge accounts for the abundance of technical achievements in our times. Why is this method so important to nursing? What is the method? How do we develop it? Certainly, one of the most important aims of nursing education is to develop the ability to think critically and to use the problem-solving process in the daily activities of the nurse. These two actions cannot be taught in a void or vacuum but require repetitive practice in a method that ensures intelligent, safe nursing care. At the same time, it forms the basis for an entire future professional life in that it will constantly demand and allow growth and development. The constant use of the problem-solving approach leads to the skilled practitioner of the science of nursing.

When we use the word "problem," what do we mean? Perhaps the best answer comes from Webster's definition: "A question raised for inquiry, consideration, or solution."‡ Actually, it is derived from two words meaning "something thrown forward." We, therefore, are thinking in terms of com-

---

*Dewey, John: How we think, Boston, 1933, D. C. Heath & Co., p. 9.
†Frederick Lamson Whitney, *The Elements of Research, 3rd edition.* © 1950, By permission of Prentice-Hall, Inc., Englewood Cliffs, N. J.
‡By permission. From Webster's Seventh New Collegiate Dictionary, copyright 1963 by G. & C. Merriam Co., Publishers of Merriam-Webster Dictionaries.

plex situations that we can move forward to resolution by utilization of the steps in the problem-solving process.

Meyer and Heidgerken identify the steps in problem solving as follows:

"1. The appearance of a problem—'a felt difficulty'
"2. The location and definition of the problem
"3. The determination of solutions
"4. The testing and elimination of solutions by reasoning
"5. The testing of the remaining solution in actual practice"*

What does this mean in terms of nursing? The patient's nursing problems represent the "felt difficulty or difficulties." His health problem, his reaction to the health problem, and the possible complications in ordinary daily activities are potential sources of difficulty. One of the most significant aspects of providing nursing care to patients with health problems is the second step in the problem-solving process—the location and definition of the problem. A question well asked is a question half answered; the question itself points toward the answer. The same fact applies to the location and definition of the patient's nursing problem. A clear-cut identification of the problem points toward the nursing care to be given the specific patient. The identification of the patient's nursing problem is often called "making a nursing diagnosis."

A nursing diagnosis is somewhat different from a medical diagnosis, the latter being based upon the pathological process which constitutes the patient's specific health problem or problems. The nursing diagnosis is arrived at by sifting information concerning the patient's medical condition, information concerning relevant sociological facts about the patient, and information concerning the patient as an individual person. The nursing diagnosis is a dynamic diagnosis, since it can and usually does change from day to day with change in degree of illness, with change in attitude, and with change in the current situation which can be initiated by almost anything.

What are the sources of relevant information about patients which can be used in making a nursing diagnosis? The sources are many: the patient, his chart, the Kardex, the patient's relatives or visitors, hospital personnel, and the nurse's own knowledge.

The patient himself constitutes a primary source of information. His signs and symptoms related to his health problem and his description of subjective complaints are important. Probably of even more significance, because it often cannot be obtained anywhere else, is the patient's reaction to his health problem. How he feels about his illness, what problems it poses for him financially and socially, and what it means to his concept of himself as a person are all factors in arriving at a nursing diagnosis. How the patient's problems appear to him constitutes important information in planning nursing care.

The patient's chart also constitutes a primary source of information. The

*Meyer, Burton, and Heidgerken, Loretta E.: Introduction to research in nursing, Philadelphia, 1962, J. B. Lippincott Co., p. 18.

patient's name, age, occupation, address, religion, socioeconomic level, and cultural background can usually be determined provided that writing on the chart is legible. The diagnosis, results of physical examination, vital signs, laboratory reports, therapeutic treatments, progress, and prognosis are found in the chart.

The Kardex offers a secondary source for quick reference. On the Kardex can be found the diagnosis, treatments, medications, diet, date of admission, and age. Sometimes the Kardex may include suggested approaches to and measures of nursing care.

The patient's relatives and/or visitors represent another source of information. They are *particularly* valuable for several types of information: clues about the patient as a person and his individual likes and dislikes, how his behavior differs now from the past, where he fits into the family constellation, what he means to others who are significant to him, what his cultural background is, and to what he is returning when he recovers.

Other hospital personnel constitutes another source of information about the patient. Doctors, other nursing personnel, social workers, occupational therapists, and any other health team members may have knowledge about the patient which can be useful to the nurse.

In addition to sources of information, the nurse brings her own knowledge to the situation and it is the collection of information sifted through her knowledge of the biological, physical, social, and nursing sciences that lead to the development of a nursing diagnosis and the hypothesis, or nursing care plan. Throughout the experience of the student, where the development of knowledge is in process, the instructor in nursing serves as a resource person in helping to arrive at the diagnosis and the hypothesis. In addition, where there are gaps in information, available sources of knowledge, such as textbooks, can be consulted.

Having made the nursing diagnosis, or identified the patient's specific nursing problems, the next step involves determining solutions, i.e., considering the possible ways and means of providing nursing care. The intellectual process of reasoning through which measures or approaches seem most likely to be effective follows. This becomes the nursing care plan. The nursing care plan can also be equated with the hypothesis (tentative supposition provisionally adopted) of the scientific method. Then the selected solution, or nursing care plan, is tested in actual practice, i.e., the nursing care is given.

After nursing care is completed, the effect is analyzed and the plan revised. It is often necessary to revise the nursing care plan while it is being carried out. The interpretation and evaluation of the tested solution for the patient's nursing problems are essential. How could the plan of nursing care have been improved? Was the original solution or hypothesis correct, or did it have to be changed or altered radically? Was the tested solution successful, i.e., was nursing care adequate and safe? Was the patient cared for and left as comfortable as the problem would allow? If the nurse were assigned to the same patient the next day, how much more would she observe or learn? Would she, in other words, repeat the nursing care given? Or, on the basis of this experience, would she change the nursing care plan?

In the evaluation and interpretation of results, the next step is to move from the specific nursing care of a specific patient to the implications for the nursing care of other patients. Can they be generalized? Is there perhaps a better method of proving the hypothesis? Of what value is the result? Would you repeat the same process? Can this be added to our general store of knowledge, or is it on the periphery and of little future value in work? Does it call for repeating, extension? Can it be applied in some other area?

"Nursing is concerned with helping patients solve health problems. It is, therefore, a problem-solving process related to health. A nursing problem is defined as 'a condition and/or situation faced by a patient, or his family, which the nurse can assist him to meet through the performance of her professional function.'[*] The following list of nursing problems is to be used in identifying patients' specific nursing problems in clinical practice."[†]

The nursing problems are classified as overt or covert or as having aspects of both. Overt problems are the obvious ones that can be identified readily. Such problems present themselves openly, such as the flushed face or the blue tinge in the nailbeds that can easily be seen, or the laboratory report indicates a bood sugar well beyond normal levels. The covert nursing problem is hidden, more difficult to elicit. The patient who is critical of his nursing care because he is apprehensive is an example. The patient's apprehension is the covert nursing problem.

"*Group I:* The nursing problems are basic—they are presented to some degree by all patients regardless of the specific health problem that may confront the patient. Such problems are apt to be both overt and covert, and identification of the problem may call for direct and/or indirect methods of approach.
  "1. To maintain good hygiene and physical comfort.
  "2. To promote optimal activity; exercise, rest, and sleep.
  "3. To promote safety through prevention of accident, injury, or other trauma and through prevention of the spread of infection.
  "4. To maintain good body mechanics and prevent and correct deformities.
"*Group II:* This group of problems relates to normal and disturbed physiological body processes. The major problems here are usually overt, and the identification of such problems usually involves a direct approach, i.e., observation of color, cardinal signs, position, skin, etc.; and specific questions designed to elicit relevant information, i.e., character, extent, and duration of pain.
  "5. To facilitate the maintenance of a supply of oxygen to all body cells.
  "6. To facilitate the maintenance of nutrition of all body cells.
  "7. To facilitate the maintenance of elimination.
  "8. To facilitate the maintenance of fluid and electrolyte balance.
  "9. To recognize the physiological responses of the body to disease conditions—pathological, physiological, and compensatory.
  "10. To facilitate the maintenance of regulatory mechanisms and functions.
  "11. To facilitate the maintenance of sensory function.

[*]Abdellah, Faye G.: Methods of identifying covert aspects of nursing problems, Nursing Research, 6:4, June 1957.
[†]Abdellah, Faye, Beland, Irene L., Martin, Almeda, and Matheney, Ruth V.: Patient-centered approaches to nursing, New York, 1960, The Macmillan Co., p. 80.

Table 2. *The relationship between the problem-solving process and the process of providing nursing care*

Problem-solving process	Providing nursing care
1. Appearance of a problem	1. The patient and his health problem
2. Location and definition of the problem	2. Reviewing chart, visiting patient, using resource people—identifying patient nursing problems, i.e., making a nursing diagnosis
3. Determination of solutions	3. Reviewing intellectually all possible steps in providing nursing care
4. Testing and elimination of solutions by reasoning	4. Developing a nursing care plan for the patient
5. Testing of the remaining solution in actual practice	5. Giving nursing care
6. Interpretation and evaluation	6. Interpreting and evaluating nursing care

"*Group III:* This group involves mainly emotional and interpersonal difficulties. The problems are usually covert and require indirect methods, i.e., listening, reflecting, open-end questions, etc., for identification.

"12. To identify and accept positive and negative expressions, feelings, and reactions.

"13. To identify and accept the interrelatedness of emotions and organic illness.

"14. To facilitate the maintenance of effective verbal and nonverbal communication.

"15. To promote the development of productive interpersonal relationships.

"16. To facilitate progress toward achievement of personal spiritual goals.

"17. To create and/or maintain a therapeutic environment.

"18. To facilitate awareness of self as an individual with varying physical, emotional, and developmental needs.

"*Group IV:* This group involves sociological or community problems as well as individual ones. They may be overt or covert and, therefore, require either direct or indirect approach.

"19. To accept the optimum possible goals in the light of limitations, physical and emotional.

"20. To use community resources as an aid in resolving problems arising from illness.

"21. To understand the role of social problems as influencing factors in the cause of illness."*

The broad nursing problems indicated are designed primarily as guides in locating and defining patients' specific nursing problems and the process to be used in the problem-solving process.

In the summary presented in Table 2, the relationship between the problem-solving process and the process of providing nursing care is indicated.

---

*Abdellah, Faye, Beland, Irene L., Martin, Almeda, and Matheney, Ruth V.: Patient-centered approaches to nursing, New York, 1960, The Macmillan Co., pp. 80-82.

BIBLIOGRAPHY

1. Abdellah, Faye G., Beland, Irene L., Martin, Almeda, and Matheney, Ruth V.: Patient-centered approaches to nursing, New York, 1960, The Macmillan Co., pp. 1-19, 75-84.

2. Chambers, Wilda: Nursing diagnosis, American Journal of Nursing **62**:102-104, Nov., 1962.
3. Dewey, John: How we think, Boston, 1933, D. C. Heath & Co.
4. Meyer, Burton, and Heidgerken, Loretta E.: Introduction to research in nursing, Philadelphia, 1962, J. B. Lippincott Co., pp. 14-20.
5. Scheerer, Martin: Problem-solving, Scientific American **208**:118-128, April 1963.

Chapter 3

Roles of the registered nurse

A role is a pattern of behavior expected of a person in a certain position. Everyone fills many roles in the society in which he lives. The executive in an industry is expected to display certain patterns of behavior that are peculiar to social expectations of executives. The same man as a father may be expected to behave like a father—he must love his children, educate them, and provide behavior examples for them. He must discipline his children when they need it. Society in general and his next-door neighbors in particular expect this of him in his role as a father. Like everyone else in society, a student nurse may be cast in many roles. For example, she may fill the role of student, sweetheart, sister, sister-in-law, and several other specific roles as well as the generalized role of being a good citizen in a specific city in a specific country at a specified time in history. Turner defines role as follows:

> "By role we mean a collection of patterns of behavior which are thought to constitute a meaningful unit and deemed appropriate to a person occupying a particular status in society (e.g., doctor or father), occupying an informally defined position in interpersonal relations (e.g., leader or compromiser), or identified with a particular value in society (e.g., honest man or patriot)."*

Society has imposed the expectations of behavior for each role. In simple situations, the conduct norms are clearly defined. For instance, small children have little difficulty in fulfilling their role as the "loved one" in a family group. Or a new army recruit wearing a nice new uniform with shiny buttons is certainly the "hero" to his girl friend. After capping ceremonies, was there ever a "probie" not certain that she was walking directly in the footsteps of Florence Nightingale?

However, when one thinks of what various members of society expect of nurses and nursing, another picture emerges. How do laymen look on the

---

*Turner, Ralph H.: Role-taking, role standpoint, and reference group behavior, American Journal of Sociology **61**:316-39, Jan. 1956 (University of Chicago).

nurse and what do they expect of her? It is perhaps the layman who has the greatest variety of expectations. He sees her in the public image, whatever that may be, depending on the culture in which he lives. The cultural patterns of behavior expectations vary throughout the United States, but there are certain very definite things the average American expects from a nurse. First, he expects her to be in a white uniform with a cap, to be technically skilled, and to be interested in and have some degree of understanding of him as a person. He expects her to know about what is wrong with him and to know what to do about it. In addition to expecting her to be intelligent, neat, kindly, pleasant, quick, and efficient, the patient will also bring with him an experience of patterns of relationship with others into which he will fit the nurse. These patterns of relationships are as varied as the number of patients with whom any one nurse will come in contact. The average nurse can anticipate being cast in almost every social role there is by the various patients to whom she gives nursing care.

To the doctor, the nurse is an able assistant. She must be there to assist him when needed and must carry out all of his instructions meticulously during the long hours he is separated from the patient. At all times, she must relay to the patient, by word and deed, her absolute trust in the doctor's integrity and ability.

What do hospital administrators expect of the nurse? She must be the protector of the hospital and custodian of expensive and elaborate equipment. She must be responsible for the conduct and safety of auxiliary personnel. She is the link between the patient, his relatives and friends, and the hospital, which in itself demands skills in interpersonal relationships and adroit public relations. The nurse controls the hospital environment in a variety of ways. Finally, in many instances, if something breaks down or the hopper overflows, she must have the mechanical ingenuity to repair the plant! As Cottrell has pointed out, satisfactory role adjustment depends on the "clarity with which a role is defined."[*] At this time of transition in nursing practice, if the nurse seems uncertain of her role or role expectation, it would be normal.

Historically, nursing has been subordinate to medicine over the years. That is, many of its acts and functions were almost directly under the instruction, supervision, and direction of the medical profession. However, because of the vast expansion of medical services in the past fifty years, and new knowledge in the medical sciences, along with the development of the basic sciences and their delineation from the functions that are peculiar to nursing, the over-all functions and corresponding roles are changing. Lesnik and Anderson list seven areas of professional nursing as follows:

> "1. The supervision of a patient involving the whole management of care, requiring the application of principles based upon the biologic, the physical, and the social sciences.

---

[*]Cottrell, Leonard: The adjustment of the individual to his age and sex roles, American Sociological Review 7:617, 1942.

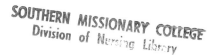
SOUTHERN MISSIONARY COLLEGE
Division of Nursing Library

"2. The observation of symptoms and reactions, including symptomatology of physical and mental conditions and needs, requiring evaluation or application of principles based upon the biologic, the physical, and the social sciences.

"3. The accurate recording and reporting of facts, including evaluation of the whole care of the patient.

"4. The supervision of others, except physicians, contributing to the care of the patient.

"5. The application and the execution of nursing procedures and technics.

"6. The direction and the education to secure physical and mental care.

"7. The application and the execution of legal orders of physicians concerning treatments and medications, with an understanding of cause and effect thereof."*

In the first six functions, the nurse acts in the role of an independent agent. It is only in the seventh role that she still remains in the old, traditional, dependent role of giving assistance contingent upon direction, supervision, or both. Even the dependent function of the nurse has changed over recent years, and more independent function requires extensive use of judgment. Medical directions are not so specific that they can be followed without questioning or understanding. For example, although a patient may be ordered out of bed, the nurse is expected to observe any signs or symptoms that may contraindicate this order.

The role of independent agent implies unlimited responsibilities. The nurse must exercise judgment in applying the basic principles of nursing based on the biological, physical, and social sciences. For example, the exercise of judgment in the entire management of patient care is implicit in the role of nursing supervisor. As an independent agent, the nurse must also formulate with care a "nursing diagnosis" when observing signs and symptoms. Should the judgment of the diagnosis warrant action, it must be taken within the scope of nursing measures. How would this apply? If a patient is having an adverse effect from an infusion, it should be discontinued; if he is having an adverse reaction to heat or cold, its application should be withdrawn; if he is displaying irrational behavior, this should be reported; if he shows signs of having a possible coronary attack, he must be placed under medical supervision and nothing done to aggravate the condition. Finally, the patients' safety at all times must be maintained. This includes a range of activities from protecting a child from a radiator burn to securing screens in a psychiatric ward to prevent the patient's self-destruction by jumping out of the window.

As stated previously, society prescribes the roles for specialized groups, such as the nurses. When a patient is admitted to a hospital ward, what are some of the roles he designates for nurses? In this complex interpersonal exchange between patient and nurse, how does the patient look at the nurse? Hildegarde Peplau, in her interesting book, *Interpersonal relations in nurs-*

---

*Lesnik, Milton J., and Anderson, Bernice E.: Nursing practice and the law, ed. 2, Philadelphia, 1955, J. B. Lippincott Co., p. 259.

ing, lists five or six major roles into which the nurse is cast: stranger, teacher, resource person, counselor, and surrogate.

It is rather startling at first to think the nurse is a stranger to the patient. But at first meeting, they are certainly two unacquainted individuals having only one thing in common—to return the patient to health. What is expected of the nurse in the role of a stranger? How differently would she receive the patient if they were introduced at a friend's party or if he was received in her own home? Can she be nonjudgmental and accept the patient exactly as he is? Can she overcome cultural and social biases and understand his right to be different?

The roles of teacher, resource person, and counselor demand identification and interpretation individually and seemingly present no difficulties. But what of the surrogate roles?

Webster defines surrogate as follows: "To put in the place of another: to appoint as successor, deputy, or substitute for oneself."* How can this happen to a nurse? If the nurse listens carefully to patients, she will hear it happening almost every day. Outside of their conscious awareness, patients will often view nurses as someone else. The nurse may represent a mother figure, a sibling, a daughter, a significant person in the patient's life outside the family circle such as an old friend, a religious leader, a teacher, or a kindly aide met on a previous hospital admission. Patients often make remarks such as the following: "You remind me so much of my aunt." "When you bathe me like this, I feel just like a baby being cared for by mother." "I have a daughter just your age and when I'm not looking, you sound just like her." "Your actions remind me so much of Dr. Strauss." "Did you attend a religious school? You are as kind as my second grade teacher." "Your laugh is just like Uncle Philip's, and he's so pleasant to have around." "Do you know Miss Wilson? She cared for me two years ago so nicely, and you must have gone to the same school."

Being aware of the role a patient places one in can obviously help in the approach to the patient and his nursing care, but does it have any other value? As much as one might like, the nurse cannot get inside the patient's mind and remove these illusory figures so that the patient will recognize her as Shirley Smith, and not Uncle Philip. However, as the reader will discover in the chapter on nurse intervention in covert nursing problems, with the use of proper interviewing techniques, the acceptance of this surrogate role at first can be a source of security for the patient that will allow for freedom of communication later, perhaps on a higher level. Eventually, the nurse can help the patient learn differences of identification by merely being herself.

By being herself, the nurse is always aware of her own behavior in relations with patients. Having identified the illusory surrogate roles in which the nurse is placed should ensure that the process is not reversed. The

---

*By permission. From Webster's Seventh New Collegiate Dictionary, copyright 1963 by G. & C. Merriam Co., Publishers of the Merriam-Webster Dictionaries.

nurse should not look upon patients as surrogates out of the past but view each patient as a separate, distinct individual, and not a stereotype. This would certainly eliminate patients being referred to as "pop," "gramps," or "mom."

The roles of the registered nurse then can be viewed from the following several aspects: her legal responsibilities in the provision of nursing, the roles in which patients place her, the roles in which co-workers place her, and her own concept of her role as a nurse. All of these reflect varying concepts of the patterns of behavior others expect of her and what she expects of herself. There is room for conflict. The nurse needs to recognize and to utilize the varied expectations that others have in regard to her behavior.

BIBLIOGRAPHY

1. Cole, William E.: Introductory sociology, New York, 1962, David McKay Co., Inc.
2. Kurtz, Richard A., and Flaming, Karl H.: Professionalism: the case of nurses, American Journal of Nursing 63:75-79, Jan. 1963.
3. Lesnik, Milton J., and Anderson, Bernice E.: Nursing practice and the law, ed. 2, Philadelphia, 1955, J. B. Lippincott Co., pp. 380-384.
4. Peplau, Hildegarde E.: Interpersonal relations in nursing, New York, 1952, G. P. Putnam's Sons, Inc., pp. 43-70.
5. Perkins, Erline W.: The registered nurse: a professional person? American Journal of Nursing 63:90-92, Feb. 1963.

Covert nursing problems

Chapter 4

Introduction to covert nursing problems

In the provision of health services to society, at no time in history has the need for understanding and intelligent interaction with patients and clients as persons been so sharply highlighted as it is in the present. Progress in the solution of problems tends to uncover new problems that need new solutions. The impact of the explosion of scientific knowledge has produced patterns of health problems and patterns of health services that have tended to impersonalize what was once a highly personal service. At the same time, the need for a deeper understanding of the psychological and social aspects of health problems generally, as well as of the specific problems of individual patients, has increased. As a member of the health team, the nurse must be able to work effectively with patients as people, as well as with the patient's specific health problem.

Among the more important factors that have led to major changes in health services is the explosion of scientific knowledge. Since no one person can know everything, we have experienced a steady growth in the phenomenon of specialization. As a result, members of the medical profession and allied fields have an intimate knowledge of certain aspects of the individual and his illness. However, this has naturally led to fewer people who view the individual patient as a totality. The rapid decrease in the number of old family doctors who dispensed their pills and treatments with a liberal dose of understanding of their patients as human beings has been loudly decried; there is much mourning at their departure. There is, likewise, a mournful plaint at the departure of the good old days in nursing when a nurse "cared about her patients." Both groups met a need. But no one really wants to go back to the level of medical and nursing care represented by those good old days when knowledge was limited by comparison with the present, when the infectious diseases were major killers, and when hospitalization could mean financial ruin. What really is needed and wanted is not a regression in medical and nursing practice but a restoration of the individual patient to his position of worth and dignity in the provision of health services.

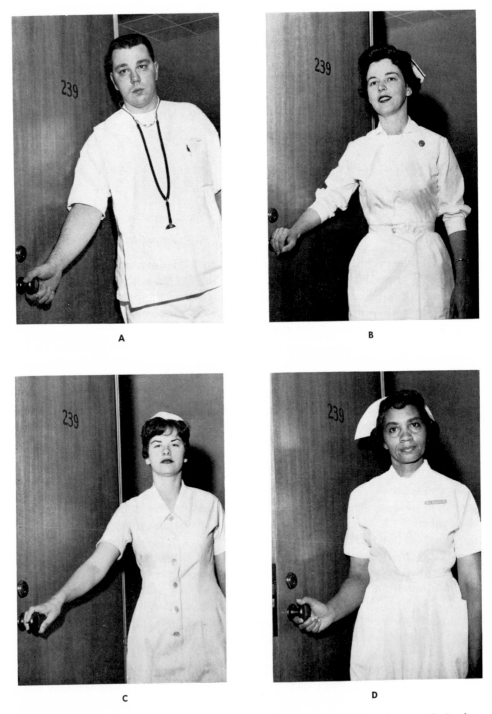

Fig. 2. The growing multiplicity of personnel: **A,** Physician. **B,** Registerd nurse. **C,** Student nurse. **D,** Practical nurse. **E,** Laboratory technician. **F,** Nurse's aide. **G,** Ward clerk.

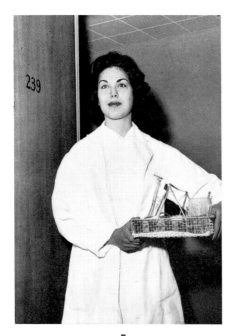

E

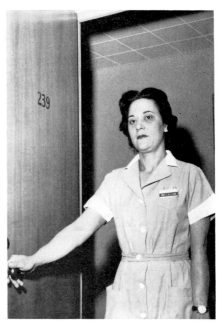

F

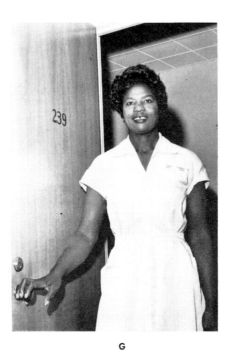

G

Fig. 2—cont'd. For legend, see opposite page.

This is not impossible, provided health workers develop skill in working with people as people.

Along with increased knowledge, and as a direct result of it, we have experienced a complete change in the pattern of major health problems presented by our population. With the control of infectious diseases (a control maintained only by constant vigilance), degenerative and long-term illnesses constitute our major health problems. Hospitalization is more often an episode rather than a circumscribed experience. The patient's need is more often for teaching, for intelligent compassion, for services that extend with continuity from the hospital back into the community. The ability to make needed adapations in health behavior and life modification is strongly influenced by the personality and cultural background of the individual. Hence, the need to work effectively with the patient as a person is enhanced in modern medical practice.

The increased scientific knowledge combined with an expanding population that is educated to demand more health services as well as better prepared to pay for them have led to a tremendous increase in the use of health services. To meet the demand, certain trends and patterns have emerged. Increasingly, members of the health team have delegated functions to those directly below them in the hierarchy. Doctors have turned over many functions to registered nurses. Registered nurses have delegated some of these functions to practical nurses, who, in turn, have delegated some functions to aides. There has also developed an increase in the number of kinds of personnel involved in providing health services. Registered nurses are assisted by practical nurses, aides, and attendants; dentists are assisted by dental hygienists. Physicians utilize the services of x-ray technicians, medical laboratory technicians, medical secretaries, and other supplementary groups. Dietitians and diet therapists constitute an important health service group; at one time in history, nurses performed their functions. The housekeeping department has become a separate entity, carrying out functions also once performed by nurses. Messengers and ward clerks supplement nursing service. Interestingly, attempts have been made to introduce "ward managers" to relieve nurses of some of their hospital administrative functions and free them for nursing care. This movement so far has been successfully resisted, apparently by nurses themselves. Social service, occupational and recreational therapy, physical therapy, and other related fields have expanded their personnel and services both in hospital and in community health services. The inevitable result has been a bewildering array of personnel, with a bewildering array of services, going in and out of the patient's hospital room, seeing him in the clinic, and visiting his home. Little wonder he feels lost—particularly lost as a total individual. Here again, progress and advancement have led to a need to reemphasize the worth and dignity of the individual as a human being. Compartmentalized patient care makes this need imperative.

With the number of specialists coming and going, those persons who are anchored in the hospital setting, especially the patients and the nursing service personnel, find themselves in a situation that is profoundly complex. In such a complex setting, interpersonal skills are at a premium. The increasing interdependence of the varied health teams means that communication and understanding among them are important determinants of the success of planned therapy for the patient. There are times when vested interests among certain members of the health teams untentionally militate against patient therapy. Only the cooperative and realistic working together of the various groups is in the interest of patients, and this depends on skill in working with people. In addition, as the one group constantly in the hospital setting, nursing service personnel must bear a major responsibility for making it possible for the patient to maintain his dignity as a purposeful, responsible individual. This means working with patients *as people.*

One additional factor highlights the need for skills in the psychological and social aspects of nursing—and that factor is automation. We are in the beginning of the age of automation, a technological revolution of such profound implication that it may well shake our society to its moral and ethical roots. The era has already begun in the field of health services. We have monitoring machines, including multipurpose monitoring, which continuously report the patient's condition. We have cardiac pacemakers. We have artificial kidneys. We have computers, including diagnostic computers. This is only the beginning. With the advent of electronic devices that will, in all probability, alter drastically the function of many of the groups involved in providing health services, it can be anticipated that the function of nurses will change. There can be no question that the introduction of numerous machines *can* further depersonalize health services. And any further depersonalization can only highlight the need for interpersonal skills that will help the patient maintain his sense of worth and dignity. Nurses must nurse people, not machines, if they are to provide the kind of nursing that society needs. This is fundamental.

DEFINITIONS

The psychological and social aspects of nursing care fall largely in the area of covert nursing problems. Such a nursing problem, as contrasted with an overt one, is a concealed or unconscious condition not readily recognizable by the patient and/or his family. The distinction between overt and covert nursing problems rests to a great extent on the fact that overt problems are apparent and can be approached by direct methods, whereas covert nursing problems are not apparent and are best approached by indirect or nondirective approaches. Overt nursing problems tend to fall into the category requiring physical and manipulative skills, whereas covert nursing problems require an analysis of behavior which demands that the nurse possess psychological or interpersonal skills. For example, a flushed face in a patient with elevated temperature is a physical symptom that can be directly observed and will call for specific physical measures, in the light of the patient's physical condition, that can be classified as direct intervention. It may involve reporting, alcohol sponge, change of position, medication, or similar direct action. This is an overt nursing problem. On the other hand, a preoperative patient may be extremely restless and not sleeping well the night before an operation. This is an indication—but of what? By listening and encouraging the patient to talk freely, the nurse discovers the patient is apprehensive about her small children while she is out of the home and is worried about how soon she can return and whether she will be able to cope with the situation. The nursing problem is the patient's anxiety. In such a situation the nurse requires psychological skills in allaying anxiety. This is a covert nursing problem, because the patient's real problem, anxiety, is not readily apparent.

KINDS OF COVERT NURSING PROBLEMS

This section will be concerned primarily with nursing problems that are psychological or emotional in nature. All nursing problems presented by patients are interrelated. Physical comfort cannot be maintained, for example, by physical hygiene measures alone. Psychological discomfort can produce physical discomfort, and vice versa. The maintenance of body regulatory mechanisms can be influenced by fear and apprehension. On the other hand, interference with or malfunctioning of the body regulatory mechanisms can produce fear and apprehension. For purposes of discussion, certain types of nursing problems that are met with similar nursing measures are isolated for consideration. The patient as a *total* person remains the central focus of any nursing care plan.

Certain types of covert problems confront patients who face health problems. Prominent among these problems are the following:

1. The need to identify and accept their positive and negative expressions, feelings, and reactions
2. The need to identify and accept the interrelatedness of their emotions and organic illness
3. The need to maintain effective verbal and nonverbal communication with others
4. The need to develop or maintain productive interpersonal relationships that will support the restoration or improvement of their health status
5. The need to achieve progress toward personal spiritual goals
6. The need to participate in the creation or maintenance of a therapeutic environment
7. The need to facilitate awareness of the self as an individual with varying physical, emotional, and developmental needs

None of these problems is unique to individuals who face specific health complications. They represent basic needs of all people, and specific illnesses simply tend to make progress in the area of personal maturity somewhat more difficult to achieve.

The need to identify and accept expressions, feelings, and reactions, including strengths and weaknesses, potentials, and limitations, is part of learning to know and understand oneself and is a task that confronts all of us. This task can be complicated by the advent of a health problem. The need to learn to accept the role of a patient, the ability to face the threat of mutilation or death, the need to face the modification of a life pattern, the need to face financial drain or loss of income are examples of the kind of situations precipitated by illness that necessarily arouse strong feelings. Such feelings can definitely affect the course of therapy or the realism of the patient's plan for readjustment to the community.

Most of our major health problems carry strong emotional impacts. Heart and circulatory diseases usually necessitate a change in life patterns; the diagnosis of cancer is still frightening to most people, and mental illness still carries a stigma although not so much so in recent years as in the not too distant past. In any case, feelings aroused, even though such feelings may not be obvious to the casual observer, are an important aspect in the therapy that is planned to restore the patient to health and to his home. If such feelings are not to hinder or delay the process of recovery (or to negate it entirely), then they must be treated as an aspect of the patient's health problem.

The patient must be able eventually to identify and accept his feelings. In order to do this, the nurse must be able to provide the patient with the kind of relationship that permits him to explore feelings without judgment, punishment, or rejection. She must use an indirect approach, because feelings are rarely elicited by direct or probing questions. She must have sufficient judgment to know when to and when not to encourage such expression on the part of the patient. Her goal in nursing care becomes to help the patient first *identify* feelings, since little or nothing can be done except endure them until they are identified. Her next nursing goal is to help the patient accept his feelings, for with identification and acceptance comes the ability on the part of most patients to take action. The mere ventilation of feelings can often result in a reduction of tension. The nurse's own ability to convey acceptance to a patient is a primary avenue through which the patient can frequently learn to identify and accept his own feelings, especially in regard to his health problem. Because his feelings about his illness, physical or emotional, have implications for his ultimate level of recovery, nursing therapy must include this aspect of nursing care for each and every patient.

The need to accept the interrelatedness of emotions and organic illness is one facet of the patient's learning to see or continuing to see himself as a total individual. There are certain categories of somatic diseases in which the need for the patient to come to grips with this interrelatedness is pointedly obvious. All the so-called psychosomatic disorders, that is, somatic pathology in which the psychological cause and somatic effect are directly related, provide striking examples. Peptic ulcers, essential hypertension, asthma, and mucous colitis belong in the group of diseases so classified. The somatic dysfunction may be temporarily halted or reversed with medical treatment, but unless the psychological difficulty that created the somatic problem is also treated, the patient will continue to have recurring episodes of the same physical disease. In its more subtle aspects, the interrelatedness of emotions and organic illness, although not always so obvious, is nonetheless a significant factor in planning nursing care. A patient with cancer may well have strong feelings about his illness, and these feelings may not be obvious either to the patient or to the observing nursing and medical personnel. Such feelings can well affect the course of the patient's planned therapy. Tension and apprehension can delay postoperative healing. Concern about financial problems or home situations may complicate and delay the recovery from a heart disorder. Therefore, one aspect of all planned nursing therapy for the patient with any physical disease must be the recognition of the possible impact of the patient's feelings on the disease process itself. The nurse's function relates to providing the patient with the opportunity for exploration, identification, and acceptance of such feelings. This supportive element of nursing care, based upon a recognition of the interrelatedness of emotions and organic illness, is designed to help the patient to an equal recognition which he, in turn, can use to help himself.

Man is essentially, by nature of the life he leads, a social creature. We achieve identity and a self-concept through interaction with others, under the rules and control of the society in which we live. Basic to the attainment of positive health is the existence of communication with others. Communication is effective when we can convey what we really mean to others and when we know what we are trying to communicate. Communication is not limited to verbal exchange but includes all the nonverbal methods of conveying meaning, such as facial expression, gestures, body posture, body movement, and similar means. In fact, we are often more accurate and more obvious with nonverbal communication than with verbal. And we are more likely to convey very real meanings, of which we are not aware, through nonverbal rather than verbal methods. Both aspects of communication are significant in maintaining effective interaction with others.

When confronted with a health problem, patients, who are still people, continue to need to maintain effective communication with others. Communication is a two-way street. There must be someone with whom to communicate. This latter role is one for nursing service personnel. Channels for communication must be kept open, and every effort must be made to understand what the patient is actually trying to say. Nonverbal clues must be interpreted as accurately as possible, and needs for information and reassurance must be identified and met.

In addition to keeping communication open and oriented toward patient needs, there is a need to provide the patient with an opportunity for productive interpersonal relationships. Communication, of course, is one of the basic aspects of interpersonal relationships. It is quite possible to communicate very clearly to a patient, and nurses often do, that the patient is a nuisance. Such communication is hardly conducive to productive interpersonal relationships. Productive interpersonal relationships are those through which a patient can grow. Ideally, any patient who recovers from an illness after professional therapy should understand himself and his health problem better, should be knowledgeably self-directive in dealing with his health problem, and should be able to work with his strengths and his limitations as a person more effectively. This indicates growth. Since, in all probability, the most significant part of any environment is the people in it, the patient's greatest need is for the kind of interpersonal relationships that promote his personal growth. Such relationships are not casually superficial, friendly, and social. They are goal-directed by the nurse, determined by patient needs, and based upon the use of a broad knowledge about human behavior. Just being "kind" is being inadequate. The patient's need for productive interpersonal relationships with others requires nursing service personnel who can intelligently and knowledgeably provide such relationships.

An additional covert nursing problem confronted by patients is the need to facilitate progress toward personal spiritual goals. In fact, many of our more common health problems, such as heart disease and cancer, may well provide the stimulus that brings the patient to a deeper search for the meaning of his life. The great danger in this area is the temptation for nursing personnel to provide the patient with ready-made answers. The spiritual goal must be the patient's own, identified and accepted by the patient. The function of the nurse, when the opportunity arises, is to provide the patient with the opportunity to explore and to identify his own goals.

The patient also needs to participate in and experience the maintenance of a therapeutic environment. A therapeutic environment is one that supports recovery and improvement when possible. It is an environment in which each individual retains a sense of worth and dignity and a feeling of being important as a person. There is much in hospital routine and administrative procedures that can hardly be considered therapeutic. The days when this was justifiable on the basis that "things had to get done" and that patients "really needed only good physical and medical treatment" are long gone. Such days ended with the changing pattern of health problems and the explosion of scientific knowledge.

That the environment has a definite effect on a patient's disease process, rate of recovery, and ultimate prognosis has been demonstrated over and over again. In psychiatric hospitals, it has been proved that patient symptoms are unfavorably affected by covert conflict between personnel. Anyone hospitalized who physically needs rest can testify with heartfelt conviction, upon recovery, about the impact of a noisy night shift. Observant visitors have noted the untoward effect of personnel casualness and indifference to the obvious anxiety of a preoperative patient. The impersonality of admission procedures have produced anxiety in untold numbers of patients—anxiety which compounded already existing problems. If the complications and delay in recovery resulting from medical rounds with their free and technical discussions in front of patients were computed, the results would undoubtedly be staggering. Some of the implications of the establishment of a therapeutic environment oriented toward patient needs have come from projects in psychiatric hospitals, in which it has been clearly demonstrated that a genuine therapeutic environment does lead to patient improvement and/or recovery with a high degree of consistency. The application of this concept to general hospitals is in its infancy. However, there can be little doubt of its promise.

The last of the covert nursing problems faced by patients is the need to facilitate awareness of oneself as an individual with varying physical, emotional, and developmental needs. This, too, is part of personal growth, and the need calls for skill on the part of nursing personnel who can provide the type of interrelationships and the kind of environment that encourage personal growth on the part of patients.

BEHAVIOR AND COVERT NURSING PROBLEMS

The identification of covert nursing problems is not always easy. Most adults, in particular, have a reasonably strong wall of defense behind which they attempt to obscure or hide those problems which they consider socially unacceptable or which they do not wish or know how to face. Certain signs or clues may exist to indicate the strong possibility of a covert nursing problem, but the identification of the specific problem requires considerable skill in, first, providing the patient with an opportunity to express it and, second, interpreting correctly what the patient expressed.

There are as many and varied clues to the existence of emotion and psychological nursing problems as there are patients. People are like the leaves on trees—no two are exactly alike. Considering that behavior is learned and that no two of us live in exactly the same environment, it is not really surprising that we all differ. Existence holds its own personal meaning for each of us, and literature in all languages has dealt with the theme of the depths of personal experience that cannot be communicated to others. One man's happiness may be another man's hell. And neither can understand to the fullest extent the experience of the other. Yet, the outward surface behavior of the two may be similar.

Nonetheless, certain kinds of behavior on the part of patients may reasonably be assumed to indicate the presence of a covert nursing problem. Included in this category are regression, crying, criticalness, hostility, depression, dependency, indifference, and extremes and change in behavior.

Regression, by definition, is a reversion to a pattern of behavior characteristic of an earlier phase of development. This is a common occurrence during an episode of a physical illness and can be annoying unless it is recognized and understood. Nursing jargon acknowledges the phenomenon. Commonly heard remarks include: "Men are such babies about pain." "She acts like a child when she gets an injection." "Women patients want as much attention as children." A careful ear will note the extent to which references to regressive behavior occur in casual ward conversation.

Regression, per se, is not "bad" in itself. In fact, it is usually a normal part of the earlier phases of physical illness. The continued use of regressive behavior, however, is generally recognized as a clue to the existence of a covert nursing problem. The patient who continues to respond as a child or an adolescent, or as a young adult if he is an older one, is expressing in behavior some problem with which he is not, temporarily at least, effectively coping. The nurse's problem then becomes one of identification of the patient's covert nursing problem.

The crying patient is one who, while having problems of her own, tends to present real problems for nurses because of the discomfort and uneasiness aroused in personnel. Again, crying is not always "bad." In fact, most of us recognize the ventilation and release of crying through the oft-given advice to "go have a good cry and get it off your chest." To be noted, however, is the fact that we advise others to go somewhere out of our own sight to have their good cry. The patient who cries, however, does give us a clue that a covert nursing problem exists although the actual problem may not be easy to identify. The crying signals a need for indirect nursing approaches and for intelligent supportive nursing care.

The patient who is constantly critical is a patient who is spelling out the existence of emotional or psychological difficulty. The patient who complains about the noise, the food, the doctors, the nurses, and the weather, is basically a person on the attack, and the person who needs to continuously attack the environment and everyone in it is not a happy person. This may be a temporary pattern associated with the specific health problem, or it may be a consistent life pattern for the individual. Such a patient tends to rank high on the rejection list. Actually, the patient is communicating a need for understanding and support. But communication is a two-way street, and the nurse must have the knowledge and skill to get beyond the immediate reaction to the patient's behavior, to understand its meaning and its significance, and to use this understanding in planning nursing care that meets the patient's expressed needs.

Closely related to the critical patient is the hostile patient. In fact, criticism is one way of expressing hostility. Hostility may be expressed in other ways, such as causing personnel a great deal of difficulty, by being demanding, by interfering with therapeutic measures, by placing blame on others, by supercilious and superior attitudes, and by using other devices to make people uncomfortable and insecure. A person who is hostile is a person with a covert nursing problem. Rather than needing a direct reaction to their hostility, such patients need from nurses a recognition that the covert, underlying cause for the hostility is the nursing problem the patient has identified. The nurse's own problem may be the patient's hostility—but the hostility is actually the obvious symptom of a covert nursing problem of the patient.

Depression is another indication that a patient is having emotional or psychological difficulties. Depressions are not always pathological. There are many situations confronting patients with health problems in which the total absence of any degree of depression would be unrealistic. Whether justified or not, in any case, the patient is not very likely to respond to blithe assurances that "all will be well in this best of all possible worlds where the omnipotent medical and nursing teams know best and will do their best." The patient's depression is an expression of feeling, a negative feeling that the patient needs to explore, identify, and accept before he can change it. He *may* be able to do this for himself, or he may not. If the former is true, nurses can facilitate the process by providing the patient with the needed opportunity. If the latter is the case, the nurse represents one of the patient's few chances for help with his problem. The depression the patient experiences is a clue for nursing action in the area of using techniques appropriate to covert nursing problems.

Dependency is a kind of behavior that hospital personnel all too often attempt to force on patients. Dependency, like regression, is often a temporary part of any physical or emotional illness during which the patient is forced to seek skilled help upon which he must depend. However, submissiveness and dependency that are prolonged or completely dominate a patient's behavior pattern are indications of a probable covert nursing problem. Again, the clue is one for nursing action. As usual, the response that is indicated is less a direct response to the dependency as such than a response that seeks to understand the basic nursing problem, which may well be anxiety or fear.

Another type of behavior that leads to a suspicion of the existence of covert nursing problems is indifference. The patient who utterly lacks concern about his symptoms or his progress is very likely to be denying what is happening to him. This is an unrealistic response at best. Underlying such denial are psychological factors that make it difficult or impossible for the patient to face the reality that confronts him. The underlying factors constitute the basic nursing problem, and the indifference is the outward indication or symptom of the underlying difficulty.

Another pattern of behavior which indicates a psychological difficulty is a preoccupation with the physical body function which some patients show. Such a focus upon body function tends to exclude aspects of existence that are important and that are, in a sense, denied by the patient. Such denial suggests that parts of existence are so painful and arouse so much anxiety that the patient must reject this very existence. The rejection of significant aspects of experience limits growth and the attainment of maturity. The patient's behavior is an outward indication of internal difficulties.

Extremes in behavior almost always indicate some degree of emotional or psychological difficulty. Extremes in behavior tend to develop to hide the unacceptable existence of their actual opposites. The patient who is too "sticky sweet" to be true is often a very hostile person who cannot accept her own hostile feelings. The patient who is too happy and too full of jokes is often a person who is depressed and who cannot face her own depression. Whenever extremes in behavior occur, it is wise to look for the opposite theme as an underlying factor in such behavior.

A sudden change in behavior is also an alert signal that the patient may be experiencing emotional or psychological problems. The classic example is the convalescent psychiatric patient who suddenly became relaxed, comfortable, and at ease, with tension disappearing. The patient had made up her mind how to commit suicide. Not all sudden changes in behavior are the result of such dramatic decisions, but certainly a sudden change in any patient's behavior is worthy of serious consideration as a potential indication of emotional problems.

The kinds of behavior that have been presented are samples of clues that patients provide to alert nurses to the existence of covert nursing problems.

UNDERSTANDING AND COVERT NURSING PROBLEMS

One of the fundamental tools needed by the nurse who is caring for patients with covert nursing problems is an understanding of human behavior. Understanding is a higher intellectual skill than knowing. To understand we must know, but we can know without understanding. To understand is to interpret, to apply, to see relationships, and to make judgments. The nurse must accurately observe behavior, correctly interpret its meaning, and be able to predict with some success how what she does will affect the patient's behavior. This constitutes the basis for intelligent intervention in patient behavior. Granted that the element of the unpredictable in human behavior makes it impossible to predict behavior with complete accuracy, skill can be developed in the observation and interpretation of behavior, in using open-end questions and reflection, in giving information, in conveying acceptance, in listening, in setting limits, and in teaching and in counseling, all of which are techniques used in working with patients with covert nursing problems.

Behavior has meaning. The nurse's observation and interpretation of patient behavior should be directed toward seeking that meaning. If a patient is critical of everyone in his surroundings, "why"? What does it mean to the patient? If a patient is dependent, what does he accomplish with this behavior and what does it mean to him? If a patient is resistant to therapeutic procedures, "why"? Why is the "why" important to the patient—what does it mean to him? If the patient treats me like a child, "why"? What do I mean to the patient in this situation? What does the patient's illness mean to him? How and why does he see it differently than I do? On the basis of the "why's" and their meaning, hypotheses as to how the patient will react to the nurse's behavior can be formulated. Such hypotheses can then be tested in action. If they are successful, "why"? If they fail, "why"? It is only through the habit of constant analysis that skill in observation and interpretation of behavior and skill in nursing intervention are developed. And the understanding of human behavior is a fundamental intellectual skill demanded by nursing.

BIBLIOGRAPHY

1. Abdellah, Faye G.: Methods of identifying covert aspects of nursing problems, Nursing Research 6:4-33, June 1957.

2. Abdellah, Faye G., Beland, Irene L., Martin, Almeda, and Matheney, Ruth V.: Patient-centered approaches to nursing, New York, 1960, The Macmillan Co., pp. 1-19.
3. Hassenplug, Lulu Wolf: The world of nursing—2000 A.D., American Journal of Nursing 62:100-102, Jan. 1962.
4. Matheney, Ruth V., and Topalis, Mary: Psychiatric nursing, ed. 3, St. Louis, 1961, The C. V. Mosby Co., pp. 69-77.
5. Mullane, Mary K.: Proposals for the future of nursing, Nursing Forum 1:73-84, Fall 1962.
6. Simmons, Leo W.: What is the potential role of the nurse in patient care? Nursing Outlook 10:103-105, Feb. 1962.
7. Charles Marie, Sister: Nursing needs more freedom, American Journal of Nursing 62:53-55, June 1962.
8. Taylor, Carol Dickinson: Sociological sheep shearing, Nursing Forum 1:78-89, Spring 1962.

Chapter 5

Personality development

Human behavior is not readily understood because of its complexity. Although a certain identifiable consistency in repeating certain patterns of behavior appears in each of us, we are, at any given moment, the sum total of all that we have experienced in the past, all that we are experiencing at the present time, plus all we hope and plan to experience in the future. And experience does not have the same meaning for any two persons. In addition to the complexity of our past, present, and future experiences, another complicating factor in understanding behavior is the fact that a great deal of our mental activity occurs on the unconscious level of the mind, outside of personal awareness. We are often unaware of our actual motivations, our real ambitions, and our true feelings. Because we may not recognize these, we can hardly communicate them to others. Nonetheless, the study of human behavior can be both fascinating and rewarding, because we can learn to identify repeated patterns or themes in behavior and we can sharply improve our ability to find meaning in and to predict behavior with increasing accuracy. Not that we are likely to achieve perfection, but we can try to improve. Improvement in understanding and predicting behavior is based upon the use of knowledge about personality and its growth, development, and change.

DEFINITIONS

Personality is used in its technical rather than popular sense. Common usage equates the word with a favorable social impact on others. One has, or has not, "personality" in everyday conversation. Technically, however, personality means the sum total of all that the individual thinks, feels, and does, as manifested in his interaction with his environment. It includes his characteristic patterns of adjustment, his beliefs, his sense of values, his failures and his successes—all that he is.

In the technical sense, personalities can be placed on a continuum of health ranging from completely healthy to seriously ill. The mentally ill would constitute the latter group. With the changing definition of the word "health," the number of persons who could be classified as having completely healthy personalities is probably reduced. At one time health was equated with the absence of disease. From this concept we moved toward a more positive concept of health, a concept which emphasized improved functioning of the individual even though he suffered from no actual disease process, physical or psychological. Recently the concept of a high-level wellness has been introduced; this approach stresses an integrated method of functioning, on the part of the individual, that is oriented toward progressively higher levels of adaptation and that aspires toward full utilization of the individual's potential. Such a concept of health is a far cry from the concept of health as the absence of disease. Such a concept of health has implications for members of the health service team, because it indicates functions and responsibilities in working with "well" people, a group who receive comparatively less attention than "sick" people.

FACTORS INFLUENCING PERSONALITY DEVELOPMENT

One of the most characteristic attributes of human nature is its plasticity. Man can and does learn from his environment, especially from the significant people in it. He can learn to make loyalty to others his highest value, or he can learn to make competition with others his highest value. He can learn to use communication constructively, or he can learn to use it destructively. He can learn to aspire to one wife and one family, or he can learn to aspire to many wives and many families. What an individual will learn and what kind of personality he will develop depend upon many factors. The development of the personality of any given individual is profoundly influenced by where he is born, the kind of society and family in which he lives, and how he learns to see himself as a person.

Cultural factors provide the setting and determine the broad basis upon which personality is developed. Society provides a range of acceptable kinds of behavior, along with controls for enforcing conformation of behavior within certain limits. Society provides us with institutions, each with its organized pattern of behavior; it also provides us with roles, each with its defined acceptable patterns of behavior. We do not have to explore the role of father, son, or daughter. These roles and the expected behavior that goes with them are already defined for us. The role of the doctor and the role of nurse carry certain behavior expectations with them; part of the student's education consists of learning what these expectations are. Society provides us with goals and defines the road for achievement of these goals. For example, the society in which we live places a high value on the possession of academic degrees. As a result, the personal ambition of an increasing proportion of the population in the United States includes higher education. Our society places a high value on success and monetary reward. So, more and more of our population seek success and monetary reward.

The culture in which one lives also provides subdivisions or classes, with acceptable patterns of behavior defined for each class. If the class system is rigid, upward mobility on the part of individuals in the lower classes is almost impossible. If the class system encourages mobility, then the individual may aspire to upward changes in status, but he must also learn to change behavior patterns to fit or to belong in the new group. A society may also encourage upward mobility in class and, at the same time, make it extremely difficult to achieve. As a result of this, many of its citizens will experience frustration, and this, in turn, will have a definite effect upon their personality development.

One aspect of understanding behavior, then, is understanding the cultural background of the individual being observed. What is the value system of his society? What are its accepted behavior patterns? What are its eating habits? What does health mean and what is accepted health behavior? What are the subdivisions within the society? Where does the pattern fit into this organization? The recognition that cultural differences do exist, and especially exist in attitudes and behavior toward health and health problems, is the first step. The second step is to seek information concerning particular cultures from which patients come. And the third step is to understand, or to use the knowledge gained to recognize that behavior which is culturally determined, even though it may differ from what our own culture has taught us to expect. Our culture does not, for example, generally expect men to moan, groan, or complain too much about pain; however, there are cultures that do.

Differences also exist in health behavior within cultures. In America, socioeconomic status influences the existence of health problems and the kind and the amount of health services that are sought and received. For example, the incidence of tuberculosis is higher in the lower socioeconomic group. In psychiatric institutions, there is a tendency for patients of lower socioeconomic status to receive more somatic treatment, such as shock and chemotherapy, and less psychotherapy than patients in higher socioeconomic levels. Although socioeconomic status is probably most closely related to variations in patterns of using health services, other variations are related to level of education, age, sex, and race. One would hardly expect the same health behavior from a sharecropping farmer and a banker. Sensitivity to differences in accepted behavior patterns among cultures and within any specific culture helps in understanding behavior.

One of the major factors in setting limits upon the extent to which personality development for any individual will approach its maximum potential is the family into which an individual is born. It is in infant and early childhood experiences that some of the most important aspects of personality are determined. The experience of being unconditionally loved and wanted contributes profoundly to the ability to grow and to mature. Family behavior patterns provide models for learning. Family attitudes, feelings, and values are deeply significant for the growing youngster, for these are the attitudes, feelings, and values he incorporates. The number of children in the family and the placement of the individual in the family constellation are also factors. Rejection, neglect, isolation, oversolicitousness, and rigid discipline with frequent punitive measures can severely limit personality growth and development in later years. It is within the confines of the family, or within its substitute, that the child learns to identify himself as an individual and to recognize the kind of individual he is. Although the general pattern of family function is culturally determined, the personal interrelationships within the specific family are the determining factors that significantly mold the matrix of the beginning personality.

The biological equipment with which any individual begins life will also have an impact upon his personality and its development. The integration, coordination, and control of behavior rest essentially in the central nervous system and other regulatory mechanisms of the body, and if these are functionally adequate to the task, they provide the physical background for personality growth and development. If most of the energy available to the individual must be used to maintain life itself, the energy needed for expanding into and exploring the environment is simply not available. If a congenital heart deformity requires that an infant be maintained at rest to survive, the process of socialization will necessarily be delayed. One obvious example is the "hospitalitis" developed by infants who spend, for one reason or another, their first couple of years as hospital patients. Such infants do not develop socially at a normal rate of growth, and this delay in growth becomes more obvious as the child becomes older. This does not mean that people cannot surmount limited hardships, such as blindness and deafness. However, organic hardships of sufficient nature to restrict the ability to relate with others can make personality development difficult.

Cultural attitudes toward physical appearance can also influence personality development. Most societies, including our own, have very definite likes and dislikes concerning what constitutes acceptable and unacceptable personal appearance. The individual whose looks and build bring him approval from those around him holds a distinct advantage over the individual who consistently meets distaste and revulsion from others.

INFANCY

During the period of infancy, the growing youngster probably learns more and gains more significant knowledge than he ever will in any other equal amount of time in his entire life. He begins as an apparently helpless mass, not even able to distinguish himself from his environment. His responses are limited and his physical being immature. He is capable of experiencing feeling tones communicated by others but cannot relate them to his own behavior since he does not know who he is. He needs to be fed, to be kept free of pain and discomfort, and to move about as far as he is capable. His tool of communication is crying, a means of communication he learns rapidly to use to manipulate his environment. He is monarch of all he surveys—or is he?

He needs the warmth and physical contact and the feeling exchange that takes place between him and his mother. He learns to differentiate himself from his environment and to know, physically, where he begins and ends. He cannot communicate verbally, but he slowly improves his ability to let others know when he is comfortable and when he is not. He expands his universe as he learns to respond to others in the immediate family, and he goes from these to responding to frequent visitors. His physical coordination improves, and he can move about more widely and explore his environment more freely, widening his range of experience. He responds with increasing accuracy to satisfaction and pleasure on one hand and to pain and discomfort on the other. He repeats pleasurable experiences and tends to avoid unpleasant ones. He begins to have a concept of "I" and "myself," and the kind of "I" he thinks he is is defined in relationships with others through their approval and disapproval of him.

He is sensitive to tension and anger and disliking and liking, and he is somewhat contagious where feelings are concerned, because he reflects those of the significant people around him. He learns to know anxiety, that diffuse feeling of discomfort, although he cannot identify it. For a while he is a delightful hedonist, governed only by his own pleasure. But, as he grows and his ability to differentiate experience increases, he is placed under increasing pressure, through the use of approval and disapproval, to conform to certain demanded behavior patterns. Toilet training introduces a period

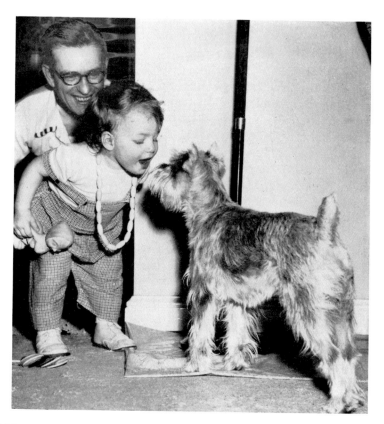

Fig. 3. With parental support, the young child freely explores the environment.

of deliberate frustrations designed to promote his socialization. Reality has more meaning; he responds to outside influences, tempering and changing his behavior in the search for approval that means security and the avoidance of anxiety. He is also learning to talk, although he uses language pretty much as his own personal tool. If he has been loved and wanted, he will feel that he is lovable and worth wanting. If he has been hated, he will hate himself. If he has been rejected, he will reject himself. If he has been threatened, he may well restrict experiences that he needs to grow on, because he is threatened. He has also learned to be more selective in his response to the many stimuli that impinge upon him in his environment. Aspects of day-by-day living that have become significant are selected for response. He is not aware of everything about him, but he is aware of those events, things, and people that have acquired particular meaning. He is particularly responsive to attitudes that are important to him. If his environment has been hostile, he is sensitive to hostility. He has also begun to build a backlog of experiences and feelings that he has forgotten and that may well remain outside conscious awareness for the rest of his life. If such experiences and feelings are painful, they are most likely to remain in the unconscious, from which site they influence personality and behavior. He would not be able to identify this feeling, but his behavior would be affected by its presence.

EARLY CHILDHOOD

During the period of early childhood, the growing personality moves, not always steadily, from his autistic world toward a world more closely approximating reality and a world more shared with others. He continues the process of differentiating himself and his identity. He makes progress in the use of language as he becomes more capable of handling symbols. However, he does go through a period of negativism when it seems his language skills are limited to the use of the word "no." Approval and disapproval of significant persons in his environment continue to be very important to him and are major motivating factors in behavior change. Increasing physical coordination is reflected in a wider range of play activities and a change in the type of such activities.

During this period of life, the child tends to adopt whole patterns of behavior from adults or siblings significant to him. He does not question the attitudes, beliefs, or standards involved, but adopts them without question. He applies these standards literally to others, and his comments and evaluations can sometimes be cruel.

As the child continues this growing self-identification, he continues to derive and strengthen his self-concept through his relationships with adults significant to him, who are usually his parents. The general direction of his self will follow the pattern they establish for him. If he is loved, he will be oriented positively toward others. If he is disliked, he will be apt to dislike others. If he is constantly asked to do more than he is capable of at this period of development, he will be oriented toward and sensitive to failure.

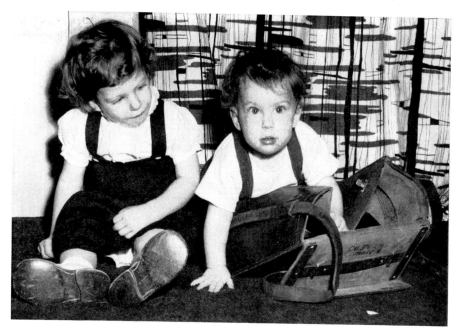

Fig. 4. Children define themselves in relation to each other.

Increasingly he will respond to those experiences and relationships which reinforce the growing self-image. If he is treated as though he were ugly, it will make little difference if he is handsome, for he will behave as though he were ugly.

LATE CHILDHOOD

The period of late childhood is a period of social expansion and growth. The child needs the companionship and interchange with a widening range of people, especially those of his own age group. If such playmates do not exist, he creates them in phantasy. He goes through a period of learning how to compete with others. He tests and develops new social skills in his play activities with his peers, learning new roles, establishing his status with others, and learning to delay satisfactions.

The road of progress is not always smooth, and the child may often regress to patterns of behavior that were appropriate to and successful in earlier phases of development. Slowly the sense of belonging widens, and the child becomes less dependent on the home situation. Much depends upon the self-concept brought to this period of life. The more secure the child, the easier is this period of growth and its successful completion.

This is also a period fraught with certain peril for parents and adult friends. Quarrels are frequent and quickly forgotten. "I'll never speak to you again" usually means just until tomorrow. Mortal enemies one day can be bosom friends the next. "I wish you would die" only means disappear temporarily. Learning to get along with others and still retain a sense of

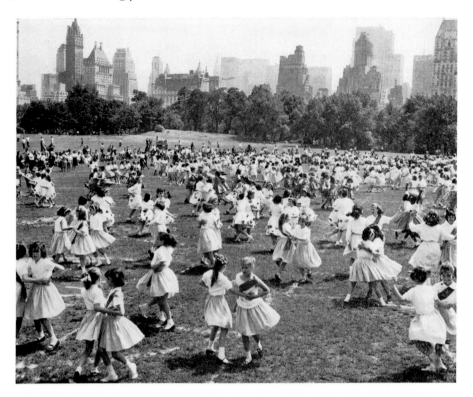

Fig 5. Play with peers is a process of developing and testing new social skills.

well-being and self-respect takes a long time. Some people never manage to learn.

ADOLESCENCE

Following childhood, the growing personality moves into what is probably its most trying period in our culture, the period of adolescence. This period is characterized by a rapid but uneven physical growth that produces an awkwardness and introduces the psychological theme of ambivalence.

The transition from childhood to adulthood is a difficult one. The maturing sexual drive with its accompanying physical changes produces problems, because there is a physical readiness for sexual activity and a cultural block in the way of its achievement. The desire for independence is accompanied by relatively immature judgment, which results in some interesting and embarrassing episodes. Parents tend to resist some of the behavior forms that the expression of independence may take. The adolescent likes to be like, and to be approved of by, his peers, which may well bring him in conflict with parental demands. Although needing to be with and like his peers, the adolescent also yearns to be alone and to develop his own set of values. The need to establish oneself as attractive to the opposite sex encourages

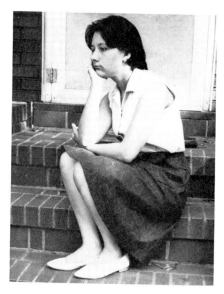

Fig. 6. Adolescence is a difficult and often a lonely period in our culture.

both many dating partners and the steady dating of one partner. Adult privileges appeal while adult responsibilities may not. Parents can appear pretty old-fashioned at this point; yet, the need for their approval continues. The approaching adulthood and eventual independence of the adolescent may cause the parents some discomfort and precipitate difficulties in family relationships.

How much the turmoil of adolescence is due to cultural patterns is uncertain. In any case, the greater the degree of security the developing individual brings to the period, the greater his chances of completing it without too much difficulty.

ADULTHOOD AND MATURITY

Having passed the adolescent period and reached adulthood, the individual may or may not achieve a mature personality. Much depends upon the developmental pattern and the methods of adaptation or adjustment upon which the person has learned to rely. A mature personality is one that is positively oriented toward others, is capable of placing the interest of others above his own, can deal constructively with his own problems most of the time, and can have enough energy left over to contribute to society.

Personality continues to grow and to change throughout life. And most persons struggle toward improved mental health continuously. While early experience may build personality handicaps that present difficulties, such handicaps can be overcome by later corrective experience in relationships with others that help the individual concerned build a more realistic and more acceptable self-concept.

DEVELOPMENTAL STAGES

In the process of reaching psychosocial maturity, as pointed out by Erikson, every person goes through certain developmental stages, each featured by a developmental task that must be successfully completed if the succeeding tasks are to be resolved in turn. Although any given developmental task may be successfully completed at its appropriate stage, it is never completed for all time, since regression may occur or stress may arouse again an interplay between the positive and the negative outcomes inherent in the task.

During the period of infancy one of the major tasks confronting the new individual is the development of trust—trust in oneself, in the environment and the people in it, and in the meaningfulness of existence. Such a sense of trust is derived through the close and intimate association with mother or mother surrogate. A continuous and consistent warm and supportive relationship results in a basic and essential sense of trust. The sense of trust rests on a feeling of inner goodness that is an outgrowth of the relationship. A mother-infant relationship that is inconsistent, cold, or rejecting or that provides little or sporadic support provides experience that builds mistrust into the basic personality of the infant. The relationship is most sensitive at the period when the child experiences a sense of loss as he discriminates himself from his environment and recognizes his mother as a separate entity. The inability to trust the self and its environment can cripple personality development and deprive the growing individual of those interpersonal relationships and experiences which are essential to growth and self-realization.

The second developmental stage occurs in early childhood, and the developmental task at this age is a sense of autonomy. It is a result of the need to establish a differentiation between the self and its own will and the pressures of outside influences. It begins with the period of "I," "we," and "no," being a period of concern with self and with resistance to outside pressures. The favorable outcome of this crisis is a development of a sense of autonomy on the part of the growing child. The negative outcome is a sense of doubt and shame, usually the result of a consistent loss in the battle of "no's" with people who are bigger and stronger.

The third developmental stage is the play age, and the developmental task is the establishment of initiative. The freedom to explore and to reach security in taking the initiative in action comes as the child moves out of the home and the family and into his immediate community. The curiosity and the exploration and the accompanying fantasies can also lead to feelings of guilt with its resulting anxiety. If the guilt is reinforced rather than the curiosity and the exploration and initiative in action, the negative outcome of guilt may result, and the growing personality may develop a sense of "badness," with restrictions on his initiative in later stages of development. This is also the period of the development of conscience.

The next developmental stage is the school age, and the growing personality confronts the task of developing the trait of industry that is essential to the capacity to enjoy work. In this stage, the world expands again, and the skills and tools in working and relating to the world are developed. The child learns to work with others and to produce things, both individually and with others. It is important for the growing personality that the initiative in action developed in the preceding stage amount to something—that what results reflects competence and worth. The danger in this period is the development of a sense of inferiority and mediocrity, usually a result of lack of recognition for efforts.

The fifth developmental stage occurs in puberty and adolescence, and the developmental task is the achievement of a sense of identity. Rapid physical development and the advent of sexual maturity precipitate the crisis of concentration or diffusion—the sense of one's own identity or the diffusion of identity that results from attempting to be too many things to too many persons. The dangers of this period are either diffusion of identity or a negative identity, an attempt to become what others do not want the adolescent to become.

The sixth developmental stage is young adulthood, and the developmental task is the ability to establish intimate relationships with others. The negative alternate choice is isolation. Having established a sense of his own identity and some degree of harmony within himself, the young adult becomes capable of investing some of himself in others. This means the establishment of friendships and eventually a satisfying and satisfactory marriage. If close relationships with others threaten a weak sense of self-identity, isolation ensues and restricts individual ability to achieve self-realization.

The seventh developmental stage is adulthood, in which the developmental task is generativity, and the negative resolution is self-absorption. Generativity is reflected in the individual's establishment and guiding of the next generation. Self-absorption is again a restricted factor in self-realization and results in a sense of stagnation.

The last developmental stage, and the last adult crisis, comes in the late middle or late years of life in which man sums up his personal balance. The result is either a sense of integrity or a sense of despair and disgust. Integrity is achieved when the individual accepts responsibility for what his life has been and finds it has both internal and external worth.

IMPLICATIONS FOR UNDERSTANDING BEHAVIOR

The use of certain specific knowledges can be extremely helpful in understanding behavior. One of the more important is the need to know something about the specific cultural background of a patient. What may appear to be incomprehensible in the light of our cultural behavior may make excellent sense when seen in the perspective of the patient's own culture. The number of visitors who descend upon an acutely ill patient may appear to us to be a hardship on the patient, but in the light of family patterns in his own culture, the patient might well be more upset by their failure to visit. For example, there is a considerable cultural difference in sanitation measures between the United States and some foreign countries, a fact that may be useful in understanding some of the behavior of foreign patients that might otherwise bring censure.

It is also useful to recognize differences in health behavior in the subdivisions of a specific society. It is well to keep in mind that people in the lower socioeconomic groups in the United States are less likely to identify symptoms of illness in need of treatment, and if a symptom has been identified, to seek treatment. Although this may clarify why some patients delay treatment when they need it, it also points out the need for teaching such patients.

A knowledge of the kinds of behavior that characterize certain levels in personality development is useful in identifying regression, a common phenomenon in illness of all types. A recognition of a certain type of behavior as an expression of regression makes it more intelligible. It also makes it easier to identify regression that is prolonged beyond a useful period for the patient.

In observing patient behavior, it becomes important to identify the patterns of recurring behavior that the patient presents rather than trying to interpret behavior on the basis of a single incident or a series of dramatic incidents. Especially significant is identifying the patient's self-image, how he sees himself in relation to others. The general direction of his self-concept will determine those elements of experience to which he is most likely to respond selectively. If, for example, the patient is hostile, he is likely to respond to and to note especially any approach, comment, or suggestion that might imply hostility toward him. Any understanding of the patient's self-image is a valuable tool for determining his nursing needs and for avoiding situations toward which he is likely to be particularly sensitive.

The recognition that personality change and growth is always possible and that a strong tendency to seek the achievement of health is a characteristic of human beings provides the basis for hope and effort in working with patients who have emotional and psychological nursing problems. People can grow and do continue to grow. We can provide at least part of the opportunity.

BIBLIOGRAPHY

1. Dunn, Halbert L.: High-level wellness for man and society, American Journal of Public Health 49:786-792, June 1959.
2. Erikson, Erik H.: Childhood in society, New York, 1950, W. W. Norton & Co., Inc., pp. 219-234.
3. Farnsworth, Dana L.: Mental health—a point of view, American Journal of Nursing 60:688-691, May 1960.
4. Hollingshead, August B., and Redlich, Frederick C.: Social class and mental illness, New York, 1958, John Wiley & Sons, Inc., p. 442.
5. Kariel, Patricia E.: The dynamics of behavior in relation to health, Nursing Outlook 10:402-405, June 1962.

6. Matheney, Ruth V., and Topalis, Mary: Psychiatric nursing, ed. 3, St. Louis, 1961, The C. V. Mosby Co., pp. 27-40.
7. Sullivan, Harry Stack: Conceptions of modern psychiatry, Washington, D. C., 1947, William Alanson White Psychiatric Foundation, pp. 1-42, 119-147.

Chapter 6

Anxiety and stress

ANXIETY

Anxiety is a universal human experience. From the moment of birth, man is capable of feeling anxiety, and the methods he learns to cope with his anxieties will form a central core of his continuously developing personality. Such learning begins very early and is closely related to relationships with the significant persons in the infant's environment. As growth takes place, its limitations or its expansiveness are to a great extent determined by the kinds of experiences that produce anxiety, the depth of anxiety produced, and the methods developed by the growing individual to handle his anxieties. All of these are learned.

Webster defines anxiety as a "painful or apprehensive uneasiness of mind usually over an impending or anticipated ill."[*] The word is derived from the Latin *anxius,* meaning "to cause pain, to choke." It is subjectively experienced as an uncomfortable feeling of apprehension or dread, vague as to cause, and accompanied by physiological responses that are physically uncomfortable. These include such feelings as muscle tension, nausea, increased perspiration, tremor, "lump in the throat," diarrhea, and changes in pulse and respiration rates. Feelings of uncertainty and varying degrees of helplessness are usually concomitant.

The degree of anxiety that constitutes the anxious response may vary from mild to the extreme of panic or terror. In a mild response there may be only a vague discomfort, producing changes in voice tone and posture, accompanied by a feeling predominantly of uncertainty rather than helplessness. As the degree of anxiety increases, the response may progress to the symptoms of a hyperactive sympathetic nervous system. As anxiety mounts beyond this stage, interferences with personality function and effective adaptation to reality become evident. Further anxiety can lead to the development of mental symptoms, including full-fledged psychoneuroses and psychoses. The symptoms of mental illness represent both an expression of and

---

[*]By permission. From Webster's Seventh New Collegiate Dictionary, copyright 1963 by G. & C. Merriam Co., Publishers of the Merriam-Webster Dictionaries.

a defense against anxiety. When anxiety becomes unbearable, panic and terror result. The individual focuses his entire energy on escape, and, if escape fails, the personality becomes totally disorganized.

Anxiety can be expressed in almost as many ways as there are people to express it. As is usually true, it is easier to identify the presence of anxiety in a person when the anxiety itself is more severe. Panic leaves no doubt in the observer's mind. The symptoms of psychotic patients, the obvious and rather glaring deviations from the acceptable social behavioral norms, are easily understood as expressions of anxiety. The symptoms of the psychoneurotic patient are not always so easily recognized, perhaps because of the anxiety aroused by the feelings of helplessness they tend to raise in health service personnel.

It is, of course, the milder expressions of anxiety on the part of relatively well-organized patients that are most difficult to identify and understand. These constitute the indirect expressions of anxiety, and such expressions are highly individualized. Criticism, excessive "sweetness," sullenness, crying, withdrawal, indifference, sarcasm, demandingness, and what is often erroneously labeled "uncooperativeness" can all be presenting symptoms of underlying anxiety. These have been discussed before as presenting symptoms indicating the existence of covert nursing problems. Muscular tension, posture, facial expression, physical restlessness, physical rigidity, level of activity, amount of rest and sleep, and many other physical aspects of behavior provide clues to the existence of underlying anxiety. Anxiety is chameleonic in its expression.

Constructive aspects of anxiety

Anxiety is not always "bad." As a matter of fact, there is a question whether the human race would have survived without this universal phenomenon. Anxiety can serve as a danger signal that stimulates constructive activity to deal with the danger. It can also serve as a stimulus to personal growth and learning and to effective thought and action. In such instances, anxiety is a constructive experience.

Anxiety is constructive when uncertainty is aroused and the accompanying feelings of helplessness are not overwhelming. This is most likely to occur when the individual's personality is strong enough to tolerate anxiety, so that the personality remains sufficiently organized to take action against the threat that arouses anxiety. Another instance in which anxiety is constructive is one in which the individual can realistically externalize the cause of his anxiety. Suppose, for example, a college student can translate his vague apprehension about his ability to succeed in college into passing the final examinations that are due a few weeks hence. With this focus, he then maps out an effective study program in preparation. The anxiety provides sufficient stimulus to lead him to carry out the program of study. In such instances, anxiety is constructive.

Anxiety that is mild, of course, is the anxiety that is most likely to be constructive. The degree of anxiety that is aroused is determined by several

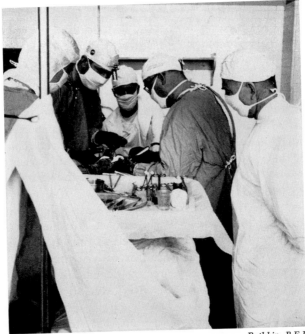

Rothkin, P.F.I.

Fig. 7. Tension and some degree of anxiety can have constructive results. (Courtesy Charles F. Pfizer Co., New York, N. Y.)

factors: the degree of external threat, the personality structure and strength of the individual, and the extent to which the anxiety is individual or shared with others. Mild anxiety is most likely to occur when the source of anxiety is external, shared by others, and experienced by a relatively healthy person.

Destructive aspects of anxiety

Anxiety becomes destructive when it interferes with the realistic adaptation of the individual to his environment, with satisfaction to both individual and environment. The healthy person can effectively utilize his own abilities with satisfaction and security, using his freely chosen system of values that are consistent with the realities of the world in which he lives. To the extent that anxiety interferes with this, it is destructive.

Anxiety lies at the roots of many maladjustments, from the minor to the very severe. It is apparent in the apprehensive person who has trouble making decisions; it is apparent in the person who is afraid to take a vacation for fear he will be replaced; it is apparent in the compulsive person who *must* follow a certain routine; it is apparent in the neurotic person who builds a restricted life around physical complaints; and it is apparent in the mental patient responding to accusing voices. In such patterns, anxiety is destructive because it limits the individual in the full use of his own skills and abilities.

Development of anxiety

There is general agreement among students of human behavior that anxiety is caused by the existence of inner feelings, thoughts, desires, actions, and drives that are unacceptable because they imply or risk disapproval or the loss of love of significant persons or because they imply punishment, separation, or isolation.

Most significant in the development of anxiety are early infant and childhood experiences and relationships with parents and family or their surrogates. Approval and disapproval are the tools used in the early education or socialization of the individual. Within the pattern of such relationships are laid the groundwork of the person's later relationships with others as well as his concept of himself as a human being. The security of undemanding love and wanting, of a sense of personal worth, is a basis for a reaching out, with trust, to the fullest self-realization through relationships with others. If, however, early interpersonal relationships build doubt and mistrust, or hostility, or a warped concept of what other people are like and what to expect from them, or a warped self-image, then the background for a low anxiety tolerance is built. In such instance, in self-defense, the growing and learning child dissociates and keeps from awareness many experiences and many aspects of existence. Because the self-system, or self-image, operates to attain security without too much anxiety, such dissociations and repression are necessary. When any such repressed and unacceptable thoughts, feelings, or action approach awareness, anxiety results. The self-system operates to defend itself by denial and rigidity, which produces conflict with the innate tendency to growth. Some degree of awareness of the inability to grow, the inadequacy of the self-system in a world of reality, produces further anxiety. Thus the pattern of actions, feelings, and thoughts identified as unacceptable in relationships with early significant people, and pushed out of awareness by the self-concept, forms the basis for anxiety. The more limited the sense of personal worth, the more infantile the pattern of interpersonal relationships, and the more unrealistic and rigid the self-system, the greater the significant aspects of existence that are kept from awareness, and the greater the potential for anxiety to reach destructive outcomes for any given person. It must be remembered that people who suffer anxiety are, at best, only dimly aware of its cause.

Cultural aspects of anxiety

The age in which we live has been called the "age of anxiety." Certainly we are more aware of anxiety, and certainly its manifestations have become more overt. Many social factors have contributed both to the rise of anxiety and to awareness of its existence.

We live in a period of rapid social change, so rapid a change that it is unprecedented in human history. As a result, the social lag in cultural values is also unprecedented. Old values, including ethical and moral standards that gave the human race some degree of stability, have lost their status, long before new cultural values could be developed to replace them. "Right" and "wrong" have both become shades of gray. The consistent external values with meaning, which could be internalized by the growing child through his relationships with others, have gone, and there is yet no replacement. The meaning of being an individual, the sense of relationships to the rest of the universe, and relationship to the society and the family circle in which one lives are fluid concerns in a state of flux. This lack of a consistent framework of belongingness in which to grow and develop produces fertile soil for the development of anxiety.

Our society has become profoundly complex. As its complexity increases, greater organization of the culture becomes a necessity. Interdependence increases. With increasing interdependence and increasing organization, the life of the individual becomes more regulated, with less and less room for the different, the unusual, the unique individual. The balance between the man and the society becomes unbalanced and the pressure for conformity increases. With such pressures, it becomes increasingly difficult for individuals to develop a sense of self-worth and dignity and to be able to see others as persons of worth and dignity. Our novels and our professional literature are filled with a search for self-identity. Such a social setting is a background that is rich in potential anxiety.

The world in which we live has suddenly become a small world. Rapid transportation and rapid, mass communication have moved us so close together that ideological conflicts are worldwide rather than restricted to limited sections of the globe. As a result, we are in the midst of a worldwide cold war, in a period when expanded knowledge has provided us with weapons that make possible destruction on such a scale that it dwarfs the imagination. In addition to this appalling aspect of the "new world" in which we live, this smaller world has brought more closely home to the average person the very wide and very disturbing gap in standards of living among the peoples of the world. While some of us experience the highest standards of living yet achieved by any nation, the world's majority lives with poverty, disease, illiteracy, hunger, and hopelessness. As we have learned more about them, they have learned more about us, and the "have-nots" have made clear they no longer intend to remain thus. The emerging nations will have their "place in the sun." But the moral questions remain, and they are disturbing. The shrinking world contributes several sources of anxiety.

Along with the rapid expansion of knowledge, there has been an emphasis on the study of man and his behavior and increased knowledge about him. With this growing knowledge there has developed an increase in self-consciousness, a deeper concern with the inner aspects of man's existence. This greater emphasis upon awareness has brought the existence and importance of the phenomenon of anxiety into focus, and covert anxiety has increasingly become overt anxiety. Perhaps this is one reason why the present is called "age of anxiety." The needs to feel a sense of worth as an individual, to relate effectively with others, and to belong somewhere in the world have not decreased, but their achievement has become con-

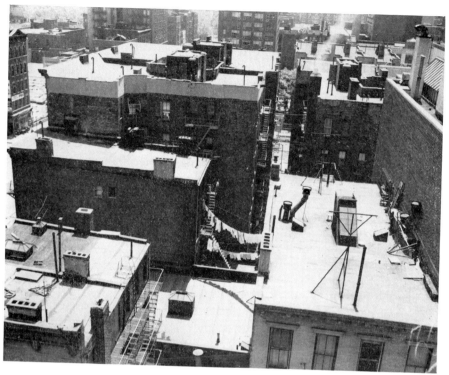

Fig. 8. In the midst of plenty, some people live in relative poverty. The discrepancy between the "have's and have-not's" is a major source of world tension.

sciously more difficult to accomplish in the cultural setting in which we live.

Defenses against anxiety

Anxiety is aroused by the unacceptable feelings, thoughts, wishes, desires, and actions that may lead to disapproval or loss of love, punishment, separation, or isolation. What these may constitute for any given individual is the result of his personal experience, especially his experience in early infancy and childhood, and his concept of himself as a person. The extent to which the behavior of all of us is determined by an effort to avoid or minimize anxiety would probably startle any of us if we were fully cognizant of the meaning or the motivation of our own behavior. We all "defend" ourselves against anxiety. How we do so is largely an individual matter. There are, however, certain patterns of defense, shared in nature if not in degree, that are common to most of us. There are the so-called "defense mechanisms."

Healthy individuals will use the defense mechanisms, but they will also more frequently use a rational attack on the cause of anxiety. For example, if a physician feels confident in treating most patients, but is anxious and feels helpless in dealing with psychoneurotic patients, he will make an organized efforts to learn to understand the "why's" of psychoneurotic behavior and the techniques of treatment.

One method of dealing with anxiety is denial, and denial is commonly used. It is rejection of things, events, or feelings as they actually are, thus eliminating any need for anxiety. A fairly easy use of denial to identify in other people (it is always easier to observe in other people) is the denial of obvious traits or characteristics that are unacceptable to the individual. People who are obviously authoritarian often deny this to themselves and think and talk about their "democratic" approach. Teachers whose actions betray their actual dislike for students talk at length about how much they "like" young people and have absolutely no recognition of their own real feelings. Mothers who have obvious favorites among their children deny favoritism and actually think they do not play favorites. They boy who is angry at his mother insists he loves her and is unaware of his concealed anger. Denial is used by everyone at some time, more frequently by some people, and can become for them a major method for dealing with anxiety.

Rationalization is a common defense mechanism for avoiding or controlling anxiety and is sufficiently well used and well known to have become part of our everyday language. It consists of finding a reason for feelings, thoughts, or actions that are acceptable, while the real and unacceptable reason is kept from awareness. An example is the wife who goes to a bridge party to punish her husband, who must prepare his own lunch, but explains it to herself and others as maintaining social contacts that will help her husband. She remains genuinely unaware of the real reason for her behavior. Rationalization is a mechanism commonly used when we indulge in responding to the pleasure principle, that is, doing what we really want to because it gives us pleasure regardless of the consequences. The employee who takes a day off to go to the races, although he can ill afford the time off or the money he will lose, but justifies it on the grounds of his need for relaxation so that he can return to work in a better frame of mind is an example. Rationalization is used by everyone, but it presents real difficulty when it becomes a major method of avoiding anxiety. It can easily be used to avoid responsibility and to perpetuate ineffective behavior and can lead to a considerable loss of contact with reality.

Displacement is another commonly used defense mechanism and occurs when emotion is transferred from one person, event, or idea to another. In most occupational settings where a hierarchy of personnel exists, this mechanism can be seen rather clearly when someone is reprimanded—the usual procedure is to take it out on someone in a lower rank, thus displacing the emotional content from superior to inferior. It is amazing how often the individual involved is unaware of what has really happened. The man who is angry at his wife and kicks the dog, the boy who is angry at his sister and kicks the table, and the student nurse who is angry at the head nurse and snaps at a patient are examples of the mechanism of displacement.

Reaction formation is an interesting defense mechanism used as a defense against anxiety. It consists of the excessive development of a trait that is the opposite of one the individual actually possesses but one that is unacceptable to him. The most common example is found in the person who is too sweet to be true. Usually underlying such behavior is hostility, which arouses anxiety since it is unacceptable to the person involved. To defend himself against the anxiety, he develops the opposite type of behavior. However, the behavior is exaggerated since constant reinforcement is needed to keep anxiety under control. Something of the same defense is found among fanatics of certain types such as the person who crusades against the use of animals in testing new drugs but who graphically describes the punishment that should be given the persons engaged in such research.

Conversion is a defense mechanism whereby the anxiety felt by an individual is converted into physical symptoms. The symptoms are both an expression of and a defense against anxiety. Conversion is not as commonly used as it once was, because the general public, through education, has become somewhat more sophisticated. Conversion hysteria, for example, was quite common in World War I, and less so in World War II. Usually the physical symptom presented is related to the actual conflict which produces the anxiety. The son who wishes to strike his father, a desire unacceptable to him and hence anxiety provoking, develops paralysis of the arm. The paralysis is both symptomatic of the anxiety and also controls it because it makes the desired action impossible.

The defense mechanism of repression, an extremely common mechanism, is the unconscious forcing of unpleasant experiences and unacceptable feelings, thoughts, and actions into the unconscious. The repressed material cannot be brought into conscious awareness. This is, in a sense, an active and continuous form of denial. While the repressed experiences continue to influence motivation and behavior from the unconscious, the process of repression serves to control or reduce anxiety. All of us are aware of the fact that there are experiences, feelings, and thoughts that we cannot recall, no matter how hard we try. The myth of the happy childhood probably rests on this mechanism. Experiences that produce severe anxiety tend to be repressed.

Regression is a defense against anxiety that is a common phenomenon both in physical and mental illness. In the former it tends to be a temporary phase, while in the latter it becomes a major mode of adaptation. It is also a common occurrence in the process of growing up. Regression is a retreat to past levels of behavior, usually those that were successful at a lower level of development. The adult who, temporarily thwarted, stamps her feet and screams has regressed to a much earlier level of behavior. All of us are guilty of this kind of lapse now and then. The teen-ager who cries to get her own way is using a regressed pattern of behavior. The adult with a physical illness who becomes dependent is regressing to an earlier stage of development. The psychiatric patient can and does regress to an infantile level of behavior. It is not unusual to see childish or adolescent behavior in adults on occasions. When, however, regression persists or becomes a predominant behavior manifestation, the underlying anxiety is sufficiently severe to constitute a major personality threat.

Identification and introjection are related defense mechanisms that serve the basic purpose of dealing with anxiety, and both are significant aspects of the process of growing. Identification is the acceptance of external ideas, values, behaviors, or persons and feeling with them as though they were part of oneself, although recognizing that they are not. One feels a personal sense of satisfaction when the home run hitter with whom one identifies connects for the circuit. Introjection goes further in that the ideals and behaviors become integrated into the individual's personality and become an integral part of him. The athletic hero with whom one identifies represents fair play, and the value of fair play becomes a part of the identifying person himself, an introjected value that will govern his own behavior without the stimulus of the hero's presence, real or fancied. This ability to identify with and introject both allays anxieties and provides a means of setting standards and goals for individual growth and development. It is through these processes, to a great extent, in relation to parents or their surrogates that the growing personality is formed.

Projection is another defense mechanism deigned to relieve a person of anxiety. Projection is the process of externalizing inner perceptions. Feelings, thoughts, and actions that originate within the individual are perceived as having their origin outside the self. All of us use projection at some time (students seem particularly prone to use it at grade time), and people whose predominant method of adaptation is projection are prone to mental illness of the paranoid varity. The student who fails an examination finds it easier to blame the instructor for failing to teach than to blame himself for failing to study. The failure is thus projected to the instructor and the anxiety of personal lack of effort or inadequacy avoided. Any personal failing or inadequacy that tends to create anxiety can thus be externalized and the anxiety, consequently, allayed. The "voices" heard by psychotic patients are actually projections of inner thoughts. Projection is a dangerous defense mechanism on which to lean to any great extent.

Sublimation is a generally constructive defense mechanism when it works to allay anxiety. The energy involved in feelings, thought, and actions that are unacceptable, individually or socially, are diverted to activities that are socially acceptable and often socially beneficial.

Transference is a defense mechanism that functions to allay anxiety and is a mechanism that lends itself well to support therapeutic processes. Basically, it consists of transferring a positive or negative emotional orientation from one object or person to another. This overuse of the response constellation has an economical aspect, because it makes the development of new sets of responses unnecessary. It also tends to reduce anxiety to some extent, since predictable responses in other situations are used. However, transference can also be used to uncover significant anxieties arising from relationships in the past when feelings that remain on an unconscious level are transferred to a therapist. Such anxieties can then be therapeutically handled. Transference is therefore of value in therapy.

STRESS

Stress is defined by Webster as "a constraining force or influence, as a physical, chemical, or emotional factor that causes bodily or mental tension."* The word is derived from the Latin *strictus,* past participle of *stringere,* meaning "to bind tight." The essence of stress, therefore, is intense strain. Stress produces anxiety, leading to a protective reaction that may or may not be appropriate and effective, and is consequently closely related to the development and the therapy of both physical and mental illness.

What constitutes stress for any given individual is a highly personalized matter. It depends upon his physical makeup, his personal experience, and the cultural setting in which he lives. Stress may be external in origin, such as an invasion by germs or noxious agents or from pressures from society. Stress may also be internal in origin and arise from the individual's interpretation of a situation as threatening to himself or from an internal physical threat such as a disturbance in fluid and electrolyte balance. There is thus a tremendous range of events, internal and external, which can constitute a source of stress for any individual.

Stress calls forth protective reaction patterns that serve to dissipate threats, avoid dangers, satisfy needs, or achieve goals. Part of this response is physiological and includes the use of all organ systems that prepare the body to respond to threat of danger. For example, if the danger is the possibility of physical assault, the body mechanisms prepare for fight or flight by accelerating or strengthening heart action, dilating bronchial tubes to increase oxygen intake, releasing glycogen from the liver to supply extra energy fuel, secreting epinephrine as a stimulant, and decreasing the activity of vegetative organs such as the stomach and visceral muscle of the intestine. The body is prepared for action. There is considerable similarity in the response of the body to stress produced by situations that are interpreted by the individual as being threatening or dangerous. Because it is the situation as interpreted by the individual that determines what constitutes a danger, almost any situation is capable of producing stress. To the psychosocial response of the individual is added the physiological response. If this combined response resolves the difficulty, the protective reaction is appropriate and effective. If, however, the response is used exclusively, or too often, or inappropriately, either physical or psychological damage can result, and not infrequently both. Personal stresses can thus activate physical disease or can present a problem in successful therapy.

IMPLICATIONS FOR NURSING

It becomes, then, part and parcel of a nurse's responsibility to know the meaning of anxiety and stress, to learn to recognize and to identify the many ways that anxiety can be expressed, and to recognize and identify the wide range of situations that can produce stress in the light of its highly personalized nature. The meaning of anxiety and stress to illness and to ther-

*By permission. From Webster's Seventh New Collegiate Dictionary, copyright 1963 by G. & C. Merriam Co., Publishers of the Merriam-Webster Dictionaries.

apy also calls for an acute sensitivity to those situations and experiences related to the nurse's own working environment that have a high potential for producing stress and anxiety.

It would be impossible to remove all stress from a hospital situation. There are, however, certain kinds of stress-producing situations in which it is possible to reduce anxiety. The change in roles that the patient undergoes as he moves from an independent role in the community to a dependent and passive role in the hospital is rife with stress. Recognition of the implications of this change, along with the anxiety that illness itself produces, can lead to a recognition of the need for orientation, the need for support from the family, the need for providing the patient with an opportunity to discuss and ventilate his feelings, the need to provide the patient with some means of retaining his identity, and the need to participate in his own therapy.

Some nursing functions are unpleasant and some are downright painful for the patient. No one likes to receive injections. Many forms of irrigation violate privacy and produce physical discomfort. A fresh look at the implications of nursing and medical procedures in terms of this anxiety potential might mean more sensitivity in their administrations, and, with this, a re-

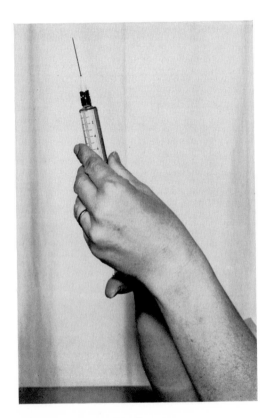

Fig. 9. Some nursing functions are sources of anxiety.

duction or avoidance of stress might considerably improve the therapeutic effect.

The recognition that physical illness itself may have been activated by stress and resultant anxiety and that the two can impede the process of recovery, if the patient is to recover, may broaden the nurse's understanding of her own role in the provision of nursing care. Good "physical care" is as inadequate in nursing as it is in medicine. The avoidance of stress and anxiety and working to reduce stress and allay anxiety are significant aspects of nursing.

In addition, there is the problem of the nurse's own anxieties. Some degree of self-understanding seems essential if the nurse is to function therapeutically. What are the kinds of patients and the kinds of situations that create the greatest anxiety for us as people? Can we learn to identify these and use the knowledge to improve our effectiveness? Can we free ourselves, to some extent at least, from the bind of our own covert problems?

BIBLIOGRAPHY

1. Bock, Walter E., and Bock, Jean K.: Society and health, New York, 1956, G. P. Putnam's Sons, pp. 238-266.
2. Fromm-Reichmann, Frieda: Psychiatric aspects of anxiety. In Stein, M., Vidich, A. J., and White, D. M. (editors): Identity and anxiety, Glencoe, Ill., 1960, Free Press, pp. 129-141.
3. May, Rollo: Centrality of the problems of anxiety in our day. In Stein, M., Vidich, A. J., and White, D. J. (editors): Identity and anxiety, Glencoe, Ill., 1960, Free Press, pp. 120-128.
4. Neyland, Margaret Prowse: Anxiety, American Journal of Nursing **62**:110-111, May 1962.
5. Simmons, Leo W., and Wolff, Harold G.: Social science in medicine, New York, 1954, Russell Sage Foundation, pp. 109-169.

Chapter 7

Nursing intervention in covert nursing problems

Nursing responsibilities in working with covert nursing problems presented by patients are almost exclusively independent functions, resting upon the use of judgment. The psychological and supportive aspects of nursing care include the use of skilled observation, conversational and interviewing techniques, conveying acceptance, teaching, constructive use of self understanding, setting limits, and developing nurse-patient relationships.

SKILL IN IDENTIFICATION OF COVERT NURSING PROBLEMS

In general, personnel in the health services have not been too skilled in the identification of covert (psychological or social) nursing problems. As pointed out by Faye Abdellah in a study that included the perception of covert problems by patients, doctors, and nurses, "It is significant to note that eighty to eighty-four percent of the emotional nursing problems described by patients were not mentioned by either nurses or doctors."[*] Physical, or overt, nursing problems are easier to identify, and their treatment is often more specific and more direct. Overt problems are also easier to elicit by direct approach, a method used frequently by health service personnel. The direct approach, however, is ineffective in identifying or eliciting covert nursing problems. Indirect approaches, including listening, paraphrasing, reflecting, and open-end questions are much more effective tools for the identification of covert nursing problems.

Patients' covert nursing problems tend to be found in the areas of negative feelings, the interrelatedness of emotions and organic illness, the maintenance of effective communication, the development of productive interpersonal relationships, the development of personal growth, and the maintenance of a therapeutic environment. These are the areas of emotional and

---

[*]Abdellah, Faye G.: Methods of identifying covert aspects of nursing problems, Nursing Research **6**:19, June 1957.

interpersonal difficulties and constitute, therefore, the guides for observation.

In observing patient behavior for the possible existence of covert nursing problems, it is unfortunate that specific kinds of behavior cannot be identified as specific indicators of a specific problem. Behavior is much too complex for this, and anxiety can be expressed in too many different ways. Nor can one rely upon interpretation of the situation in which the patient is found, for experience has a different meaning for each of us. With this caution in mind, there are certain clues that should alert the nurse to the possibility of potential covert nursing problems.

Indications of physical tension would suggest stress and anxiety. Rigid body posture, strained facial expression, or an over response to environmental stimuli are examples. Negative emotional responses to the environment and the people in it are significant clues. Hostility, criticism, over sweetness, whining, crying, and demanding attention are all symptoms of underlying anxiety. The denial of physical illness and its implications is another type of behavior that would arouse suspicion. The patient with a very recent and serious coronary infarction who insists upon going to the bathroom himself and shaving himself (and all nurses have known at least *one* such patient) is an example of the denial of the implications of illness. The patient who responds with behavior or emotional reaction that is not exactly appropriate may also be presenting evidence of a covert nursing problem. The patient with newly diagnosed diabetes who does not plan to adapt his dietary pattern to his metabolic problem would be an example. The patient deeply depressed as the result of a minor injury in an accident would be another example of inappropriate response. In almost all such instances, the patient is providing outward evidence of the existence of a covert nursing problem. The patient who talks too much and the patient who talks too little are doing the same thing. We may not always be able to identify the specific problem, but we can sharpen our ability to recognize that a problem exists. We may be reasonably certain that the immediate preoperative patient who exhibits anxiety has some fear of surgery, but that a mother dislikes her child is a fact not as easy to pinpoint. In either case, we can offer the patient the opportunity to explore *what* he feels, and this is the method of nursing intervention that is indicated.

Another clue, frequent in occurrence, is repeated reference to a certain topic. A recurring topic is one the patient should be encouraged to explore, for it is often a sensitive one. In the observation of patient behavior, the pattern of the particular patient should be sought, and judgments based on single episodes or isolated incidents should be avoided.

In the identification of covert nursing problems, certain techniques are effective, and certain techniques are ineffective. Direct questions, such as "What is bothering you?" are ineffective. Indirect, or open-end, questions that leave the patient free to express what he wishes are more effective. For example, if a patient is asked "How did you sleep last night?" he really can answer only "I did" or "I didn't." If, on the other hand, he is asked

"How did it go last night?" he is free to respond with almost anything. "Tell me more about your problems with your wife" is not as effective as "Would you like to tell me about it?" The question that is somewhat unstructured and gives the patient the freedom to respond and to talk about problems that concern him is the indirect approach.

Listening is an effective method for encouraging patients to express and to explore matters that concern them. Listening is something most people know little about. Most of us, instead of listening, are simply quiet until the other person stops talking—if we wait that long. Listening means hearing what the other person says, along with evidence that we *are* hearing manifested by facial and eye expression. A truly interested and observant listener learns many things.

Paraphrasing what a patient has said is another method of encouraging verbal exploration of topics of interest to the patient. If a patient says "I'm worried about what will happen in my job," the simple response "You're worried about your job" will frequently lead to additional discussion. It leaves channels of communication open for the patient to use as he wishes, and it indicates the nurse's willingness to listen.

Reflection is a somewhat more sophisticated response than paraphrasing and requires a bit more skill in use. In reflection, the nurse identifies and reflects the *feeling* expressed rather than paraphrasing the patient's verbal production. When, for example, the patient says "I'm afraid my boss is trying to get rid of me," the feeling expressed is worry or apprehension, and *this* feeling would be reflected by the nurse. When a patient talks about being unhappy at the loss of a friend or a family member, the unhappiness is "reflected," i.e., saying "you are unhappy?" This is an extremely effective method in identifying the existence of covert nursing problems, and its effectiveness is due to the fact that it conveys acceptance of what the patient actually expresses. The acceptance then encourages further exploration.

Another method of encouraging patient communication is the use of the incomplete sentence, utilizing material the patient has already given. For example, when the patient is talking about pain, the incomplete statement "You have pain . . ." will encourage him to continue. The incomplete sentence, ending with a raised inflection, provides a stimulus to patient verbalization.

There are certain "don'ts" in working with covert nursing problems. Don't ask direct, structured questions. Don't tell the patient what to do and what to feel; this is a means of rejection. Don't waste the patient's time discussing your own problems; this is also a method of rejection.

TALKING WITH PATIENTS

The relationship that exists between a nurse and a patient is a service relationship that exists for the improvement of the health status of patients. It is not a relationship between friends at a purely social level. Conversation, one means of communication and an aspect of the nurse-patient relationship, becomes, therefore, a tool to be used in the patient's interest.

There are several guide lines that govern talking with patients. Such conversation should be purposeful, not merely a means of passing time pleasantly. The purpose is determined by patient needs. Conversation should be focused on the patient, about the patient, and related to the patient. It is easy to fall into the trap of being held to a casual discussion of the weather or the state of the union. It is easier to fall into the trap of talking about oneself. Although questions that are personal can be answered briefly, conversation should be shifted back to the patient and his concerns. Following are some typical goals sought in talking with patients.

1. To learn more about his health problems and the factors that affect them
2. To provide the patient with an opportunity to explore his feelings and reactions
3. To identify and to *meet* needs for information and teaching
4. To provide a sense of worth and dignity to the patient

Goals such as these can be reached only if talking with patients is, to a great extent, listening to patients talk about themselves.

Since nurses and patients are strangers at their first meeting, orientation is an important first step. The patient needs to know who the nurse is and for which functions she will be responsible. The identification of the nurse's name and her registered nurse status are essential. Orientation and explanation of what is to be done and what to expect throughout the hospitalization experience are continued. The explanation of "why" as well as "what" is helpful.

Peplau* suggests avoiding the use of questions asking "why" and "how" with patients, because they call for considerable analytic abilities. "How" asks for the process by which something has occurred, and "why" asks for the reasons or explanations. Both words have been so overworked that they have lost their meaning. Most nurses who ask patients "Why are you crying?" would be quite startled if the patient responded with an actual explanation of "why."

Talking with patients, then, is a goal-directed activity, focused on the patient and designed to identify and work with the patient's nursing problems.

INTERVIEWING

Webster defines interview as "a formal consultation; a meeting at which a reporter obtains information from a person."† Interviewing, a one-to-one form of goal-directed communication, is a technique frequently employed by nurses, as well as by other professional groups, such as physicians, psychologists, and social workers. An interview is usually conducted in a relatively formal setting with the two people involved sitting facing each other.

*Peplau, Hildegard E.: Talking with patients, American Journal of Nursing **60**:964-966, July 1960.
†By permission. From Webster's Seventh New Collegiate Dictionary, copyright 1963 by G. & C. Merriam Co., Publishers of the Merriam-Webster Dictionaries.

In nursing, particularly in hospitals, this is often not the situation. Interviewing, when combined with some actual physical service, such as a back rub, provides a somewhat more intimate setting which appears to facilitate the progress of the interview. The "helping" aspect of nursing combined with interviewing mutually supports both processes.

Regardless of what member of the health team uses interviewing, the basic principles remain the same. The differences lie in the purposes. Nurses use interviewing to help to establish interpersonal relationships with patients, to provide patients with an opportunity to ventilate and explore feelings, and to intervene in emotionally charged situations that are likely to arise in relation to the patient's illness, his therapy, and his reaction to both.

Maurice Greenhill* has identified nine principles of interviewing and has related these specifically to nursing.

1. The initiative must be left up to the patient. He should be free to express those things he wants to and encouraged to introduce topics as he wishes. The significant aspect of the nurse's function in relation to this principle is to keep channels of communication open. The use of open-end questions, paraphrasing, incomplete sentences, and other means of talking with patients discussed previously serves this purpose. The temptation to cut off patients' verbalization through unrealistic or unwanted reassurance, or focusing upon specific information the nurse wants at the moment needs to be resisted.

2. The indirect approach should be used. In general, this principle is closely related to the first, for leaving the initiative to the patient is most effectively done by indirect approaches. Probing, direct questions that hit quickly at the heart of the matter are avoided. As the patient retains the initiative and moves from talking vaguely about problem areas to specific problems in the area, the nurse supports and encourages, but does not try to direct the patient beyond what he himself wishes to verbalize in the interview.

3. The interview should be kept as open-ended as possible. Again, channels of communication should be kept open, and the patient encouraged to express what he wishes. For example, if a patient is to receive a treatment such as an irrigation or an injection, the explanation given should be presented in such a way that the patient feels free to react. A finality in words or tone of voice that imply "this is it" can readily close off patient communication. The voice tone or words that imply "everything will be all right" can close off communication. Again, the use of incomplete sentences and similar techniques opens the channels for patient use if he so wishes.

4. The interviewer should use minimal verbal activity. This is not as simple as it sounds and requires considerable practice. Silence pressures most people, and as the patient's verbal activity is reduced, the inter-

---

*Greenhill, Maurice H.: Interviewing with a purpose, American Journal of Nursing **56**:1259-1262, Oct. 1956.

viewer's tends to rise. Increased verbal activity itself can be a sign of anxiety on the part of the interviewer. Minimal verbal activity, combined with non-verbal activity that encourages the patient, represents probably the best combination to support patient expression. Non-verbal activity includes leaning toward the patient, a facial expression of interest, or nodding the head. The interview is most productive when patient production is highest, and the interviewer's verbal activity is minimal.

5. Spontaneity on the part of the patient should be encouraged. Spontaneous comments should not be ignored, or the topic returned to a previous one. Spontaneous expressions, of course, are best encouraged and supported by indirect approaches and by minimal verbal activity combined with non-verbal interest on the part of the interviewer.

6. The interview should facilitate the expression of feelings. If a patient, for example, is talking about his symptoms, the nurse should avoid focusing purely on this aspect of the patient's illness and encourage the expression of the patient's feelings about his illness. Regardless of the feeling expressed, the expression should be facilitated. The rejection of the expression of feelings is usually done without thinking or realizing that it is being done. The patient who feels the nurse on night duty does not like him should be permitted to express the feeling, rather than having it rejected by the explanation that this cannot be true.

7. The interview should be focused on emotionally charged areas. In reality, the most active function of the interviewer is to focus, to indicate areas for a further discussion. Without this function of focusing, indicating topics of interest, the interview can produce little or nothing. To paraphrase, to reflect, or to use a similar method, selecting from the patient's own topics introduced those areas that, judging from tone of voice, pressure of speech, or facial expression, appear to be emotionally charged focuses the interview in this direction. This is an important function of the interviewer.

8. To produce movement in the interview, the interviewer must respond to leads and clues provided by the patient as to what constitutes an emotionally charged area. Body tension, grimacing, sudden stops, recurring topics, change in the tone of voice, and similar clues constitute the leads that are significant and call for focusing activities on the part of the interviewer.

9. Data must come from the interview content. If the interviewer begins with a preconceived plan for securing information and sticks to it, if he ignores leads and clues provided by the patient, if he uses a completely structured approach with questions that are direct and restrict responses, then the interview will rarely accomplish the purposes that are inherent in the nursing situation.

In looking back over the principles that guide interviewing as a technique, it is easy to see why these principles are effective in accomplishing nursing purposes such as establishing productive nurse-patient relationships and providing the patient with opportunities for ventilation of feelings. The principles are based upon respect for the individual as a person of worth and dignity in his own right. The principles recognize the potentiality for individual growth and for the individual's ultimate responsibility for his own development. They also place the nurse in a relationship that emphasizes helping the patient to help himself.

ACCEPTANCE

One of the important functions of the nurse in working effectively with patients' covert nursing problems is to convey acceptance of patients as persons. Acceptance is not to be confused with a laissez-faire approach that permits a patient to do as he pleases with complete approval. Nor is it to be confused with always agreeing with a patient. Acceptance is an active process that requires effort and practice to achieve. The heart of acceptance is being non-judgmental and non-punitive toward patients while maintaining one's own sensitivity, sincerity, and integrity. It is being able to like people while we do not agree with them. It is respecting people for their potential while not necessarily admiring their achievement. It is understanding the many factors that influence human behavior while not superimposing one's own sense of values as a criterion for standards of behavior for others.

In giving nursing care to patients with covert nursing problems, acceptance serves two different functions: it reduces the need for the patient's defenses because he is not judged or punished for his feelings and behavior, and it makes it easier for the patient to actually face and recognize his own feelings and behavior. Rejection, which can be quite subtly expressed, blocks this process and increases the patient's need for his defenses. Before behavior or feelings can be changed, they must first be identified. Acceptance facilitates such identification.

The actual process of conveying acceptance is done through many of the functions discussed previously in this chapter. Listening, reflection, open-end questions, encouraging patient initiative and spontaneity, the use of minimal verbal activity, focusing on emotionally significant areas, and facilitating the expression of feelings all contribute to conveying acceptance. To be effective these must be combined with a nonpunitive and a non-judgmental approach.

TEACHING

Teaching is another function of the nurse in providing nursing care for patients with covert nursing problems, and this is an area in which there is often confusion between "telling" and "teaching." When a teaching need is identified, the usual impulse is to tell a patient what he needs to know and then to assume that the patient has acquired and will use the knowledge. Many teachers suffer from the same approach to teaching.

The purpose of teaching is to help someone learn. Learning is evidenced by changes of behavior in the learner. To assume that knowledge produces change in behavior is fallacious. And this is especially true in the area of covert nursing problems. Many of us know, and know why, we should not feel as we do, but the knowledge does not produce changed feelings. Therefore, teaching in the area of covert nursing problems uses much the same indirect approach that has been presented. In fact, a better job of teaching patients by nurses might be done in all areas, including the physical, if this indirect approach were used. If nurses restrained themselves from pouring forth knowledge when a patient indicated a need for it and spent more effort helping the patient to recognize his own need for gaining knowledge, the number of readmissions to hospitals might drop sharply.

The first step in teaching patients is to identify the teaching need. This may be evidenced by the patient's verbalization of the need, by inference from something he says or does, by data from his chart, by information from his family or from his co-workers, or from knowledge of his health problem and his social and cultural background. In any case, once the nurse has identified the need, the next step is to help the patient identify the need also. If the latter step is ignored, as it so often is, teaching is not likely to be very successful. Encouraging patient exploration of the area through the indirect approach and through focusing back to the area when the opportunity occurs is most effective. Perhaps the hardest part of teaching is getting the potential learner to recognize and accept the need to know.

Once the need to know is jointly agreed upon, the nurse must make decisions as to motivational factors, cultural patterns, educational background, socioeconomic level, and similar facts that will influence the content presented and the method chosen to teach. In any case, the patient is encouraged to participate and to express his feelings (as well as his accumulation of facts) throughout the procedure. And every effort to assess the patient's level of knowledge and *how he plans to use it* should be made. In planning the teaching of the patients, Hilgard has identified fourteen points on which there is general agreement among the varied theories of learning that are of value to the nurse in planning and implementing teaching plans.

"1. In deciding who should learn what, the capacities of the learner are very important. Brighter people can learn things less bright ones cannot learn; in general, older children can learn more readily than younger ones; the decline of ability with age, in the adult years, depends upon what it is that is being learned.

"2. A motivated learner acquires what he learns more readily than one who is not motivated. The relevant motives include both general and specific ones, for example, desire to learn, need for achievement (general), desire for a certain reward or to avoid a threatened punishment (specific).

"3. Motivation that is too intense (especially pain, fear, anxiety) may be accompanied by distracting emotional states, so that excessive motivation may be less effective than moderate motivation for learning some kinds of tasks, especially those involving difficult discriminations.

"4. Learning under the control of reward is usually preferable to learning under the control of punishment. Correspondingly, learning motivated by success is preferable to learning motivated by failure. Even though the theoretical issue is still unresolved, the practical outcome must take into account the social by-products, which tend to be more favorable under reward than punishment.

"5. Learning under intrinsic motivation is preferable to learning under extrinsic motivation.

"6. Tolerance for failure is best taught through providing a backlog of success that compensates for experienced failure.

"7. Individuals need practice in setting realistic goals for themselves, goals neither so low as to elicit little effort nor so high as to foreordain to failure. Realistic goal-setting leads to more satisfactory improvement than unrealistic goal-setting.

"8. The personal history of the individual, for example, his reaction to authority, may hamper or enhance his ability to learn from a given teacher.

"9. Active participation by a learner is preferable to passive reception when learning, for example, from a lecture or a motion picture.

"10. Meaningful materials and meaningful tasks are learned more readily than tasks not understood by the learner.

"11. There is no substitute for repetitive practice in the overlearning of skills (for instance, the performance of a concert pianist), or in the memorization of unrelated facts that have to be automatized.

"12. Information about the nature of a good performance, knowledge of his own mistakes, and knowledge of successful results, aid learning.

"13. Transfer to new tasks will be better if, in learning, the learner can discover relationships for himself, and if he has experience during learning of applying principles within a variety of tasks.

"14. Spaced or distributed recalls are advantageous in fixing material that is to be long retained."*

USE OF SELF-UNDERSTANDING

One of the more important tools a nurse employs in working with patients with covert nursing problems is self-understanding. How a nurse feels about a patient or a situation can influence to a marked degree the quality of nursing care given. Because patients cannot be assigned to nurses on the basis of the latter's likes or dislikes, except in unusual circumstances, the nurse must learn to identify her own feelings and sense of values in order to be able to prevent their negating the quality of nursing care given.

Many situations are difficult to handle without being dominated by the nurse's own emotional response. Almost any type of patient can arouse anxiety, hostility, or anger within the nurse including crying patients, hostile patients, whining patients, and depressed patients. When negative responses are aroused, the common tendency is to reject the patient and approach him only when necessary. This limits the extent and the quality of his nursing care.

Nurses, like everyone else, are human beings with feelings, goals, ambitions, likes and dislikes, and individual value systems. They cannot be expected to like everyone, and there is really no need for them to feel guilty if they do not. No one can dictate how a nurse ought to feel in any

---

*Hilgard, Ernest R.: Theories of learning, ed. 2, New York, 1956, Appleton-Century Crofts, Inc., pp. 486-487. (Copyright © 1956, Appleton-Century-Crofts, Inc.)

given situation, and it would be useless to try. But the nurse, too, can learn to identify how she feels, can ventilate her feelings to remove some of their control over her behavior, and can learn how to give good nursing care to patients whom she does not adore. This involves expressing her feelings to the proper persons at the proper time, and the student nurse must learn who these persons are. They may be found among instructors and nursing service personnel and sometimes psychologists and physicians individually or during group sessions.

The statement is often heard that nurses should satisfy their emotional needs away from nursing, and not at the expense of patients. This statement is hardly accurate. Nursing is a satisfying occupation, and it is a shame for nurses to miss this satisfaction. A more accurate statement would be that nurses should not satisfy their emotional needs in an immature fashion. Mature satisfaction of emotional needs, in which the nurse does not sacrifice the patients, is found in nursing. Such maturity implies that the nurse has some degree of knowledge about how she feels and still is able to give quality nursing care to all patients.

One bit of knowledge the nurse needs to master is an understanding of what she is really saying or implying by what she does say.

"Bernstein, Brophy, McCarthy, and Roepe have classified types of verbal responses as evaluative, hostile, supportive, probing, or understanding. Evaluative responses are those in which the nurse makes a judgment (good or bad) about the patient's feelings and may go on to imply what he ought to feel or do. An example would be a response to a patient's complaint about nursing care in this manner. 'Most patients seem to think the nursing care around here is pretty good. You will get better faster if you have a little more faith in us.' Here the nurse implies that the patient is wrong and that he ought to change his attitude for his own sake. Such a response contributes little to patient care. A hostile response is one that rejects the patient through ridicule or blame or denies him the right to have any feelings on the subject at all. An example would be a nurse responding to a patient's complaint about an aide with, 'You have no right to complain about her. She's underpaid and overworked, and you take up too much of her time with your constant demands.' This type of response can hardly help even an irritated nurse feel better. In the supportive response, based on a misguided conception of what constitutes reassurance, the nurse denies that the patient really has a problem and implies that his concerns or worries are unnecessary. An example would be a nurse telling a patient who has expressed fear about a forthcoming operation that, 'Everybody is afraid of operations, but you have a good doctor, and we have a good staff, and everything will be all right.' This should accomplish little except to shut off any opportunity for the patient to face and deal with his fear. A probing response is one in which the nurse seeks further information and implies that she has the correct answers if she only can get enough information. An example would be a nurse who, in response to a patient's complaint that her husband was unfaithful, says, 'Let us find out about this. What makes you sure he is?' This probing approach is ineffective in dealing with patient feelings. An understanding response is one in which the nurse tries to understand what the patient is saying from his point of view. An example would be a nurse who replies to a patient's expressed concern over a pending operation with, 'You are worried about your operation.' This leaves the door open for the patient to explore his feelings further in an atmosphere in which it is safe 'to feel.' He is 'understood.' Students need practice to learn how to analyze their own verbal responses, to recognize what they are really saying to patients, and, especially, to develop skill in using the understanding response."°

Nurses must also learn to identify their own value systems and the sources of their values. What aspects of life are most significant to them and how these rate in priority are derived from their cultural background their families, and their personal experience. Other persons, with variation in these factors, may well hold value systems that are different. The tend ency to equate difference with inferiority is strong, although there is n scientific basis for such a judgment. Understanding cultural differences a differences and not as a degree above or below a certain standard can b valuable in providing nursing care to patients from different cultura backgrounds.

SETTING LIMITS

The difficult problem of setting limits to relationships with patients i one function assumed by nurses in providing nursing care to patients wit covert nursing problems. In conveying acceptance and in using an indired or nondirective approach, some concept of limits must be defined and con sistently enforced.

Certain guide lines apply in almost any nurse-patient relationship. These are as follows:

1. The time spent with a patient is focused on the patient.
2. The patient is not permitted actions that endanger himself or other
3. The relationship is limited to goal-directed activity in the patient interests.
4. The determination of limits is jointly reached by those concerne with the patient's therapy and consistently carried through by all.
5. Limitations are enforced, accompanied by acceptance of the *patient* rejection if he feels this way.

Although the general atmosphere of permissiveness and acceptanc with the facilitation of the expression of feelings, forms the matrix of th nurse-patient relationship, limitations in the interest of the patient are al an important aspect in such a relationship.

DEVELOPING NURSE-PATIENT RELATIONSHIPS

Although much of this chapter relates to the basic considerations establishing productive nurse-patient relationships, certain aspects, suc as the developmental stages, are singled out for emphasis in this discussio It should be clearly understood that the nurse-patient relationship bei discussed is that relationship with the so-called "normal" patient. The ki of health problems that currently represent our major threats demand ps

---

°Matheney, Ruth V., and Topalis, Mary: Psychiatric nursing, ed. 3, St. Louis, 1961, T C. V. Mosby Co., pp. 83-84.

chological skills of as high an order as the physical and technical skills demanded. Good physical nursing care alone is no longer adequate.

The nurse-patient relationship, as pointed out previously, is a therapeutic tool, not a casual or superficial relationship on a mild popularity contest basis. It is goal-directed to meet patient needs.

A relationship is something to be developed and goes through developmental stages, each with its own characteristics. The first stage of the nurse-patient relationship is the beginning period, characterized by orientation, explanation, and limit setting during a period when the patient and the nurse work toward a goal of mutual trust. The nurse bears a heavy responsibility at this period, for she must, during this stage, set the atmosphere and the direction the relationship will take. For example, she should approach a patient for the first time armed with all the possible knowledge she can glean that will help her to know and to understand the unique individual she will meet. Age, religion, cultural background, health problem, marital status, degree of illness or health, and medical orders are samples of the kinds of information she may collect as part of her own orientation. In addition, she will encourage the patient to talk about himself to add to her information. As part of the patient's orientation, she makes clear who she is and the extent of the services she will offer. If the patient is new to hospital setting, she tries to interpret what he can expect in such a setting. Also, during this beginning phase she begins setting limits. For example, she makes clear to the patient that the time spent with him will be focused on him as a patient, that he is free to express his feelings, and that he will be expected to participate in his own therapy to the extent that he can.

During this period the patient can be expected to test the growing relationship. He may, for example, try to get the nurse to talk about herself, attempting to find out whether she is really more interested in herself than in him. He may try to set the tone of the relationship at a social friend-to-friend peer level. Such exploration is to be expected. Simple factual responses without elaboration and a returning focus on the patient are usually successful.

Also during this phase, the nurse can observe clues to discern the role in which the patient places her, as well as deciphering her own interpretation of the role of the patient in general and the role in which she casts this particular patient. Stereotypes on both sides of the relationship should be identified. Too often, many elderly male patients have had their identity constantly assaulted by the hospital personnel's familiar greeting of "Hello, Pop." The identification of the role in which the patient tends to cast the nurse is useful in understanding the way in which he behaves toward her.

In setting the stage during this beginning phase, the indirect approach, using reflective and accepting techniques discussed previously, is most effective. It makes no difference what the patient's presenting problem may be, either overt or covert in nature.

When the patient and the nurse have developed a feeling of mutual trust, the working phase of the nurse-patient relationship has arrived and the patient will begin to talk more freely about himself. In general, he can be expected to begin around the periphery of a problem and move toward the center. He is more likely to talk about actions before beginning on thoughts or feelings. During this working phase, the continued use of nondirective or reflective technique is important. Certain "don'ts" become important:

1. Don't interpret to the patient.
2. Don't deny or belittle the patient's feelings.
3. Don't make assumptions.
4. Don't use approval or disapproval.
5. Don't threaten.
6. Don't advise.
7. Don't take over responsibility for the patient.
8. Don't probe.
9. Don't demand the patient get better as a result of your help.

During the working phase, alertness to clues provided by the patient is important. What patterns or themes appear in the patient's behavior? What happens as a result of interaction between patient and nurse? What makes the patient appear to relax? What makes him uneasy? What does he avoid? What brings about change in his behavior and what kind of change? What is the pattern of progression in the type or depth of problems discussed? In addition to observing the response of the patient to the nurse-patient relationship, his behavior pattern with other groups should also be observed.

The goals of the working phase of the nurse-patient relationship are patient growth in self-understanding and in self-responsibility.

The last phase is the termination of the nurse-patient relationship. This comes as a result of the patient's discharge, as a result of change in the nurse's assignment, or as a result of an unsatisfactory relationship which is obviously not therapeutic. Some preparation for this is advisable, and the time of the termination may be indicated in the beginning phase of the relationship. A patient, for example, who knows when he enters the hospital that he will probably be discharged within a week knows that termination of the relationship will closely follow its initiation. The nurse who knows her assignment will change the next Monday should not simply disappear, but should prepare the patient for the termination of a working relationship. This phase may present some difficulties, depending on the individual patient. In any case, a relationship in a working phase that must terminate should not come to an abrupt end without some explanation.

LIMITATIONS OF THE NURSE'S ROLE

As health services and their multiple categories of personnel become increasingly interdependent, the differentiation of functions and responsibility among the groups involved become more difficult. There are overlappings in these areas among categories of nursing personnel and between doctors and nurses. Many groups use the same techniques, such as interviewing, but usually for somewhat different purposes. In any case, the patient is better served by the coordinated effort of the groups. And in the complex setting of medical care, there are certain limits in the role of the nurse that must be accepted.

A nurse cannot, by law, diagnose and prescribe. She cannot substitute, through her own work, for what she considers to be incompetence on the part of the physician. In the instance of patients with covert nursing problems, she cannot assume the role of the psychiatrist. Under the direction of a psychiatrist, she may administer therapy through individual interviews or group therapy sessions. She cannot, however, initiate depth psychotherapy individually, however much it may be needed.

Another problem in limitation that is often difficult is the short stay of patients and the limited time that a nurse may be in contact with a particular patient, especially in the modern general hospital. The same general approach discussed here is used, however, even though the only realistic goal may be not to increase the patient's anxiety or covert nursing problems. A relationship that opens the channels for a little patient growth in areas of need is some contribution.

Nurses are often caught in situations in which, although attempting to provide therapeutic interaction with patients, they receive little support from others in the working situation, including nurses and doctors. Although this may restrict or limit the scope of her effectiveness, she is under obligation to continue her efforts. The quality of individual nursing care should not be sacrificed to the mediocrity of other personnel.

Another limitation placed on nurses is by the patient who rejects help or who denies any difficulty. Patients cannot be forced to help themselves, and there is only acceptance to be offered the rejecting patient. Hopefully, at some later day, repeated experiences of acceptance will help the patient to know himself better. However, no nurse can expect complete success.

BIBLIOGRAPHY

1. Bernstein, Lewis, Brophy, Mary, McCarthy, Mary Jane, and Roepe, Ruby: Teaching nurse-patient relationships, Nursing Research 3:80-84, Oct. 1954.
2. Connolly, Mary Grace: What acceptance means to patients, American Journal of Nursing 60:1754-1757, Dec. 1960.
3. Copp, Laurel, and Copp, John Dixon: Look to the pattern of relationships, American Journal of Nursing 60:1284-1286, Sept. 1960.
4. Davis, Anne J.: The skills of communication, American Journal of Nursing 63:66-70, Jan. 1963.
5. Eldred, Stanley H.: Improving nurse-patient communication, American Journal of Nursing 60:1600-1602, Nov. 1960.
6. Greenhill, Maurice H.: Interviewing with a purpose, American Journal of Nursing 56:1259-1262, Oct. 1956.
7. Hilgard, Ernest R.: Theories of learning, ed. 2, New York, 1956, Appleton-Century-Crofts, Inc., pp. 486-487.
8. Hofling, Charles K., and Leininger, Madeliene M.: Basic psychiatric concepts in nursing, Philadelphia, 1960, J. B. Lippincott Co., pp. 27-68.

9. Ingles, Thelma: Do patients feel lost in a general hospital, American Journal of Nursing **60**:648-651, May 1960.
10. Kachelski, M. Audrey: The nurse-patient relationship, American Journal of Nursing **61**:76-81, May 1961.
11. Martin, Harry W., and Prange, Arthur J.: The stages of illness: a psychosocial approach, Nursing Outlook **10**:168-171.
12. Matheney, Ruth V., and Topalis, Mary: Psychiatric nursing, ed. 3, St. Louis, 1961, The C. V. Mosby Co., pp. 69-99.
13. McCabe, Gracia: Cultural influences on patient behavior, American Journal of Nursing **60**:1101-1104, Aug. 1960.
14. Meadow, Lloyd, and Gass, Gertrude Zemon: Problems of the novice interviewer, American Journal of Nursing **63**:97-99, Feb. 1963.
15. Orlando, Ida Jean: The dynamic nurse-patient relationship, New York, 1961, G. P. Putnam's Sons, Inc., p. 91.
16. Peplau, Hildegard E.: Talking with patients, American Journal of Nursing **60**:964-966, July 1960.
17. Rogers, Carl R.: A counseling approach to human problems, American Journal of Nursing **56**:994-997, Aug. 1956.
18. Suhrie, Eleanor Brody: The importance of listening, Nursing Outlook **8**:686-687, Dec. 1960.
19. Travelbee, Joyce: What do we mean by rapport, American Journal of Nursing **63**:70-72, Feb. 1963.
20. Van Sant, Genee E.: Patients' problems are not always obvious, American Journal of Nursing **62**:59, April 1962.

Chapter 8

Therapeutic environment in a nonpsychiatric hospital

Every patient entering a hospital is faced with anxiety from several sources. As Esther Lucile Brown[*] points out, the patient is certain to have some anxiety about himself, some fear of the hospital itself, and some anxiety arising from the change to the "sick" role in the hospital. In addition, he may bring with him many anxieties, exacerbated by his illness, about his family, his job, his friends, or almost any aspect of his daily existence. The patient's medical problem alone, therefore, cannot be the sole determinant of therapeutic plans in any instance. The patient's anxiety adds to the need for effective therapeutic plans in the area of emotional and supportive care. In addition to the use of skilled interpersonal relationships, the social setting of the hospital itself can be used to contribute to therapy.

THE HOSPITAL AND THE SOCIAL THERAPY SETTING

There is perhaps no more neglected aspect of medical and nursing therapy than the social setting in which it is given. One of the basic purposes of skilled interpersonal relationships is to help the patient maintain his sense of personal integrity and worth. As pointed out in the chapter on anxiety and stress, a major problem in our increasingly complex world is for the individual to develop and maintain a sense of self-identity with the assurance that he and his life have meaning. Most hospitals are organized and operated for efficiency, but, in their efficiency, make it difficult for the patient to maintain any sense of self-identity or importance. Room numbers and diagnoses serve as substitutes for names. Admission procedures are cold-blooded, highly impersonal, and usually insensitive. Visitors are

---

[*]Brown, Esther Lucile: Newer dimensions of patient care. Part I. The use of the physical and social environment of the general hospital for therapeutic purposes, New York, 1961, Russell Sage Foundation, pp. 11-13.

restricted to certain limited hours. Explanations are withheld. Responsibility for himself is taken from the patient, and numerous people make decisions for him without bothering to tell him what the decisions are, let alone consulting him in advance. His clothes and personal belongings may well be removed, and he may be dressed in gowns or pajamas that have little relationship to his taste or even to modern attire. He may be moved from bed to bed within a unit or from unit to unit without warning. He may be aroused at 5, 6, or 7 o'clock in the morning and be told to brush his teeth and wash his face and hands. His coffee and his toast may, and probably will, be served cold. He may have to sit on his bed to eat his meals. He may be ambulatory, with nowhere to go and nowhere to sit. His complaints may be brushed aside with reassuring comments that "everything will be all right." He may be placed up in a wheel chair and situated in a dim corridor with no view, lined up with a group of patients all facing the same direction. His privacy is casually and routinely invaded. If he complains about the hospital, he is considered to be "uncooperative." He may have been considered competent to administer cortisone to himself at home—but if he wants an aspirin in a hospital, the doctor must order it and someone holding a license to practice nursing must administer it. The rather obvious assumption underlying the social setting and organization of most hospitals is that all patients on admission either are or become incompetent.

Such routines and organization present a totally different life pattern from that which most human beings are accustomed to following. Sometimes they reduce the individual patient to the lowest possible level of self-identity and security in any belief that he can possibly have worth and dignity. In addition, the need to adapt to a pattern so different from his previous social experience, and during a period of stress, can hardly accomplish much except increase anxiety.

The social setting of the hospital, as has been demonstrated, can be adapted to more nearly approximate the social setting in which patients have developed some sense of security and adaptability. In reducing the discrepancy, the hospital setting can be used as social therapy to support medical therapy and to improve its effectiveness. This means merely paying attention to the things that matter to people in the normal setting of their lives. Although hospital architecture may need revision to provide for a more flexible and more nearly realistic routine, there are many steps that can be taken even now.

An important factor is learning to use patients' names correctly and, even more important, to *think* of patients as people with names rather than diagnoses and room numbers. It would be at least one concession to the fact that patients are people and some support for the idea that, as people, they are important. Attention to the use of "Miss" and "Mrs." correctly and, in the light of the patient's age and cultural background, sensitivity to the use of the first name are also helpful. The use of stereotyped responses to age groups, such as "Pop," "Mom," "Grandma," and "Son" is to be avoided. A name is an identification and is important to the person who owns it.

Routines can certainly be more flexible than they are at present. Rigid enforcement of all existing rules and regulations under all circumstances reduces individuals to nonentities, to cogs in wheels. Although fire regulations should always be rigidly enforced, does this necessarily hold true for other rules and regulations? Is it always necessary that every patient be awakened at the same time? If a picture or some other prized possession is wanted by the patient, why shouldn't he have it? If a patient is happier looking out a window, why must his bed be kept in a military line with other beds in the same room? If a patient likes to wear his own pajamas, why shouldn't he? If he has a battered old bathrobe of which he is especially fond, why not let him have it? If he wants his bed turned around because he is tired of looking at the same cracks in the wall, why not? What are the things that are important to him? Is there really any reason why he can't have them?

Eating together is a common practice in everyday life. With many patients ambulatory in the average general hospital, this joint activity could be encouraged. Where dining rooms do exist on units, personnel can encourage their use. Where dining rooms are not in existence, someone with interest and ingenuity can surely find a way to get at least several patients together for meals. One young student moved several bed-side stands together to form a table. It was not the most comfortable setting in the world, but the patients enjoyed it. There is another aspect of eating that is significant—serving food that is hot when it ought to be and cold when it ought to be. Too often trays are served and left sitting where patients cannot reach them or are all prepared at the same time and then served, with the result that the food on the last trays served is at room temperature. Such careless routines indicate a lack of concern for people. "Hot" coffee, served hot, does much to bring comfort and warmth to the average person.

If the patient has difficulty with the hospital diet and if the family is willing and able to bring in food that he likes and can eat, not only should they be encouraged to do so, but they should also be provided with facilities to heat hot food and chill cold food. It may also be helpful if members of the family sit with patients while they are eating. Where the method of family participation in preparing food and being present at meal time has been tried, it often improves the patient's appetite.

Interest in individual patients as persons, expressed through listening *and hearing*, through encouraging patients to vocalize feelings, through paying attention to complaints and to individual likes and dislikes, and by learning to know and use knowledge of the patient as a person, could contribute much to softening the cold impersonality of the hospital setting.

An additional contribution of the social setting to the patient's sense of worth could be made by treating him as a responsible individual who is consulted about and can participate in his own therapy. While this *must* be done when the patient is in his own home, it tends to be neglected in the hospital. The patient certainly has the first right to know what is wrong with him and what is being done about it. And he most certainly deserves an explanation of what *is* being done and *why,* always given so that he can comprehend.

Patients can also be encouraged to help and to accept help from each other. Perhaps one of the best illustrations of this is the extreme usefulness of the patient who has had a laryngectomy (removal of the larynx) and has learned to speak again with patients who are about to undergo or have recently undergone a laryngectomy. Where this practice has been followed, patients have testified to its very real contribution to their own therapy. Such contributions need not always be so dramatic or so directly related to the patient's health problem. Patients can read to each other, can form discussion groups, can exchange experiences or recipes, can knit socks for other patients with cold feet, and any such joint venture can contribute to the sense of usefulness of both the giver and the recipient. This is a resource in patient care that is relatively untapped.

The pattern of permitting visitors in the units of the hospital could be reassessed and in an increasing number of hospitals is being reassessed and administered more flexibly. Increasing recognition of the personality damage that can result to young children due to the separation from parents has led to open visiting hours in many pediatric units. Some hospitals make provision for one or both parents to stay overnight. The rigid restriction of children from visiting hospitals at all is under serious question. There are times when children *need* to visit parents, siblings, or other significant persons in their lives. There are times when patients *need* visits from children. An additional difficulty with rigid visiting hours is that they are not always convenient or even possible for some persons. The restriction of the visiting hours to a two-hour time span, selected to suit the work load on the patient care unit, also tends to increase the number of visitors within that time span, regardless of regulations that may say only two visitors at a time. Such restrictions also fail to take into account the cultural differences that occur in the meaning of visiting the sick. Certainly the criteria that determines "when," "who," and "how many" visitors and "how long" they stay, ought to be suited, first to the patient's needs and second to the needs of family and friends who wish to visit. Such criteria imply a great deal more flexibility in visiting patterns within institutions than exists at present. The contribution of family and friends to supporting patients through therapeuic plans have often been overlooked, and it represents a real potential in social therapy.

The expectations concerning patient behavior and the concept of the patient role in the hospital held by hospital personnel, including nurses, could be revised to contribute more effectively to social therapy. There is always pressure on the patient to conform to the pattern of the "good" patient, and the use of approval and disapproval, grossly or subtly expressed, is a major weapon. The good patient, of course, is docile, does as he is told, appreciates everything done for him, does not complain of pain if he feels it, gets well, and goes home grateful to the hospital. The expectations that personnel hold for patients does influence the behavior of many patients. If nurses expected patients to be human beings, with differences and uniquenesses of their own, with feelings and patterns of likes and dislikes, patients might feel more free to be themselves.

Another step that might contribute to patients' maintaining or developing a sense of being respected as individuals would be for nurses, as well as other hospital personnel, to retain, or to develop, or to redevelop an acute sensitivity to how it feels to "be on the other side of the fence." Although it is discouraging to walk down a corridor with patients lined up in wheel chairs all facing the same direction, it is even more discouraging to see nursing personnel and physicians walking down the same corridor completely insensitive to the whole scene. For medical personnel who have been patients, there should be a high degree of sensitivity to how the hospital looks to patients. For those who will listen and who desire to know, there is much to be learned that will sharpen the ability to be sensitive to patient reactions to the environment.

In regard to the physical aspects of what could be a therapeutic environment, progress has been made in many new hospitals and in many hospitals that have been renovated. The use of pastel colors on the walls, the addition of patient lounges and dining rooms (which are often sacrificed to educational needs for conference rooms), and the use of colorful drapes and bedspreads have become widespread. Patient rooms, however, even though colors and modern furniture have been added, still tend to be regimented in the amount of furniture and its placement and in the decoration. Neatness tends to be more important than comfort and the expression of individuality.

Other factors in the physical environment that need attention are cleanliness, and, above all, control of noises. There are few hospital patients who do not complain of noise—not necessary noise, but *un*necessary noise. Two main sources of loud conversation are the nurses' stations and the utility room, particularly at night. Another is the banging of equipment.

THE VALUE SYSTEM OF HOSPITAL PERSONNEL

The medical and social therapy of patients will be strongly influenced by the social structure and the value system of hospital personnel in the hospital setting. The expressed goals of nursing service and the goals indicated by actual behavior of nurses may be and frequently are in conflict. Although nurses may say they are interested in providing the best possible nursing care for patients, their behavior on the hospital unit may indicate greater concern with patient control. Nurses may refuse special requests to avoid "spoiling" patients, may stay away from "difficult" patients except when they have to approach them, or may use approval or disapproval to reward "good" patients and discourage "bad" patients. Certainly, such behavior would indicate that a major nursing goal on the unit is control of patients. Nurses and other nursing personnel should try to analyze the real goals in nursing care that are in operation. Change to a positive direction cannot take place until real goals are identified.

It is true that an undesirable hospital setting is not always the fault of the nursing service or other personnel involved. Students of the social structure in the hospital setting have indicated that, existing outside the formal organizational structure of the institution, there are unofficial but effecive organizations designed to protect the security of the groups involved. The hospital itself is an anxiety-laden situation. In addition, we are in a period of changing patterns of responsibilities and functions and a period of multiplication of categories of personnel. Doctors have delegated functions down the hierarchy, and each succeeding level has done the same. There is considerable overlapping of functions and distinctions, and definitions of levels are not yet clear. Delegated responsibility has not often been accompanied by authority delegated sufficiently to cope with the responsibility. Such a situation increases the anxiety of all concerned. In addition, old stereotypes stand in the way of adaptation. Doctors sigh for the old handmaiden, and nurses for the lack of support they once received from physicians. As registered nurses move upward in status, they struggle to rise further and establish their contribution more clearly. Practical nurses are undergoing the same process. Doctors see encroachment in their area. None of this inevitable development provides a solid bedrock of security from which any one of the groups can operate, thus creating the potential for anxiety and conflict over responsibilities in patient care. The patient's medical and nursing care must necessarily suffer where any such conflict exists. The use of the hospital setting demands thorough study of the interrelationships among personnel involved in health care and that steps be taken toward resolution of the difficulties identified.

Among all groups, including nursing, there are needs for social approval, for a sense of accomplishment, for a sense of importance of the job, for security, and for support in anxiety-producing situations. The factors in relationships between doctors and nurses, between registered and practical nurses, and between other groups that block the achievement of these goals for any group must be identified and removed in the interests of patients.

CHARACTERISTICS OF THERAPEUTIC GROUPS

Much of the social therapy aspect of the hospital is related to group situations, involving more than one-to-one nurse-patient relationships. Groups that tend to be therapeutic in nature have characteristics that are distinctly different from groups that are prone to develop or to support neurotic behavior. These characeristics are significant for the kind of group setting or atmosphere that needs to be developed in the general hospital.

Destructive groups are directive and characterized by authoritarianism. Decisions are made for patients, and the direction and selection of topics and routines are usually determined by authority figures. Authority is equated with position, and not with competence. Approval and disapproval are typical methods used for bringing patient behavior into a preconceived, acceptable pattern, such methods being imposed by the authority figure with other members of the group following suit. In such groups achievement is important; in other words, the patient must show signs of getting well or appreciating what is done for him. In destructive groups, also, the intellect and its operations are stressed. Typically, such groups tend to react with repression of significant emotions or emotionally charged subjects, such an anxiety, fear, anger, sex, or death. Members of the group judge each other and are judged by authority figures, with right and wrong used to encourage feelings of guilt. Many parts of experience are isolated and kept secret, and major concern is focused upon the conscious aspect of life.

Such a pattern is characteristic of many hospital and nursing service personnel groups of the not too distant past, and many nurses will recognize in the preceding descriptions institutions in which they studied or were employed. Many such hospitals still exist. Considering the recent, strongly military and religious background of nursing, this fact is not difficult to understand.

On the other hand, study of effective group therapy functioning has revealed a totally different set of characteristics. Permissiveness promotes therapy, and groups in a permissive setting with clearly established limits tend to develop self-direction rather than being subordinate to the imposed direction of authority figures. The group values honesty in identifying and facing problems above intellectual achievement and values the expression of feelings above facts and intellectual exercises. Acceptance and the encouragement of the expression of feelings develop. The group tends to be matter-of-fact about the many facets of experience and to be frank and open in discussion. A sense of belonging characterizes the group. Concern with the conscious aspects of life is broadened to concern with the unconscious aspects of life as well. In other words, a therapeutic group has many of the characteristics of a therapeutic interpersonal relationship.

Groups, like relationships, undergo development. They go through the beginning phase of orientation, exploration, and setting limits. They also need democratic leadership. Group members assume roles within the group, such as the conscientious objector, pacifier, summarizer, "idea man," or similar roles. Groups need leadership to focus, to summarize, to suggest new approaches, and to encourage expression of feelings and similar functions. Groups also reach a working phase and a termination phase.

Although the groups of patients and personnel in patient units in general hospitals usually are not so structured or so continuous as groups in therapeutic sessions or in committees, they do have some similarities. New members go through the orientation phase, and groups terminate as members change. A single project on which the total group works is not always present, and the membership is characterized by change. Nonetheless, it would appear that the permissive atmosphere, the encouragement of the expression of feelings, the value in facing problems honestly, and the matter-of-fact frank and open approach would have value for the less cohesive, less structured group of patients and personnel in a hospital unit. Leadership would inevitably rest with personnel. And this approach should contribute to the social therapy value of the hospital.

THE NURSE AND THE THERAPEUTIC ENVIRONMENT

The nurse constitutes part of the patient's hospital environment and, of course, has a significant contribution to make to social therapy as well as to individual patient therapy because she is a factor in the social setting. She also represents an authority figure in the hospital and occupies as a consequence a position of leadership in setting the social tone of the patient care unit.

The nurse can exert her influence on the unit in the direction of a therapeutic group atmosphere. She can exemplify and encourage among patients a permissive attitude toward the expression of feelings and the frank and open facing of problems. She can accept and encourage self-direction on the part of both patients and personnel.

The nurse can also exert leadership in adapting routines to patient needs. She can serve a genuine purpose by developing the habit of *questioning* routines in terms of their contribution to or interference with the patients' therapy and the patients' sense of worth and dignity. Many routines in hospitals have long lost their usefulness and meaning but continue to exist because no one has raised any questions concerning their value. For example, if baths are routinely given in the morning and if the patient has been accustomed to bathing before going to bed and is more comfortable and sleeps better this way, this routine could certainly be adjusted in the light of patient needs. Many such simple changes could be made with benefit to the patients' welfare.

One major contribution to a therapeutic environment that nurses could make would be to focus on patients and not on tasks, things, or routines. Nursing care plans can be more than a list of tasks; they can be made in terms of goals to be accomplished with a patient. A nurse can "make a patient comfortable," rather than "giving a bath." Assignments can be to a person, rather than to a room number or a diagnosis. Names can be used when talking about patients. The patient's likes and interests can be used to indicate that he *is* important.

The nurse can also make a contribution by involving the patient in decisions concerning himself whenever and wherever possible. She can orient him to what goes on about him and explain what she and others are doing and why. In either case, she also needs to permit the patient to react honestly to what is done for him and to him.

The nurse can also promote patient interaction and can particularly encourage patients to help and to accept help from each other. Although this has been done in psychiatric hospitals, the practice has tended to be negated in general hospitals. Several patients in wheel chairs can be grouped together in front of a window rather than sitting in their separate rooms. Special talents or interests of patients can be made known to other patients who might well be interested. The promotion of patient interaction represents one underdeveloped resource in social therapy.

Visitors, particularly families or others of significance to the patient, may have a real contribution to make to patient therapy. They usually know a great deal more about the patient than nursing personnel and can often provide information that can be extremely useful. They, too, are usually under some degree of stress and have some degree of anxiety and, therefore, will frequently talk if given the opportunity. As a rule, all many of them need is a good listener.

Nurses also can make a contribution to a therapeutic environment through control over the physical environment. Noise, odors, cleanliness, removal of safety hazards, placement of beds, toleration of prized possessions, and similar factors can be controlled and manipulated in terms of using the environment for the patients' welfare rather than maintaining the environment in a preconceived *status quo.*

In working with others in the patient care unit, the nurse can use her knowledge of the basic needs of most workers to improve the therapeutic environment. The most common contacts of the nurse are with other nurses, practical nurses, aides, doctors, orderlies, supervisors, and other groups such as social workers and messengers. Guiding her contact with such persons by a recognition of the need for social approval, for a sense of importance and accomplishment in the job, and for support in anxiety-producing situations would contribute to a more therapeutic environment. The nurse, however, cannot do this simply by repression of her own feelings—she must find a place for expresson and clarification of her own feelings.

The nurse also needs, in the development of a therapeutic environment, to coordinate her functioning with other groups involved in patient therapy —the doctor, the dietitian, the social worker, the hospital administrators, and others. She should know and support their efforts, and she has every right to expect their support. Conflicts should be brought out in the open and resolved, rather than being permitted to linger on covertly.

The nurse also needs to analyze and study the social structure and the value system that exists in the hospital and in the patient care unit. Although changing such a structure can rarely be accomplished by a single nurse, it is certain no change will take place if the need for change is not first identified by someone and if there is not a prime mover to initiate change. The nurse can serve one or both functions.

The nurse can also encourage and support, and sometimes initiate, any change that will make the hospital environment more nearly approximate the realities of the social situation as it exists outside the hospital. There are many undesirable aspects of the sick role that are not really necessary. A patient need not be deprived of all the symbols that identify him. A doctor could "prescribe" in the hospital as well as the home. Children could see a sick parent if it were good for them both. A patient could be led instead of being told. A patient could make many decisions for himself. Routines could be subordinated to patient needs. And hospital construction and renovation *could* make provisions for movies, swimming pools, and many other utilities of everyday living. The social environment of the hospital *can* be used to promote the patients' sense of identity and worth.

BIBLIOGRAPHY

1. Abdellah, Faye G., Beland, Irene L., Martin, Almeda, and Matheney, Ruth V.: Patient centered approaches to nursing, New York, 1960, The Macmillan Co., pp. 185-187.
2. Brown, Esther Lucile: Newer dimensions of patient care. Part I. The use of the physical and social environment of the general hospital for therapeutic purposes, New York, 1961, Russell Sage Foundation.
3. Brown, Esther Lucile: Newer dimensions of patient care. Part II. Improving staff motivation and competence in the general hospital, New York, 1962, Russell Sage Foudation.
4. Fullinger, Walter F., Jr.: Remotivation, American Journal of Nursing 60:682-685, May 1960.
5. Johnson, Dorothy E.: Consequences for patients and personnel, American Journal of Nursing 62:96-100, May 1962.
6. Merton, Robert K.: Status orientations in nursing, American Journal of Nursing 62:70-73, Oct. 1962.
7. Prange, Arthur J., Jr., and Martin, Harry W.: Aids to understanding patients, American Journal of Nursing 62:98-100, July 1962.
8. Willie, Charles V.: Patient and nurse: members of a group, Nursing Outlook 5:585-587, Oct. 1957.

Chapter 9

Meeting religious needs of patients

The sense of values by which man lives frequently has its roots in religious beliefs, and such beliefs, whatever their version, constitute a significant aspect of any man's existence. The patient who enters the hospital or is seen in the clinic or in his home will bring with him his own religion and his own spiritual needs. Part of a nurse's responsibility is to be sensitive to such needs and to understand and support their significance to the patient.

Although not directly responsible for religious or spiritual ministration, the nurse has certain obligations in relation to patients' religious or spiritual needs. One aspect is respect for the religious beliefs of patients, regardless of what that religion might be. Although the major religious faiths in the United States are Roman Catholic, Protestant, and Jewish, contact with patients from other major world religions is no longer unusual because of present-day communications and patterns of travel. For our major religious groups, priests, ministers, or rabbis are usually on call and within reach; for the religious groups of the Near East and Far East, this may not be true. If a patient is admitted whose faith is not one with which the nurse is familiar, it would seem in the interests of nursing care for the total patient that she investigate the basic beliefs and the significant symbolic rituals of the particular religion. Respect for the patient's religion could then be more intelligently demonstrated.

It is also the nurse's obligation to understand the significance of religious rituals of the major religions of our country. For example, in the Jewish religion baptism is not desired, in the Protestant religion baptism is sometimes optional, in the Roman Catholic religion baptism is necessary for salvation. The nurse, therefore, must know enough about the really significant obligations of our three major faiths.

Another obligation of the nurse is to notify the chaplain of the proper faith at the times determined by religious beliefs and by the accepted pattern of the institution in which the nurse is employed. This is a responsibility normally delegated to and assumed by nursing service personnel. Such notification usually includes admission, impending surgery, patient request, critical illness, or impending death.

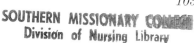
SOUTHERN MISSIONARY COLLEGE
Division of Nursing Library

In addition to the usual specified times for notification of the clergy, special other circumstances may arise when the priest, minister, or rabbi may be called, or at least be kept informed. Such circumstances might include expressions of guilt, expressions of suicidal wishes or threats, over-dependency on the hospital and resistance to discharge, and psychoneurotic or psychotic behavior. If the patient is rational and makes clear a desire to be left alone, the patient's wishes must be respected, but the chaplain should be made aware of the situation.

The nurse should also do all that is possible to provide privacy when the chaplain visits a patient. Procedures that are not emergency measures may be delayed, screens provided, personnel discouraged from intruding, and similar measures taken.

When a patient makes a specific request for spiritual assistance from the nurse, such request should be honored. If the patient, for example, asks a nurse to pray with him, the nurse should, to the best of her ability, comply. If the patient requests religious literature, it should be obtained. If such literature is not readily available, the request should be relayed to the nursing service administration. If the request is one with which the nurse feels she cannot comply, every effort should be made to find someone who can.

It is the nurse's obligation to make the best possible use of the clergy as resource persons who can contribute to the patient's welfare, especially when the patient is under stress.

In the Roman Catholic faith, baptism is necessary for salvation. In all instances, if baptism is indicated, the services of a priest should be obtained if at all possible. If a priest is not available in case of emergency, whoever is present may perform the baptism, having witnesses present if possible. In emergency baptism, the following three conditions should be met:

1. If the patient has reached the age of reason, and is able to so indicate, he must indicate the intention to be baptized.
2. The correct words should be used: "(Name), I baptize you in the name of the Father, and of the Son, and of the Holy Ghost. Amen."
3. Water must be poured over an area of skin, preferably the forehead, while the words are being said.

In cases of doubt, where, for example, the patient may be unconscious or there is doubt as to whether the patient is alive, conditional baptism may be administered by prefacing the usual words with "If you are capable." In instances of sudden death, the baptism may be performed up to a period of three or more hours after apparent death, or a period of thirty minutes following death from a lingering illness.

The baptism should be recorded in duplicate, including the patient's name, the date of his birth, the date of the baptism, the place of the baptism, the name of the person who performed the baptism, and the signature of the witnesses.

All Roman Catholics are required to receive the Last Sacrament when in danger of death. The nurse should promptly notify the priest whenever this situation arises.

In general, the nurse should call the priest when a patient is critically ill, again when the patient appears to be dying, when a patient is found recently dead, before a patient undergoes major surgery, and when a patient has received an emergency baptism.

In the Protestant faith, no religious ministration is considered absolutely necessary in instances of serious illness or death, because the Protestant religion, with its many variations, rests on the belief that each person is capable of direct communication with God. However, the clergy should be notified when a patient is critically ill or dying or before a patient undergoes major surgery. Patients' wishes, of course, should be respected. Since baptism is optional, if a patient expresses a wish for baptism and a member of the clergy cannot be present, anyone who is present may perform the baptism.

The Jewish religion is composed of three groups: Orthodox, Conservative, and Reform. The Orthodox group follows the traditions that have existed since ancient times. Important among these traditional practices and laws are the dietary laws. The Orthodox group may not eat pork in any form or sea animals without scales; they also do not eat game, such as quail. Meat or meat derivatives, such as soup or gravy, are not eaten at the same meal with dairy products, such as butter and milk. The meat that is eaten by Orthodox Jews is prepared in a certain manner in keeping with religious laws, and it is the special preparation that makes the meat kosher. While Orthodox Jews are excused from adherence to their dietary laws during illness, most of them will not violate the laws under any circumstances.

When a person of Jewish faith is in danger of death, the rabbi should be summoned to pray with the patient, because a patient should not be left alone from the moment death is imminent.

In summary, the nurse's responsibility rests primarily in respecting the patients' religious beliefs and in using the clergy as resource persons when the patient faces stress situations.

BIBLIOGRAPHY

1. Ballinger, Reverend Malcolm B.: Religious care for hospital patients, Bulletin: American Protestant Hospital Association, vol. XVI, no. 3, July 1952.
2. Catholic Hospital Association: Routine spiritual care procedures, St. Louis, 1950, pp. 1-20.
3. Phillips, Clare: Meeting your patients' religious needs, RN **22**:1-12, March 1959.

Basic needs of patients

Chapter 10

Approach to nursing care

The nursing problems encountered in this unit are basic. They occur in all patients regardless of the specific health problem that may confront the individual. Essentially such problems are centered in the needs of patients, and are directly related to the individual security of a person in the physical, psychological, and sociological sense. The consideration of these needs is developed in line with problems 1 to 4 in Group I of the twenty-one nursing problems (see pages 29-30) and problems 6 and 7 in Group II, the latter viewed from the aspect of their relationship to the first four. Presented are principles and techniques of nursing care that will enable the nurse to assist the patient in resolving nursing problems of this nature.

Group I:
1. To maintain good hygiene and physical comfort
2. To promote optimal activity, exercise, rest, and sleep
3. To promote safety through the prevention of accident, injury, or other trauma and through the prevention of the spread of infection
4. To maintain good body mechanics and to prevent and to correct deformities

Group II:
6. To facilitate the maintenance of nutrition of all body cells
7. To facilitate the maintenance of elimination

The development of content is not sequential with the original statement of the problems but is organized and presented in a pattern intended to foster a concept of approach to patient care that evolves from an understanding of what constitutes safety in nursing.

The approach to understanding technical aspects of nursing care for patients is built on the foundation of personal past experiences of the nurse. During the various developmental stages in life, the individual acquires and uses knowledge that is drawn from many sources. These sources may be classified under the general headings of hygiene, sanitation, health, sociology, and psychology, even though at the time of learning the individual is often unaware of the source and classification of such knowledge.

At a relatively early age the person is made aware of the importance of personal cleanliness, of measures to maintain and to promote physical well-being, and of specific measures to control infections through the safe disposal of wastes. As the person grows such learning is generally extended beyond personal needs and develops into the social conscience of a responsible member of the community. Also, at an early age man acquires a recognition of and knowledge about the complexities of social interaction and its effects upon individual and group behavior. He quickly learns the order of personal importance in family constellations, feels the impact of his own need to be accepted by family, friends, and superiors, and develops a strong sense of gregariousness and need for companionship and sharing.

With progressive individual growth in knowledge and social skills, one might assume that the usual individual is able to make satisfactory adjustments at each level of development. However, the uniqueness of each person makes such an assumption open to question when that person is a patient in need of nursing care. When viewed in terms of the variety of factors that may thwart the achievement of complete maturity in the life situation, such an assumption is unrealistic in an approach to patient nursing care. Actually, everyone is aware of the numerous conflicts which complicate the full achievement of personal goals. Not the least among these is illness or injury. Regardless, however, of personal level of development, everyone has acquired some knowledge of the facts of life by the time adolescence is reached.

The beginning understanding of what is fundamental in nursing care lies in the application of learning gained in previous personal experience to the recognition of nursing problems presented by patients. Scientific knowledge gained through formal study and structured experience, and the resulting intellectual growth, promotes the development of scientifically based understanding. Many of the behaviors the nurse has used in past experiences are appropriate to use in providing nursing care. The major difference acquired through study and related clinical experience consists of building a scientific basis that underlies the nurse's behavior and provides her with a background on which the use of judgment rests. For example, every one is accustomed to observing other people. However, in the basic nursing school curriculum, the nurse learns to use scientific observation, evaluative, purposeful, and broad in range and scope. Such scientific observation leads to judgments about patient needs and consequently what the nursing care plan will be. It is a basis for and contributes to the full understanding of planning and implementing nursing care designed to help the patient function at his optimum potential. Therefore, any approach to the patient's nursing care must evolve from an understanding of individual needs related to the specific health problems confronting the patient.

From the basic standpoint there are three areas of learning on which the nurse structures the knowledge requisite to understanding the fundamentals of nursing: the rationale of medical management of health problems, the technique of observation, and the measures and methods of nursing intervention.

Recognition of the rationale of medical therapy promotes understanding of the technique of scientific observation, especially when the problem-solving process is combined with the use of judgment in the total clinical assessment of patient needs. The collection of scientific data, including physical examination, laboratory analysis, physiological signs, and the observation and interpretation of symptoms are the sources of the rationale of medical treatment. Medical treatment is primarily aimed at the restoration of physiological homeostasis or the maintenance of optimal function.

Medical treatment is commonly classified in four categories: prophylactic, diagnostic, therapeutic, and palliative. In all areas of health and health problems, prophylaxis, or measures to prevent the occurrence of disease, is a continuous ongoing process from the beginning of life until the end.

The practice of instilling silver nitrate solution into the eyes of the newborn infant is a specific preventive measure against gonorrheal infection. (This particular practice is mandatory in many states because of the danger of blindness in such infections. It is done routinely without consideration of whether or not the mother has, has not, or ever has had gonorrhea.) Through the early stages of life children are inoculated against the common communicable diseases. Vaccines and toxoid injections are given to stimulate the production of antibodies which provide partial or total immunization. Prophylactic treatment is not only concerned with maintaining wellness, but it is also designed to prevent further complication of an existent health problem. Many of the procedures instituted before surgery is performed are done to prevent potentially dangerous complications during or immediately following operation. For example, food and fluid are withheld to lessen the threat of aspiration of vomitus during and following the period of anesthesia and surgery.

There is a great variety of other situations in which prophylactic medical treatment is employed in conjunction with other types of treatment, and in each instance the premise upon which such treatment rests is the *prevention* of either disease or possible complications.

Specific knowledge of precisely what evidence the multiple kinds of tests and procedures will demonstrate enables the nurse to function adequately in the preparation for and implementation of the medical procedures. Whether directly or indirectly involved in the actual performance of the test, the nurse is inevitably involved in preparing the patient physically and mentally and providing emotional support in a variety of situations that involve testing or therapeutic measures. Regardless of explanations given by doctors, technicians, or therapists, it is not unusual to find that the patient turns to the nurse for additional explanations. Whether the nurse's function in this setting is that of a synthesizing or a catalyzing agent, it is nevertheless an extremely important one.

Obviously the medical therapy prescribed will depend upon the results of diagnostic measures. It becomes self-evident that unless the patient is accurately and totally ready for the diagnostic procedure, it either will not be successfully implemented or the results will lack integrity. Because of the tremendous resources available, the physician uses every available diagnostic measure to ensure the accuracy of a diagnosis or determine the cause of the patient's health problem. Once a diagnosis is established, related therapeutic measures are instituted. Selection of therapy is based on scientific evidence that it is curative and restorative and on evaluation of the individual patient's capacity to withstand and/or respond to the therapy. Although therapy is usually specific, it is not always successful.

Palliative medical treatments are designed not to cure disease but to relieve signs and symptoms and make the patient more comfortable. They alleviate physiological and psychological stress resulting from health problems. They encompass a wide selection of supportive measures. Of themselves, palliative measures cannot eradicate permanently a specific pathological process, but they do alleviate temporarily the signs and symptoms of physical and mental discomfort due to the process. In this way they promote the physical and mental rest essential to reparative body processes and, eventually, a return to homeostasis. When restoration of homeostasis is not possible, palliative measures provide for patient comfort in accord with the concept of human dignity.

For example, prescription of hypnotics to relieve sleeplessness is a palliative measure when sleeplessness results from mental discomfort. A specific somnifacient cannot directly reduce anxiety or apprehension, but it can alleviate the insomnia. Similarly, analgesics prescribed for pain due to trauma or pathological processes in body structures cannot directly reverse physiological stress, but they can relieve pain and thereby foster natural reparative processes. When pain is intractable, analgesics and narcotics ensure at least optimal comfort, especially when the patient's clinical prognosis is doubtful.

TECHNIQUE OF SCIENTIFIC OBSERVATION

Scientific observation is a comprehensive term used to indicate a complexity of methods used to study any given subject. The reference here is to the independent nursing function of assessment and evaluation of the patient. As a nursing responsibility, observation is a common factor in all areas of nursing care in all nursing problems with all patients. It is prerequisite to the nursing care plan that is intended to provide for total patient needs.

The word "scientific" is used to indicate that observation must be knowledgeable and meaningful. It is not casual or incidental but structured and deliberate. It implies that observation or the process of noting is not sufficient but that the processes of evaluation and disposition of factual data gained through observation are also involved. The technique of observation is concerned with four facts: what to observe, how to observe, the implications of observation, and action following the observations.

What to observe

Observation as a clinical skill is essentially concerned with the patient's overt and covert manifestations of a positive or negative nature. Because covert patient problems have been discussed in a previous chapter, this section will be confined to exploration of the overt physical symptoms and signs that are determinants in planning and in implementing nursing care. The signs of disease constitute the evidence of anatomical change that can be elicited by examination or diagnostic test; the symptoms are the evidences of altered function and the body's effort to compensate and restore equilibrium. The break in the integrity of lung tissue produced by an invasion of the tuberculosis bacillus and revealed by x-ray is a sign of disease. The rise in temperature, the body's attempt to drive out the bacillus, is a symptom.

A sign or symptom is an indication of disturbance in health. It may be vague, or it may be strongly positive. The degree of intensity is usually relative to the degree of disturbance in homeostasis. A symptom is defined as objective when it is sensible to the observer; i.e., it can be perceived by sight, touch, hearing, or smell. Thus, a nurse actually perceives color and temperature of the skin, identifies audible respirations, and detects significant, characteristic odors in body secretions or excretions. A symptom is defined as subjective when it is not directly sensible to the observer but is described by the patient. Thus a nurse intellectually perceives pain, nausea, vertigo, malaise, weakness, visual defects, and the like. Although there is often objective manifestation of the existence of subjective symptoms, frequently there is not. For example, the threshold for pain is an individual factor in each person. The severity of pain must be determined on this factor, not on the degree of disturbance projected by the patient. *The nurse's observation of subjective symptoms must be totally objective.*

In order to recognize digression in health, it is necessary to have a concept of the normal. From the physical standpoint, there are certain factors which characterize the "well person." The most obvious and yet the most critical of these are skin color, temperature, pulse, and respiration. In addition, possession of a relative degree of physical energy and of effective body mechanics as well as freedom from distress due to nausea, vomiting, or pain are health norms. Still other indicators of health status relate to interest in and tolerance for food intake as well as ability to eliminate the waste products of metabolism through the urinary and intestinal tracts. Although specific consideration of the urinary and gastrointestinal systems will be undertaken in subsequent chapters, it is important to note here that observation of body secretions and excretions and recognition of the significance of deviations from the norms in them are significant. Thus it would be obvious that the amount excreted, the quality of excretions, the facility of excretion, and the presence of abnormal constituents in urine or stool are least common denominators in evaluating health status. Likewise, anorexia or loss of appetite, food aversion, or inability to masticate, ingest, and digest food points up a disturbance in homeostasis that has implications for the nurse in planning patient care. It is obvious, therefore, that any approach to patient care must consider the particular aspects of critical observation in each individual patient.

How to observe

In varying circumstances, observation may be done with the patient being fully cognizant, or it may be done unobstrusively with the patient being unaware of it. Actually the latter type of observation is important only when the patient's anxiety or apprehension is increased by any method of scrutiny. Regardless of whether the approach is deliberate or casual, observation must be a continuous process during all phases of the patient's illness. The nurse must utilize every opportunity available to make accurate and full observation of physical symptoms without unduly inconveniencing the patient.

The administration of a bath affords an excellent opportunity for general assessment of skin condition and total physical capacity, as well as eliciting the existence of subjective symptoms. Beyond this, in all aspects of giving direct nursing care to patients, the nurse can make observations of general and local manifestations that are significant. Feeding, giving medications,

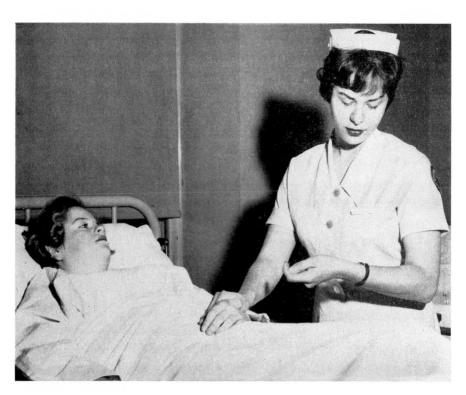

Fig. 10. The nurse counts the pulse obviously while counting respirations unobtrusively.

changing dressings, and administering irrigations are instances of giving direct care that afford opportunity for critical observation. Objective symptoms are detected by deliberate acts of inspection (looking at, seeing, visualizing), palpation (feeling and touching), manipulation (moving, as in body motion or joints in full range of motion), and identification of odors (smelling). Inspection establishes critical facts related to general or local skin color, presence of rashes or lesions, and status of wound healing. In addition, it verifies characteristics of body discharges and excretions. Palpation reveals heat, swelling, and tenderness. Manipulation pinpoints limited mobility, immobility, and pain on motion. Smelling identifies specific aspects of deviations in homeostasis related to elimination of waste from the respiratory and alimentary tracts as well as discharges from other body cavities or wounds.

Implications of observations

Physical symptoms are categorized as being toward (positive) or untoward (negative) indications. In essence they are indicative of a return to

Table 3. *Meaning of specific symptoms related to body appearance and function*

Area of observation	Symptom	Possible implications
Skin		
1. Color		
(a) General	Flushed	Fever
	Pallor	Malnutrition, syncope, anemia
	Cyanosis	Cardiac or respiratory distress
	Jaundice	Liver or gallbladder disease
(b) Local	Erythema (red)	Congestion, inflammation, infection
	Ecchymosis (blue)	Trauma, interstitial bleeding
	Necrosis (black)	Devitalized tissue
	Gangrene (black)	Massive death of tissue as in digit, foot, or extremity
2. Temperature and turgor	Warm, moist, or dry	Fever
	Warm, dry	Dehydration, acidosis
	Cold, clammy	Hemorrhage, shock
3. Abnormalities	Rash, urticaria	Sensitivity (drug, food, or contact), communicable disease
Physical capacity and status		
1. Activity	Malaise	Weakness
	Lethargy	Debilitation
	Loss of function	Inflammation, fracture, central nervous system disturbance
	"Self-splinting"	Pain
	Hyperactive	Disturbance in body regulatory mechanism, anxiety
	Cachexia	Malnutrition
2. Rest and comfort	Tension	Apprehension
	Restlessness	Discomfort, hemorrhage, anoxia
	Sleeplessness	Anxiety, pain, lonesomeness

Continued on next page.

Table 3. *Meaning of specific symptoms related to body appearance and function—* cont'd

Area of observation	Symptom	Possible implications
Orientation	Loss of consciousness	Central nervous system Disturbances or intercranial hemorrhage
	Syncope	Anemia
	Disorientation	Toxicity, brain damage, delirium, mental illness
Communication	Aphasia	Brain damage
	Hearing loss	Auditory or acoustic nerve destruction, middle ear pathology
	Apathy	Emotional disturbance
Intake of food and fluid	Anorexia	Fever, anemia, malignancies, emotional disturbances
	Dysphagia	Obstruction of pharynx, esophagus
	Polydipsia	Dehydration, diabetes mellitus
Output of waste		
1. Amount and consistency	Diaphoresis	Fever, shock, heat prostration
	Polyuria	Diabetes mellitus
	Oliguria to anuria	Renal failure, obstruction in ureters, bladder, or urethra, retention
	Diarrhea	Infection, colitis
	Constipation to obstipation	Obstruction, Poor dietary habits, impaction
2. Color	Hematuria	Calculi, tumors, infection
	Tarry stool	Duodenal bleeding
	Frank blood in stool	Rectal bleeding
3. Abnormal output		
(a) Vomitus	Undigested food	Gastric tumor, ulcer, obstruction
	"Coffee ground"	Duodenal ulcer
	Hematemesis	Gastric ulcer
(b) Sputum	Hemoptysis	Pneumonia, tuberculosis, congestive heart failure
	Pus	Lung abscess
(c) Bleeding	Frank blood from any body cavity	Varices, tumors

homeostasis or indicative of a deviation from homeostasis. Recognition and identification of these reactions are fundamental to observation. It is not only sufficient to recognize them, but it is also necessary to identify their implications. Symptoms may be simple and obvious or complex and subtle. From the standpoint of fundamental nursing care, patient safety is dependent upon the nurse's ability to identify the significance of what is observed. The outline presented in Table 3 is designed as an example to provide beginning knowledge of the meaning of specific symptoms related to body appearance and function.

The implications of symptoms are broad in scope. Pinpointing their meaning scientifically is the function of the physician. The nursing responsibility is essentially involved with recognition of symptoms, awareness of their implications within the framework of patient safety, and communication of significant data to all members of the health team.

Action following observation

The use and sharing of knowledge gained through scientific observation fulfills the purpose for which observation is undertaken, i.e., to identify changes in the patient's health status in the light of health processes, therapeutic measures, and all aspects of total nursing care. It is therefore not only necessary to know that something exists and why it exists, but it is also necessary to know what to do about it. Knowing when to act requires an understanding of the priority of the patient's needs in order to ensure total safety. Knowing what action to take requires also the ability to use the right resource personnel and the ability to relate effectively with all people involved. Knowing how to act requires the capacity to communicate vital data verbally, reporting to and consulting with members of the health team, including non-nursing personnel. In addition, it requires the ability to make accurate, precise, and concise notations of critical data on patients' records.

Priority and urgency of action

Recognition of the existence of conditions that are a potential or an immediate threat to patient safety directs the nurse to do something about it immediately. When a patient hemorrhages twelve hours postoperatively, a patient who is convalescing from a coronary heart attack suddenly complains of severe chest pain, or the motor of an oxygen tent supplying oxygen for a patient who has congestive heart failure stops running, there is no doubt that immediate action must be taken. Such situations constitute an emergency. On the other hand, if a patient complains of some difficulty in dietary adjustment or if a patient experiences constipation related to inactivity or diet, action may well be deferred until the physician sees the patient.

What action to take

Knowing the right resource personnel to use and being able to relate effectively with all people involved are essentially tied up in orientation to a clinical setting and using the proper channels of communications. Relating this to the emergency situations mentioned in the preceding paragraph, the course of action is obvious. When a patient hemorrhages or suffers acute cardiac distress, the physician must be called at once. When the motor of an oxygen tent stops running, obviously the services of a technician must be secured promptly.

Another aspect of action that is fundamental is the use of supportive nursing measures in states of acute distress. Specific aspects of such nursing care are more suitably dealt with in subsequent chapters. However, as a point of illustration here, the need for action other than reporting should be recognized. When a patient receiving oxygen via tent is suddenly cut off from the supply because the motor fails, the canopy should be removed so that the patient will have access to the source of supply in the free air.

Knowing how to act

Effective communication of knowledge is dependent upon the ability to think clearly and upon fluency in using language. In the hospital setting this requires scientific knowledge related to health and disease as well as a technical and general vocabulary. Whether observations are reported verbally or recorded on the patient's record, accuracy of facts and their significance are ensured by correct use of technical terminology. Notations on the clinical record should be concise to avoid excessive use of time spent reading and precise to avoid error due to misinterpretation of words.

One final point must be made. Although it would seem theoretically unnecessary, in view of actual practice, emphasis on legibility of notations has become crucial. Clinical records function as resource data about patient's health status for medical and nursing personnel, as sources of learning for students, as invaluable sources of public health statistical data, and as legal documents supporting the rights of patients, medical and nursing personnel, and the hospital. If data recorded cannot be read, records are useless, and an invaluable source of information designed to benefit society in general and patients in particular is lost to all concerned.

VITAL SIGNS

In addition to the utilization of sensory function, of skilled observations, and of intellectual skill in interpretation, nurses are responsible for a variety of procedures involving scientific assessment. However, regardless of the significance of a multitude of tests in a variety of situations, the most constant and critical of all observations is the assessment of the status of vital signs.

The term "vital signs" includes the body temperature, pulse, respiration, and blood pressure. Assignment of the term vital to these manifestations is based upon the physiological fact that all of them tend toward a state of relative constancy within a norm related to age, sex, physical size, occupation, and activity. Deviations from established norms with this pattern indicate a threat to patient safety. Therefore, nursing care of patients involves continuing assessment of these vital signs because of their critical role as indicators of general health status.

Temperature

Body temperature has been defined as the balance of heat maintained between that which is produced and that which is lost from the body. Thus, a "well person" maintains a body temperature that can be registered as 98.6° F. (37° C.) on a clinical thermometer. This is an approximate norm. Deviations within a reasonable number of degrees above or below this reading must be evaluated in light of activity, rest, and disease processes, among other factors, in the individual patient. Understanding of the implications of deviations from the normal is based on the following three scientific facts:

1. How heat is produced in the body
2. How heat is lost from the body
3. How body temperature balance can be disturbed

Normal heat production and heat loss involve the physiological factors related to food ingestion, assimilation, and excretion of waste. Such functions naturally involve muscle action as well as that of ductile and ductless glands. When there is interference with natural physiological function because of disease processes, the resultant disturbance in homeostasis is a measurable deviation in body temperature above or below the established norm.

Nursing intervention

Body temperature is determined by means of an instrument known as a clinical thermometer which is calibrated according to the Fahrenheit or Centigrade scales of measurement. Because it is scientifically indicative of homeostatic disturbance, body temperature is measured at regular intervals in the hosiptal setting, as well as in any patient setting. The most meaningful clinical differentiation in temperature is that between morning and night. Hence, the nurse is commonly required to keep note of the registrations at specified time intervals: i.e., 8 A.M., 12 NOON, 4. P.M., 8 P.M., 12 A.M. Variations in temperature related to time of day are grossly significant to the physician in view of disease processes and individual response to physiological or emotional stress.

Body temperature is commonly measured orally or rectally. The selection of site is determined by several factors. Rectal temperature readings are scientifically judged to be the more accurate. Therefore, when deviations from normal temperature are critical in view of the patient's disease, rectal temperature readings are indicated. On the other hand, when the patient's health problem contraindicates taking temperaure rectally, then oral temperature readings are acceptable. Conversely, when patients are convalescent or afebrile, oral temperature readings are commonly accepted as norms. However, when a patient's use of reason is impaired by age or illness or his oxygen intake is limited, use of an oral thermometer constitutes a threat to safety.

The actual procedure of taking temperature involves specific measures to ensure patient safety. These measures relate directly to protection from physical and microbiological danger. The instrument selected must be intact, i.e., free of superficial cracks or chips, and it must be clean, i.e., free of any possible source of infection. An additional aspect of patient safety requires scientific accuracy in measurement. The efficiency of the thermometer must be established; the mercury must be shaken down below normal range of temperature before it is placed in the mouth or rectum, and it must remain in place for the required period of time.

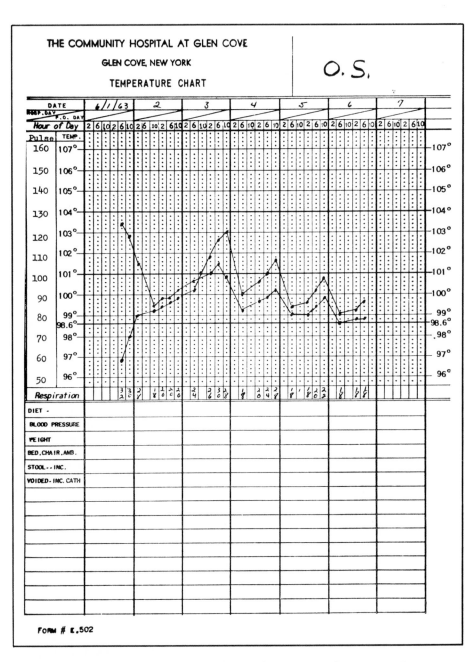

Fig. 11. The pattern of temperature, pulse, and respiration deviation is diagnostically and therapeutically significant.

Table 4. *Safe practice in taking temperature*

	Time in place	Indications	Contraindications	Critical points

Oral	3-5 minutes	Convalescence
		Rectal conditions
		Obstetrical and
		  gynecological
		  conditions
			Dyspnea
			Unconsciousness
			Disorientation
			Children
			Senility
				1. Do not use for ½ hour after oral cavity has been exposed to extremes of temperature (hot or cold beverage, irrigations, smoking)
				2. Insert sublingually
				3. Mouth must be closed

Rectal	3 minutes	Fever
		Upper respiratory
		  conditions
		Cardiac conditions
		Central nervous
		  system disorders
		Psychiatric dis-
		  orders
		Children
			Rectal hemorrhage
			Rectal surgery
			Gynecological
			  surgery
			Labor and post-
			  partum stages
				1. Lubricate bulb
				2. Insert bulb beyond external anal sphincter
				3. Hold distal end in situations in which patient's condition requires securing safety

A guideline for establishing a pattern of safe practice in taking temperature is presented in Table 4.

After the reading has been taken, the thermometer should immediately be washed in cool water and soap, rinsed, dried, and stored in a dry, covered container. Several methods of chemical disinfection are employed in various clinical settings. The results of many research studies raise serious question as to the efficiency of such techniques. However, regardless of the use of chemical agents, the specific cleansing, washing, and drying are fundamental to safety.

Body temperature may also be measured in the groin, axilla, and vagina. However, it is taken in these areas only when oral or rectal measurement is not possible because of specific pathological states.

Pulse

As a direct echo of the heartbeat, the pulse is a valuable and readily accessible indicator of the state of vital function. For this reason, observation of the pulse is probably one of the most continuously and continually employed methods. Meaningful observations are based upon knowledge of the normal characteristics of a pulse and recognition of the existence of abnormalities in the pattern perceived. Normal pulse characteristics are generally equated with chronological age groups in light of sex, physical size, weight, and activity. Identifiable characteristics include rate (beats per minutes), rhythm (regularity of tempo), volume (intensity of beat), and the condition of the wall of the artery.

Nursing intervention

The pulse is taken by compression of an artery by the first three fingers. Although the radial artery is most commonly used, the pulse may also be taken by compression of the temporal, facial, carotid, femoral, or dorsalis pedis arteries when the radial area is not accessible. Because deviations in quality of pulse rate are vital in all patients and critical in many, it should not only by taken at regular intervals daily, but also as often as there is a change in patient activity or whenever there is overt manifestation of physiological change. When the pulse is being taken, the patient should be at rest and the arm and hand supported in natural alignment in relation to posture. When arterial pulsation is felt, notation of the rhythm, volume, and condition of the artery is made before counting rate.

A normal heart rate is characterized by a fairly consistent number of beats per minute. When there is no directly related pathology, there is a regularity of rhythm and the heart beats the same number of times in each quarter of a minute. When patients have no primary disease of the cardiovascular or central nervous systems or when they are not in an acute state as a result of surgical or medical intervention, the pulse may be taken for a quarter or half a minute and multiplied accordingly. However, in specific circumstances such as heart disease or disease of the nerves that regulate heart action, the pulse must be counted for the full minute.

From the level of fundamental critical observation, the comparison of characteristics listed in Table 5 is designed as a basis for further development.

In certain states of cardiac disease, the patient experiences auricular fibrillation. Inefficient cardiac action prevents all the heartbeats from reaching the distal arteries. When it is necessary to determine actual heart rate to treat this condition safely (e.g., prescription of digitalis preparations), the apical beat is counted by means of a stethoscope. When apical and radial rates are counted simultaneously by two people, the procedure is defined as taking an apical-radial pulse. The difference between the two rates is the actual pulse deficit. The number of impulses not transmitted is one factor the physician uses in estimating the degree of impaired cardiotonic efficiency. When a patient is receiving digitalis preparations, accurate perception of apical rate is vital. Such preparations strengthen the contractions and reduce the rate of the heart. A heart rate that is slower than

Table 5. *Comparison of pulse characteristics and deviations*

	Normal	*Deviations*
Rate	Adult, 70-90 (widely variable)	Markedly slow or rapid in relation to criteria (patient)
Rhythm	Regular	Arrhythmias Coupling Missed beats
Volume	Appropriate to size of instrument producing it (pulsation definite)	Bounding, full Thready, weak
Condition of artery	Pliable but firm	Wiry, hard Flabby, soft

60 beats per minute is usually considered dangerous to maintenance of life.

Respiration

Respiration is the exchange of gases, oxygen, and carbon dioxide between an organism and its environment. External respiration is the exchange of oxygen and carbon dioxide between the lungs and the blood, and internal respiration is the exchange of the same gases between the blood and the body cells. Respiration is controlled by three factors: the respiratory center in the medulla, the autonomic nervous system, and the chemical composition of the blood. As the carbon dioxide content of the blood rises, the respiratory center is stimulated to increase the rate of breathing in order to remove the carbon dioxide content and correspondingly increase the oxygen content of blood and body tissues. While breathing is usually involuntary and automatic, some degree of voluntary control of respiration is possible. For example, an individual can hold his breath or deliberately change the rate and character of his respirations. However, involuntary control takes over as the carbon dioxide content of the blood rises.

Significant aspects of the vital sign of respiration include rate and character, the muscle activity of the chest and abdomen, and the patient's color.

The typical respiration rate is regular, rythmic, and effortless. The average person at rest inhales and exhales about 14-18 times per minute, although individual variations in norms occur. Children breathe more rapidly than adults, and infants breathe more rapidly than children. Normal respiration rate is identified as eupnea, and increased rate as polypnea, and an absence of respiration as apnea. The depth of respiration is also significant. Breathing may vary in the direction of either shallow or deep, resulting in less or more than the approximate 500 c.c. that is usually exchanged in normal respiration.

Any factor that influences the metabolic rate or the control mechanism of respiration results in a change of respiration. Increased activity, fever, exposure to cold, fright, or drugs are examples of factors that can increase the metabolic rate and hence increase the rate and depth of respirations. Most pathology, with the exception of brain pathology, tends to increase the rate of respiration. Increased intracranial pressure usually produces a slowed rate of respiration because of pressure on the respiratory center in the medulla. Some drugs (morphine, for example) can also slow the rate of breathing by depressing the respiratory center.

Disease processes that impair oxygen intake, such as congestive heart failure with an accumulation of fluid in the pulmonary area, produce certain typical patterns of respiratory change. Difficulty in breathing is called dyspnea; hard and deep breathing is called hyperpnea. When a patient instinctively assumes a sitting or erect position to relieve marked dyspnea, the condition is identified as orthopnea. Orthopnea occurs most frequently in patients suffering with heart disease. Extremely heavy, noisy breathing is described as stertorous. A relatively serious symptom is Cheyne-Stokes respiration, characterized by a period of short and shallow breathing, then increasing rate and depth in breathing, followed by a period of apnea.

In addition to rate and character, the movements of the chest and abdominal walls are points of observation in relation to respiration. Usually both the chest and abdominal walls are used in respiration, and the presence of costal (chest) or abdominal respiratory movements simultaneouly is normal. The presence of exaggerated costal movement with reduced abdominal movement, or vice versa, usually indicates difficulty in the area of reduced activity. Exaggerated movements accompany dyspnea in its varying forms, and decreased chest or abdominal expansion is related to disease processes in the area that lead the patient to protect himself from painful movement. Shallow and/or slow respirations as a result of increased intracranial pressure or the administration of a drug that depresses respiration may be accompanied by decreased chest and abdominal expansion.

Since one of the primary purposes of respiration is the exchange of oxygen and carbon dioxide and the maintenance of adequate oxygenation of body cells, the patient's color becomes a point of significant observation. A patient with respiratory difficulty due to any cause may indicate oxygen want or lack by a bluish color of the mucous membrane, nail beds, or skin. The bluish color (cyanosis) is due to a decreased oxygen content of the bloodstream. The extent and depth of cyanosis are indications of the degree of oxygen want.

Nursing intervention

The observation, description, and interpretation of respiratory rate and character constitute a major nursing responsibility. Respiratory patterns frequently are key indicators in diagnosis and consequently in therapy. In asthma, for example, the short inspiration and the longer period of expiration are unmistakable characteristics of the disease. Therefore, the observation of respiration is often a critical area of observation.

Respiration should be observed unobtrusively since awareness of breathing leads to voluntary control and changes in rate and character. If an individual becomes conscious of the fact that he is breathing, he will find it almost impossible to let the automatic regulation of respiration function. Therefore, counting the rate and observing the character of respirations should be done without making the process obvious to the patient. Respirations may be observed while the nurse appears to continue counting the pulse. The rise and fall of the chest wall or the abdomen may be counted, or the nurse may breathe with the patient and count her own respiratory rate. Although the respirations may be counted for one-half a minute and doubled, a full minute count, repeated, is usually wise when respiration characteristics are significant.

In observing respirations, all of the factors that influence it must be considered. The character and rate of respiration are influenced by activity, disease, voluntary versus automatic control, emotional or feeling reaction,

Table 6. *Respiration characteristics and deviations*

	Normal	Deviations
Rate	14-18 per minute (at rest)	Slow Hyperpnea Apnea Cheyne-Stokes
Character	Regular Rhythmic Quiet Effortless	Dyspnea Orthopnea Shallow Stertorous Moist Wheezy Associated pain Exaggerated chest or abdominal movement Cheyne-Stokes

environmental oxygen concentration and temperature, fluid and electrolyte balance, and individual variations in norms. For this reason, the conditions under which respirations are observed are as significant as the rate and character of respiration.

In addition to the rate and character of respirations, two additional factors to be considered in the observation of respiration are position and pain. The patient may assume a particular position to make breathing more comfortable, such as the erect or sitting position in the presence of heart disease and marked dyspnea. A patient may also "splint" his chest to avoid pain; for example, holding his chest wall with his hands when he coughs. In all instances, respiratory rate and character should be related to position in evaluating observations. Pain is also a factor in such evaluation, and the relationship of pain and respiration is significant. Since pain is experienced by the patient, the determination of its extent, nature, and association with breathing is usually best described by the patient. Table 6 indicates the major points in the observation of respiration.

Blood pressure

The term "blood pressure" refers to the force of the pressure exerted within the arterial vessels during each of the phases of cardiac action, i.e., the period of contraction and the period of relaxation. The first phase is physiologically termed the period of systole (contraction), and the existent force is identified as the systolic pressure. The second phase is termed the period of diastole (relaxation), and the existent force is identified as the diastolic pressure.

Arterial blood pressure is measured clinically by means of an instrument called a sphygmomanometer. There are two types of devices in common use, the mercury and the anaeroid (spring). Because it is the more stable instrument, the mercury manometer is widely used in clinical settings.

The important scientific operational principles of the manometer may be summarized as follows:

1. Air pressure simultaneously occludes circulation in the brachial artery and causes the mercury to rise in the calibrated glass tube.
2. Release of pressure simultaneously allows reestablishment of circulation and descent of the column of mercury.
3. Release of constriction on the artery permits blood to surge through the lumen with the force exerted by systole. The beat is concurrently audible by means of a stethescope and is visible on the calibrated tube as the mercury vacillates in response to the force.
4. Diminution of the force within the artery as the heart passes into diastolic phase causes reduction and eventual cessation of audible sound and markedly less fluctuation in the mercury. Correspondingly, the reduction of air pressure within the cuff permits the total drop of mercury within the calibrated tube.

The actual blood pressure is related to the amount of force exerted as measured by millimeters of mercury at the actual points of occurrence of systole and diastole. The numerical point at which the mercury stands in each instance is the clinical interpretation of blood pressure. The readings are represented as a fraction, i.e., systolic over diastolic.

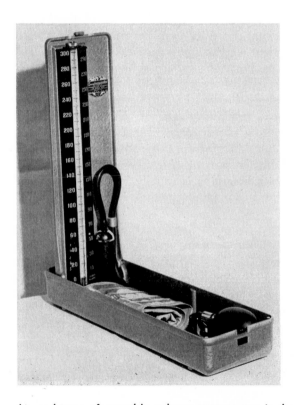

Fig. 12. A commonly used type of portable sphygmomanometer is the Baumanometer.

As with other vital signs indicative of physiological status, blood pressure is evaluated within norms. Generally, there are two normal values that are fundamental. The first includes the common factors relative to age, sex, size, and activity. The second is centered in the physiological uniqueness of the individual. However, because of the universality of common factors, medical science defines normal blood pressure in this regard. The most widely accepted normal blood pressure reading in adulthood is 120/80, with a variable of 10 to 15 mm. in either direction (in both systolic and diastolic phases) considered well within normal limits. The mathematical ratio between the two numbers is medically significant because the maintenance of diastolic pressure is dependent upon the initial systolic force and the resistance in peripheral vessels. This numerical differential represents the mean arterial pulse pressure. A marked increase or decrease in the differential is an indication of disturbed physiological homeostasis.

Nursing intervention

Critical observation of patients with a wide variety of nursing problems requires periodic estimation of circulatory stability. Although complete scientific accuracy in blood pressure readings is limited by variables related to the individual observer error, defective apparatus, and the dis-

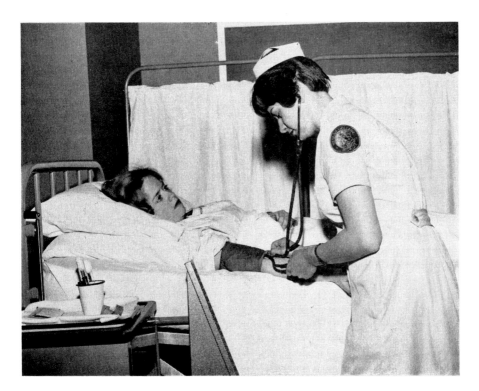

Fig. 13. Among the first steps in learning to take a blood pressure are cuff placement and locating the patient's pulse.

agreement of authorities on the exact point of reading each phase, relative accuracy is essential to patient safety. The facts fundamental to taking blood pressure have knowledgeable and technical aspects. They are summarized as follows:

1. Knowledge of the authoritative standard of the point at which systolic and diastolic pressure is read that is used in the clinical setting

   In one instance, the systolic pressure is taken at the first audible beat, and the diastolic is taken at the point of change in intensity from loud to soft. In another instance, the diastolic reading is taken at the point at which the beat becomes inaudible. Regardless of the difference in standards, the factor that is critical is that one criterion be used by all members of the health team concerned.

2. Knowledge of the previous pattern of blood pressure in individual patients

3. Knowledge of the integrity of apparatus used

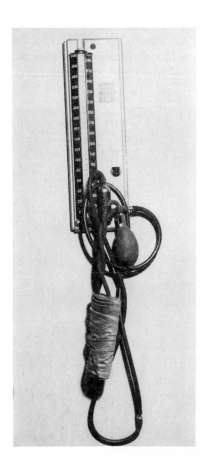

Fig. 14. In many hospitals, the sphygmomanometer is located on the wall. This has the advantages of being closer to eye level and being readily available without taking up space.

4. Knowledge relative to obtaining consistent readings if blood pressure is taken on the same extremity each time and at the same time when daily or biweekly readings are indicated
5. Technical knowledge related to the correct application of the cuff to provide efficient occlusion of the artery at a point that permits digital perception of the brachial artery and application of the stethescope
6. Technical knowledge of reading indicated pressure responses as near to eye level as possible to reduce errors of visualization
7. Knowledge basic to recording and reporting blood pressure readings with understanding of the urgency of reporting significant changes

It must be remembered that blood pressure is frequently one of the most critical of the vital signs.

MEASURES AND METHODS OF NURSING INTERVENTION

The approach to nursing care is organized around four categories of measures and methods of nursing intervention similar to that identified in the rationale of medical treatment: preventive, supportive, restorative, and rehabilitative. The measures and methods of nursing intervention are the basic knowledges and skills required to implement nursing care in each of these categories.

Preventive nursing measures are essentially concerned with maintaining total health in all aspects basic to the physical and psychological integrity of the individual. Specific methods employed may include a wide range of procedures designed as positive approaches, such as the use of bedrails, disinfection and sterilization to eliminate cross-infection, and continuous assessment of physical safety in the total patient environment.

Supportive nursing measures are directed toward sustaining normal physiological and psychological patient needs in the presence of stress. Specific methods employed may include a wide range of activities designed to provide physical hygiene, to supply fundamental needs related to nutrition and elimination, and to sustain patients' physical and psychological requirements in the areas of comfort, exercise, rest, and sleep.

Restorative nursing measures are primarily dependent nursing functions and involve prescribed medical therapeutic measures that are technically initiated by the doctor or the nurse but are commonly within the realm of nurse function in regard to maintenance of therapeutic medical treatment, aftercare of patients, or observation of immediate or subsequent response of patients to medical therapy. Examples of such nursing methods are of such wide range that they almost defy identification. However, for purposes of fundamental approach, the following are mentioned: administration of enemas, maintaining the patency of gastrointestinal tubes (or indeed any medically inserted tube), postoperative management, and implementation of medically planned infusional therapy in acute states of electrolyte and fluid imbalance. In this category there is the aspect of observation in areas involving diagnostic and palliative medical procedures such as obtaining specimens for diagnostic or palliative purposes.

Rehabilitative nursing measures are a combination of independent and dependent nursing functions, because nursing methods are partly related to preventive nursing and partly related to medical evaluation of the patient's limitations. However, emphasis at this point is placed on nursing measures directed toward restoration of the patient to full activity in so far as his health problem permits. Such methods include increasing activity and exercise within a patient's limitations, health teaching in relation to all physical, nutritional, or occupational capacities, provision for access to resource personnel in related health disciplines, and planning with family members or social colleagues for health needs within the home environment.

Each of these categories includes specific aspects of nursing function related to total safety and comfort, maintenance of and/or restoration of homeostasis to the highest possible level, facilitating return to the family and community life, and health teaching designed to minimize future health problems, new or old.

BIBLIOGRAPHY

1. Barnett, Catherine: This to me is nursing, Nursing Outlook **8:**72-75, Feb. 1960.
2. Brown, Esther Lucile: Newer dimensions of patient care. Part I. The use of physical and social environment of the general hospital for therapeutic purposes, New York, 1961, Russell Sage Foundation.
3. Larson, Virginia: What hospitalization means to patients, American Journal of Nursing **61:**44-47, May 1961.
4. Leone, Lucille Petry: Wanted: good nursing, Nursing Outlook **5:**576-578, Sept. 1957.
5. McLain, M. Esther, Gragg, Shirley H.: Scientific principles in nursing, ed. 4, St. Louis, 1962, The C. V. Mosby Co., pp. 205-243.
6. Mary Mercita, Sister: Rehabilitation—bridge to a useful and happy life, Nursing Outlook **9:**581-583, Sept. 1961.
7. Noles, Eva M.: Nursing a geriatric patient, American Journal of Nursing **63:**73-75, Jan. 1963.
8. Rockwell, Virginia Tyler: Surgical hand scrubbing, American Journal of Nursing **63:**75-81, June 1963.
9. Rogers, Martha E.: Building a strong educational foundation, American Journal of Nursing **63:**94-95, June 1963.
10. Rogers, Martha E.: Some comments on a theoretical basis of nursing practice, Nursing Science **1:**11-13, 60-61, April-May, 1963.
11. Russell, Robert B.: View from a pillow, American Journal of Nursing **61:**88-91, Dec. 1961.
12. Wilcox, Jane: Observer factors in the measurement of blood pressure, Nursing Research **10:**4-17, Winter 1961.
13. Winters, Margaret C., and Gilmer, Lee: The Nurse's judgement and the patient's understanding, American Journal of Nursing **61:**50-54, Dec. 1961.
14. Wood, M. Marian: Guide to better care—a nursing plan, American Journal of Nursing **61:**61-62, Dec. 1961.

Chapter 11

Basic safety needs of patients

Because of the immediate responsibility of the nurse for safety and because of the complexity of the concept of safety, patient safety is an area of concern in nursing care. In reality, this encompasses the total person of the patient, physical and mental. This discussion will be concerned primarily with the physical aspects of nursing care along with a general consideration of the psychological aspects as they relate to total patient care.

By definition, the word "safe" means "secure from threat of danger, harm, or loss."* In order to ensure this state, the nurse must have specific knowledge of factors that will create security in the patient's environment and ability to translate that knowledge into appropriate action. Conversely, specific knowledge of factors that militate against safety and the ability to use specific measures and techniques prophylactically and therapeutically are fundamental to safe nursing.

The promotion of patient safety is related basically to the prevention of accident, injury or trauma, and the prevention of the spread of infection. Essentially it is concerned with the creation of an environment that is physically, psychologically, and microbiologically secure.

PREVENTION OF ACCIDENT AND INJURY

Modern society has long been aware of the fact that scientific advancement has introduced certain concrete hazards in man's environment. In contrast to the advantages that technological inventions have afforded us, the inherent dangers seem relatively unimportant. Yet, it is imperative that present-day miracles such as electricity, illuminating gas, the sulfur match, and pneumatic and mechanical motion devices be viewed as inherent dangers in the environment. Such a reference may seem archaic in this era of space ships and atomic submarines, but statistics provide scientific evidence of the fact that mechanical injury and fire cause more fatalities than are justifiable in view of the presupposed advantage of technological im-

---

*By permission. From Webster's Seventh New Collegiate Dictionary, copyright 1963 by G. & C. Merriam Co., Publishers of the Merriam-Webster Dictionaries.

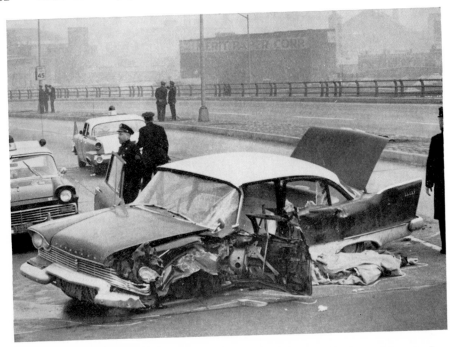

Fig. 15. Automobiles have become lethal weapons and add to the growing number of deaths by accident.

provements resulting from the explosion of knowledge. For this reason, particular consideration must be given the physical and psychological aspects of the increased incidence of injuries and accidents. For, if man in society is forearmed with knowledge and the facilities to utilize such knowledge, there should ensue a diminution in the incidence of injuries and accidents.

Scientific studies prove that the lack of knowledge and understanding, as well as psychological and emotional disturbances, contributed directly to the impairment of production efficiency in man. The implications of this in terms of hospitalized patients are readily seen. The nurse, the focus of multiple services rendered to the patient, must have knowledge and understanding related to providing for patient safety. The major hazards to patient safety are the following:

1. Accident and injury
   (a) Fire
   (b) Electrical equipment
   (c) Worn or defective furnishings and equipment
   (d) Lack of knowledge and judgment on the part of responsible personnel
2. Psychological trauma
3. Cross-infection

Careful analysis of positive measures that will protect the patient against the occurrence of physical or psychological trauma is relevant to the provision of safe nursing care.

Fire

Fire has long been one of the greatest threats to man's survival. Inherent in fire is the potential for triple hazard in the form of burns, trauma, and asphyxiation. The seriousness of the jeopardy related to fire is magnified in hospitals. Vulnerable patients who are helpless or nonambulatory, the multiplicity of patients and personnel, the number and range of combustible and incendiary agents present, and the limited physical space utilized by people and equipment combine to intensify the danger of fire in the hospital. The area of nursing responsibility is relatively simple yet specifically focused in regard to the physical safety of patients. It is the responsibility of the nurse to know and to implement the civic laws related to fire prevention in public buildings and to have complete understanding of measures to be taken in event of fire.

Despite the use of fireproofing methods in building construction, there is still a high incidence of multiple injuries, smoke poisoning, and burns associated with fires in hospitals, nursing homes, child-care institutions, and schools. Perhaps it is well to specify that philosophically, from the standpoint of safety, jeopardy to the life of one person is as serious as jeopardy to the life of many. Therefore, it is imperative that the following aspects of fire prevention be understood:

1. Conscientious enforcement of smoking regulations
2. Maintenance of electrical equipment and devices
3. Safe storage and handling of combustible agents
4. Safe disposal of refuse that ignites readily
5. Installation and maintenance of fireproof doors in halls and on stairwell entrances
6. Inservice education of personnel related to fire prevention, fire control apparatus, and action to be taken in the event of fire

Serious attention to these basic rules is essential.

Among the more common causes of fire are smoking and faulty or defective electrical equipment. Both of these factors are potential dangers in the environment of the patient. The nurse is required to have certain knowledge of measures to be taken in order to minimize the potential danger.

Many jurisdictions have laws restricting smoking in public buildings. It is virtually impossible to enforce such laws in toto in the hospital setting. A maximum degree of compliance with the law is to be expected from personnel since they are able to remove themselves from restricted areas to those areas designated by the fire department as safe for smoking. However, patients who are confined by sickness or injury may encounter personal difficulty in complying with such laws despite the validity of their existence. Consequently, although the nurse as a person directly concerned with the patient's safety must be involved with enforcement of fire prevention laws, she must also be a person aware that modification of regulations

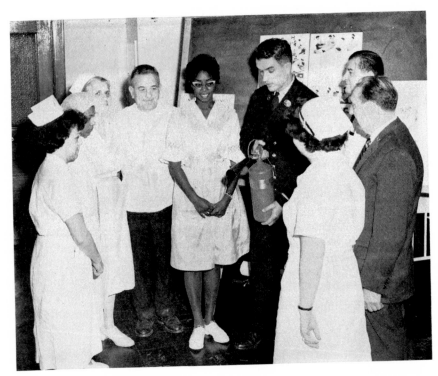

Fig. 16. A fireman teaches nursing personnel how to use a fire extinguisher. (Courtesy the New York Fire Department.)

is permissible under particular circumstances and in certain settings. The following guidelines are fundamental to safety measures related to smoking in the hospital:

1. Personnel should not smoke in the immediate environment of the patient.
2. Specific areas in which personnel may smoke with maximum safety precautions should be provided.
3. Specific areas in which patients not confined to bed may smoke with maximum safety precautions should be provided.
4. Patients confined to bed should be permitted to smoke only when under direct supervision of hospital personnel.
5. "No smoking" regulations should be enforced in toto in all areas in which combustible or combustion-supporting agents are in use.
6. Visitors to the hospital should be permitted to smoke only in designated areas provided for their convenience such as waiting or reception rooms in which maximum safety precautions have been provided.
7. Security officers should be responsible for continuous inspection of all areas in the hospital to minimize and to control the incidence of fire.

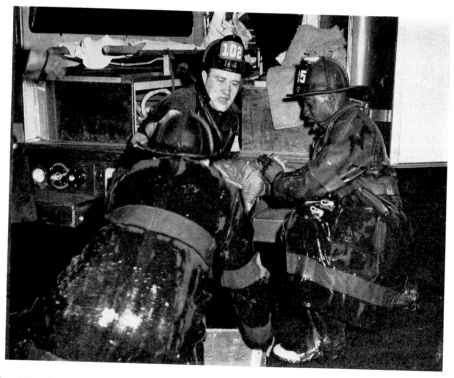

Fig. 17. The tragedy of fire is that it could usually have been prevented. (Courtesy the New York Fire Department.)

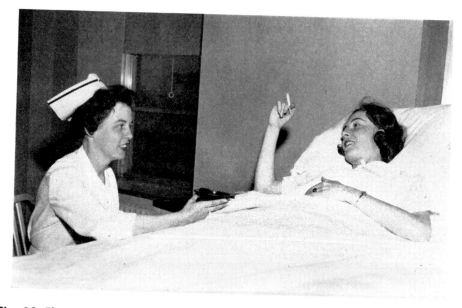

Fig. 18. The patient smoking in bed should be under supervision.

Because it is a high-ranking cause of fire in public buildings, faulty or misused electrical equipment must be considered from the standpoint of what can go wrong and how fire can be prevented. Maintenance of electrical equipment is primarily the responsibility of the hospital administration. However, once again the immediate proximity of the nurse to the patient renders her responsible for functions related to prevention. Generalizations concerning fire prevention involved in using electricity are summarized as follows:

1. Report faulty equipment and defective wiring to responsible authority.
2. Remove faulty equipment from service to avoid its use by persons unaware of the danger.
3. Never temporarily mend or "patch up" electrical equipment. Repairs must be done by competent and knowledgeable personnel and equipment used again only after safety has been ensured.
4. In areas in which combustible or combustion supporting agents are in use, electrical equipment must be handled judiciously with specific knowledge of maximum safety precautions.

In addition to being a major threat as a cause of fire, electricity is also a danger to individual life in the form of electric shock or electrocution. This aspect will be considered in the following discussion.

Electrical equipment

In present-day society, electricity has become as commonplace as running water. In a large number of households, with nothing more laborious than the flip of a switch, we can wash quantities of dishes, do a family laundry, mow a lawn, cook a meal or dust-clean a home with a minimum of effort. The miracle of electricity is even more dramatic when viewed from the standpoint of greater effectiveness in patient care. Aspiration and decompression apparatus, thermal controlling appliances, oscillating beds, cardiac pacemaker monitors, and motor-driven refrigeration units for oxygen therapy are just a few of the modern developments that afford better patient care through the use of electricity. When viewed in terms of patient comfort and security, this modern miracle brings just as great a contribution in terms of signal lights, telephones, and intercommunication systems. Yet, despite the wonder of modern electrical developments, electricity as a force remains an element which requires careful handling. In this respect, the concern of the nurse is with the knowledge and understanding of what constitutes a threat to the patient's safety and to the safety of personnel in the use of electrically-powered equipment and devices in implementing specific aspects of patient care.

A primary law related to the safe handling of electricity bears repetition here—electrically powered equipment and devices must be in sound operating condition. When used in direct contact with the patient's person, such contrivances are capable of transmitting direct electrical shock if wiring or motor parts are exposed. Insulation and coverings on all such equipment must be intact if it is to be safe in use.

A second primary law directing safe handling of electricity relates to its use in the presence of moisture. The science of physics has demonstrated that water is an excellent conductor of electricity. Because of this knowledge, present-day society learned such safety maxims as not to turn a light switch, plug in an appliance, or answer a telephone with wet hands. Over a period of years, police files have recorded innumerable accidental deaths caused by electrocution due to careless handling of electric equipment and devices in the presence of water or some other liquid agent. It is not unusual in severe storms in which electric power lines have been torn down for people to be electrocuted through direct contact with "live wires," water being a direct conductor of the electricity.

Another excellent conductor of electricity is metal. Like moisture, metal acts as a ready pathway for the transmission of electric current. Although this knowledge has been used in a variety of ways to harness power to produce good effects, it also poses a potential threat to safety if misused. A great number of tragedies have resulted in a variety of situations because of this fact. Whether it concerned a curious toddler poking into an electric outlet or an excavation worker (unaware of buried wiring) lustily using a pick, the unfortunate accidents of electrocution serve dramatically to illustrate the danger of metal in contact with electricity.

Therefore, it seems evident that scientific and factual data emphasize to the nurse the need for caution in using electrical devices or equipment directly or indirectly on patients. The ever-present menace of shock and burns demands that if the maintenance and promotion of patient safety is a fundamental concept of nursing care, then specific universal rules must be observed:

1. Equipment, devices, wiring, contact plugs, and outlets must be in sound condition before operation.
2. Only devices specifically designed and safely insulated may be used in the presence of moisture.
3. Metals, except those parts scientifically designed to conduct power from source to desired area, must not come in contact with parts of apparatus or patients.
4. The need to avoid handling electricity with wet hands must be emphasized.
5. The nurse must be aware of her role as a teacher in regard to safety and give specific information regarding these rules to patients and the public.

In summation, scientific, technological achievements have reached a remarkable level of advancement in providing facilities which make possible the more effective implementation of therapeutic measures in hospitals and "better products for better living in the home." However, modern equipment requires modern know-how, and the basic safety rules require unfailing application. Extreme care in regard to this must never be confused with neurotic anxiety. In the use of modern equipment, anxiety about its safe use may be regarded as a healthy emotion.

Worn or defective equipment or furnishings

The next area of potential danger that threatens patient safety is the furniture and equipment used to facilitate nursing care. Adjustable beds, tables, bed rails, carriages, wheelchairs, and pneumatic lifts are likely to result in injury if not in proper operating condition. (It is well to note that personnel using such equipment must have a sound knowledge of how to use it.) Therefore, it is imperative that equipment used for supportive or transportation purposes be checked continually for defective or broken parts. In this instance, as in using electrical devices, "do-it-yourself" repair jobs are taboo. Temporary patching-up of furnishings and equipment is grossly unsafe. Broken and defective articles must be removed from service and referred to the person responsible for repair. Although at times this is difficult for the nurse when pressures exist in a situation and facilities are inadequate, the safety of the patient is of prime concern. Here again, the nurse's position of immediate responsibility requires the ability to act maturely and judiciously in refusing to use unsafe equipment. It requires, also, that the hospital administration assume its responsibility for providing safe and adequate facilities for implementing patient care.

Lack of knowledge and judgment

The next major area defined as a safety hazard in physical trauma is possibly the greatest threat. This is the personnel member himself. "Human error" as an element in accidents has long been scrutinized by scientific investigators from the perspective of physiological and psychological implications. "Job efficiency," "accident-proneness," and "increased productivity" are jargon phrases that are frequently encountered in publications concerned with research studies related to cause, effect, and correction in regard to safer and better living in society. Much of the knowledge gained through such research is invaluable to nursing in the promotion of patient welfare.

The elements essential to efficiency in complex action are knowledge, understanding, and judgment. Anything that impairs these increases the possibility of accident. Examined in the light of the nurse-patient situation, this fact means that there must be specific knowledge of what is safe. Some of this has already been spelled out in the previous discussion of physical safety, but in this discussion it is intended to be interpreted comprehensively to include every aspect of patient care. Through knowledge and understanding, the nurse develops concepts related to physiological status, prophylactics, therapeutic and palliative measures, and psychological disturbances that predispose the patient to physical trauma.

Deviation in homeostasis in the body, whether a cause of or a result of a pathological state, frequently impairs motor, sensory, and intellectual function. A patient thus affected must be protected from injury by positive means. The nurse must be able to assess validly the physical and mental capacity of the patient. The limitations and precautions required to assure safety must be understood. The resulting judgments will direct the nurse in appropriate action.

Judicious use of protective and supportive devices is a perennial nursing responsibility which carries serious personal and legal liability. Bed rails, restraints, body supports, wheelchairs, self-ambulation, and crutch-walking are prime examples of measures and activities to be implemented with knowledgeable understanding of the "level of wellness" of the individual and the resulting responsibility of the nurse.

Psychological disturbance has been definitely identified as a frequent causative factor in accidents through research studies. Because of this fact, the nurse must realize that emotional responses and mood variations, resulting from illness, can jeopardize patient safety. Outside the realm of organic or functional disturbances of the mind, emotional turbulence is equally capable of blocking rational mental processes, disrupting knowledge and understanding and impairing judgment. For this reason, the patient who is beset by fear, anxiety, anger, or depression because of his disease, hospitalization, or prognosis needs positive protection from physical harm. This must be considered not only from the standpoint of self-inflicted injuries or injuries inflicted on other persons, but also in relation to accidents due to errors in judgment. These incidents, commonly labeled as carelessness, actually may be the result of emotional disturbances. The nurse who is fully aware of this fact will ensure maximum safety precautions in all instances. In the light of the foregoing, it is well for the nurse to be aware of herself as a person with the same inclination to psychological disturbance. Realization of inherent danger in undertaking action while under undue emotional stress or pressure will foster the development of the nurse's capacity to assure maximum patient safety. Errors in the administration of medications and treatments of a serious nature are not unusual. Mistakes on the part of hospital personnel frequently cause grave inconvenience and injury to patients. The growing number of legal suits against hospital administrations, doctors, and nurses bear evidence to the growing public resentment of treatment received in some of our health institutions. In light of this situation, it is essential that we become increasingly competent in discharging our responsibilities related to safe practice in the management of patients and the implementation of nursing care.

PSYCHOLOGICAL TRAUMA

Reference was made in the preceding section to emotional response due to disease and hospitalization. The discussion in this section is included as a relatively basic application of a principle of safety. It involves the aspect of interpersonal relationships directed toward prevention or alleviation of trauma that can be inflicted in the psychological sense. Nursing has long been defined as encompassing the care of the total patient, body and mind. In this context, it is believed that any consideration of prevention of accident, injury, or trauma must include specific aspects of the emotional needs of the patient.

It is essential to think of the emotional needs of the patient in the light of specific aspects of nursing care directed toward alleviation or prevention of psychological trauma.

In the patient setting, the impact of human relationships can be a positive or negative force in adjustment. An environment that is harmonious and congenial is much more conducive to emotional stability than one that is fraught with personal conflicts. The patient is literally forced into human relationships he might otherwise never choose. Illness places a patient in a relatively intimate association with patients and hospital personnel whom he cannot actually consider in any sense other than strangers. The nurse who understands and empathizes will make every effort to maintain the individuality of the patient through a pattern of behavior that is acceptable to him. Work relationships among nurses, hospital personnel, and patients must create an aura of mutual interest and support. Authoritarianism and arbitrary behavior militate against feelings of worth and security. Although routines of work are of value in the sense of job accomplishment, they must never be so inflexible that they cannot be adjusted to individual patient feelings.

The nurse must be sensitive to the need to create a "psychological atmosphere" that is acceptable to the patient if the incidence of psychological trauma is to be minimized. Self-understanding will enable the nurse to be a positive force in the total adjustment of the patient to his illness.

PREVENTION OF THE SPREAD OF INFECTION

The final broad area to be considered in the promotion of patient safety is concerned with methods and techniques relative to preventing the spread of infection.

Science has long since postulated the principle that many diseases in society are communicable from person to person. These diseases are transmissible through direct contact with the source of infection. The organisms and microorganisms that may cause a particular disease are present in the secretions and excretions of the system of the body that they infect. Microorganisms that cause infectious diseases of the upper respiratory system are present in the secretions of the nose and throat. Those that cause infectious diseases of the gastrointestinal tract are found in the stool. Those that produce local infections are found in the exudate, or discharge, of the wound. In addition to these specific sources of infection, science has further postulated the continuous existence of infectious agents in the atmosphere. The virus, the many-strained menace to modern man's health, is omnipresent in the air and dust of our total physical environment.

The ability of man to survive in the presence of such threats to his well-being is dependent upon his resistance to the infectious agent or his fastidiousness in using simple measures to avoid direct contact with sources of infection. By nature, man is endowed with a relatively high capacity to resist the more common infections. However, if his "level of wellness" is lowered through neglect of physiological or psychological needs, his susceptibility to disease increases. Furthermore, where the "level of wellness" is already low because of the existence of disease or injury, there is increased proneness to still other infections. The nurse, using knowledge of the nature of the invading organism and the level of the patient's resistance, institutes and utilizes certain measures and techniques that will prevent the transmission of infections or cross-contamination from patient to patient, patient to nurse, or nurse to patient.

The basic practice of handwashing required in any consideration of controlling infection is so universally accepted that it appears elementary in a nursing textbook. However, to exclude exploration of the implications of this technique is incompatible with development of safe nursing practices. It has long been established that infections are commonly carried by contaminated hands. In view of the natural function and use of the hands, it is not difficult to accept this fact. Because of the variety of functions that the nurse performs in giving patient care, it is readily conceivable that nurses' hands are the most constant source of contamination in the patient's environment. In the course of a short space of time, the nurse may be required to provide myriad personal and intimate services to several patients with a variety of actual or potential infections. Envision the nurse involved successively in meeting basic patient needs related to cleanliness, elimination, and nutrition or in meeting individual needs related to physiological responses of vomiting, coughing, expectoration, and bleeding and draining wounds; the potential danger in the hands of the nurse becomes three dimensional.

Thorough handwashing before and after contamination by contact with each patient or with the same patient is fundamental to the prevention of the spread of infection. Effective handwashing requires the use of ordinary soap, running water, and sufficient friction to remove debris from the parts. Agents which inhibit the growth of microorganisms by creating physiologically incompatible flora are used to great advantage in many hospitals. The continuous removal of ordinary dirt and debris from fingernails is an essential ritual in effective handwashing.

Structured directly on this basic understanding of facts related to the transmission of infection through personal contact are particular techniques designed to render equipment used in the course of patient care free from contamination. Specifically, the techniques referred to are disinfection and sterilization. The meaning and methods of implementation of these technics are essential to the nurse's ability to provide a safe environment for the patient.

Before discussing the actual steps involved in disinfection or sterilization, it may be well to clarify certain facts relating to the application of concepts to controlling cross-infection in the actual management of patients. In the hospital setting there have evolved two specific techniques based

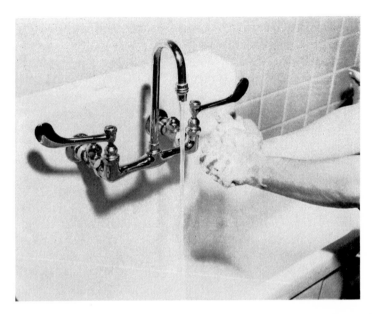

Fig. 19. Soap, friction, and running water used in sufficient quantities are basic elements in medical asepsis.

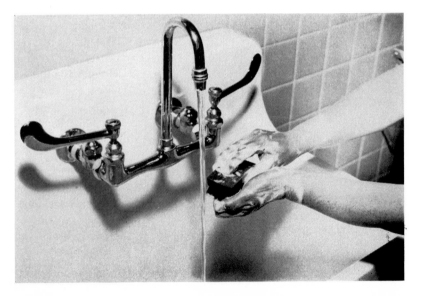

Fig. 20. In addition to handwashing, the use of a nail brush protects both patients and personnel.

on diagnostic categories. For this reason, there exists the concept of two configurations of technical patterns designed to ensure patient safety against cross-infection. One configuration is termed medical asepsis, and the second is termed surgical asepsis. Realistically, there is a marked degree of overlapping in the use of the two techniques. In order to clarify functional operation in fundamental nursing, it is well to consider each of these as they are implemented in the clinical setting.

Medical asepsis

This term generally is used to denote the precautions taken to prevent the transmission of infection, whether actual or potential, in all patients. Specific techniques employed include handwashing, disinfection, and sterilization as well as the use of gloves, masks, and gowns. The means used may be as simple as handwashing between patient contacts or as complex as the combination of many techniques in caring for a patient with poliomyelitis. The principle of operational function is focused on the patient as a source of infection, and precaution is directed toward avoiding carrying disease from patient to patient or from patient to personnel. In essence, this theory labels the patient "contaminated" and the operator "clean," or free from contamination. Although equally careful consideration is given to protect the patient from cross-infection, the major emphasis is placed on the concept of the patient as a focus of infection.

Surgical asepsis

This term is commonly used to indicate the techniques used to protect the patient against infection or contamination. It consists of a variety of methods and procedures designed to safeguard the patient in specific situations. It can run the gamut from the complex, technical ritual that is essential during surgical intervention in the operating room to the use of sterile dressings on simple wounds to the use of sterile syringes and needles when injecting medication parenterally or through the surface of the body.

Scientifically sterile techniques are employed in the recognition of the biological principle that identifies the skin as the first line of defense against microbial invasion. Therefore, in handling any wound that is essentially defined as a break in the continuity of tissue, the use of sterile equipment is mandatory. Similarly, if the surface of the body is disrupted, whether by direct incision or the insertion of a needle, the use of maximum sterile precautions is obligatory.

Another fact that is basic to understanding surgical aseptic techniques relates to the need to recognize the hands of the operator as a potential source of infection. Although broad consideration has already been given to this subject in this chapter, specific reference is made here to the unique implications when sterile procedures are involved. When the potential of danger is great, the hands of the operator are scrubbed with detergent soap in a prescribed manner and sterile gloves are worn. Modification of this technique is acceptable in situations in which the severity of danger is reduced. Thus, when a procedure such as an operative incision or catheterization (which is the insertion of a tube or catheter into the urinary bladder through the natural orifice or meatus) is to be done, careful hand-scrubbing and rubber gloves are indicated. However, it is believed to be safe to eliminate gloves when doing simple dressings or giving injections, because in the procedures, sterile instruments are used to handle dressings and syringes, and apparatus attached directly to needles are held at a point of maximum distance from the needle itself, which is the part inserted into the body. Another application of this principle is seen in the procedure of skin disinfection prior to incision, injection, or insertion to prevent carrying contamination from the external surface to the internal tissues of the body.

In contrast to the rationale of medical asepsis, this theory operates on the premise that the patient is "sterile" (literally, "clean"), and the operator is "unsterile" (literally, "contaminated"). In this framework, although equal consideration is given to protection of the operator in handling potentially or actually infectious conditions, major emphasis is focused on preserving the integrity of the patient in a "microbially free environment."

Methods of disinfection

Literally, disinfection is the process of destroying pathogenic organisms. According to present-day concepts of microbiologists, it is possible to achieve this in a variety of ways. Contaminated articles or equipment can be rendered clean or free from disease-producing microorganisms by using any of the following methods:

1. Physical means
   (a) Rinse, wash in hot soap and water solution, and then rinse thoroughly under running water.
   (b) Expose to sunlight and fresh air for a six-hour to eight-hour period.
2. Chemical means
   (a) Rinse, wash, rinse, immerse in a disinfecting solution, and then rinse and dry.

Applying these broad rules to the patient situation, the nurse is able to function effectively in handling contaminated equipment. Operating on the premise that any and all equipment used in the course of total patient care is contaminated, the nurse learns to use her knowledge of potential infection in a constructive way. Thus, dishes, bedpans, bath equipment, and the like must be rinsed and washed with hot water and detergent, rinsed under running water, and dried before being used again. The use of friction and a detergent agent that will loosen substances (secretions, excretions, food, dust, etc.) that may harbor organisms is basic to effective disinfection.

In addition to this universally fundamental method of controlling cross-infection, the use of various chemical agents is indicated for disinfection of equipment that has been contaminated by specific substances. Thermometer and rectal tubes are prime examples of equipment so contaminated. In order to increase the margin of safety, it is common practice in hospitals, in addition to washing, to immerse such articles in an appropriate solution for the prescribed period of time before reusing them.

The subject of chemical disinfection has long been a controversial one among scientists and medical practitioners. Continuous research and experimentation have uncovered new knowledge that resulted in the revision of many procedures and techniques employed in handling contaminated equipment. Scientific investigation of this nature will always be an ongoing process, and the conclusions reached will change the methods selected to prevent cross-infection. Although clinical agencies vary in the selection of specific disinfectants for specific uses, the scientific principles underlying their selection are constant. It is this knowledge that is of prime importance to the nurse. The following facts are critical in the selection and effective use of any disinfecting agent:

1. The agent must have been demonstrated as being effective against the specific microorganisms.
2. The agent must be used in the percentage strength that has been demonstrated to be effective in destruction of the pathogenic microorganisms.
3. The equipment to be disinfected must be washed clean of contaminated substances, rinsed, and dried before being placed in the solution.
4. The equipment must be totally submerged in the solution and remain for the period of time demonstrated as effective against pathogenic microorganisms.
5. After removal from solution, the equipment should be rinsed under running water and dried before storage.

In reference to the last two directives, it should be understood that unless an article is completely covered by the solution, it will not be efficiently disinfected. In addition to this, the corrosive and disintegrating effect of some chemicals on certain materials should be noted. Finally, the danger to the patient's safety through absorption or ingestion of chemicals that are residual on equipment introduced into any orifices of the body must be scrupulously avoided. Specific information related to types of chemical agents commonly used for disinfection can be found in the Appendix. Such factual knowledge is basic to safe operational function related to preventing spread of infection.

The use of sunlight and fresh air as physical means of disinfection has certain value in specific circumstances. By and large, however, it is not widely relied upon in modern hospital settings, in which newer and surer methods are available for controlling cross-infection. The principle underlying the effectiveness of sunlight and fresh air is significant in the total patient environment in relation to adequate ventilation. Furthermore, it still may be employed in rendering safe for reuse valuable articles that would be ruined by washing or chemical disinfection. This has real meaning in the home, or in health agencies in which alternates are not available. Thus, pillows, mattresses, blankets, and such fomites that are not washable may be considered free from pathogenic microorganisms if treated in this way.

At the present time, however, the need to resort to any of these methods of disinfection has been curtailed in many hospital settings. The industrial advances which have resulted in a whole new world of plastics and paper products have enlarged the margin of patient safety and have facilitated the operational factors in preventing the spread of infection. The increasingly widespread use of disposable equipment utilized in many aspects of patient care is of tremendous advantage. Primarily, the advantage is centered in increased personal protection for the patient. However, the factor involving the reduction of time spent by nursing personnel in disinfection of contaminated equipment affords more time for direct patient care. There is still a further advantage in reduction of cost to the patient, for disposable materials are less expensive in the final analysis than permanent materials when viewed from the aspects of loss, breakage, and deterioration. For these reasons, many articles used in administering specific treatments to patients are directly disposable. Prime examples of these are demonstrated by various tubes and tubing used in irrigating or draining body cavities; containers, syringes, and needles employed in introducing medication or solutions into the body; and paper cups and medicine glasses used to provide fluid, nutrition, or oral medication. Particular description of equipment is found in other chapters dealing with implementation of treatments in handling specific nursing problems and in the Appendix.

Sterilization

By definition, the term "sterilization" means the destruction of all microorganisms. Just as in the process of disinfection, there are several ways in which sterilization can be carried out. It is essential to know the methods employed and the use of those methods in specific situations.

Basically, sterilization processes can be categorized as follows:
1. Physical means
    (a) Boiling
    (b) Autoclaving
    (c) Baking
2. Chemical means
    (a) Immersion in a solution of a designated percentage strength for a prescribed period of time

The selection of method is again directed essentially by the facilities available in any given situation. Prerequisite for any method selected is the preparation of the equipment to be sterilized. Primarily, it must be free of all contaminants, and this requires washing, rinsing, and drying as a fundamental procedure when dealing with articles such as glassware, metal containers, instruments, and the like. Secondarily, consideration must be given to the specific purpose of the equipment. If the need of the situation requires that materials be sterile, then provision must be made for coverage or external protection that will maintain sterility. There are several routines used in achieving this, and again, methods vary in each setting. The critical point centers in the security of sterility, so that packages and containers must be airtight and stored in a dry area.

In reference to the specific method that is selected, particular aspects that become critical relate to degree of intensity of the agent and the duration and totality of the exposure of the articles being sterilized. From this evolves the following general operational rules for sterilization:

1. Boiling
   (a) Water must be actively boiling.
   (b) Equipment must be completely covered or submerged in water.
   (c) Equipment must remain in the actively boiling water for the period of time required.
2. Autoclaving
   (a) Steam pressure must be of the degree required.
   (b) Articles being sterilized at the same time must be made of identical materials (metal, glass, rubber, etc.).
   (c) Articles must remain under constant pressure for the period of time required.
3. Chemical agents
   (a) Agents must be specific percentage strength required.
   (b) Articles must be completely submerged in solution.
   (c) Articles must remain in the solution for the period of time required.

An outline designed to provide fundamental knowledge of a procedural approach to the problem is included in the Appendix.

Numerous modifications and adaptations of many basic techniques have been adopted in the clinical setting. As has been stated previously, the development of commercially prepared, especially disposable, equipment has been a tremendous asset in providing safe and efficient health service. Commercially prepared sterile equipment is equally valuable in widening the margin of safety as well as reducing the time spent by nursing or auxiliary personnel in cleaning and packaging articles for sterilization. The advantage, here again, is in an increase in available time to give direct patient care.

In summarizing, the successful protection of patients and personnel from cross-infection rests upon the conscientious use of knowledge of sources of infection and the effective and appropriate methods of control.

BIBLIOGRAPHY

1. Foster, Marion: A positive approach to medical asepsis, American Journal of Nursing **62**:76-77, April 1962.
2. Fuerst, Elinor V., and Wolff, La Verne: Fundamentals of Nursing, ed. 2, Philadelphia, 1959, J. B. Lippincott Co., pp. 53-98.
3. Harmer, Bertha, and Henderson, Virginia: Textbook of principles and practice of Nursing, ed. 5, New York, 1955, The Macmillan Co., pp. 125-152, 183-226.
4. Hershey, Nathan: Restrictions and safety, American Journal of Nursing **63**:124-125, June 1963.

5. Knocke, Lazelle: Crutch walking, American Journal of Nursing **61**:70-73, Oct. 1961.
6. Kummer, Sylvia B., and Kammer, Jerome M.: Pointers to preventing accidents, American Journal of Nursing **63**:118-119, Feb. 1963.
7. Lewis, Edith P.: Fire on the ninth floor, American Journal of Nursing **62**:50-55, Feb. 1962.
8. McClain, M. Esther, and Gragg, Shirley H.: Scientific principles in nursing, ed. 4, St. Louis, 1962, The C. V. Mosby Co., pp. 47-56.
9. Madden, Barbara Williams, and Affeldt, John E.: To prevent helplessness and deformity, American Journal of Nursing **62**:59-61, Dec. 1962.
10. Nordmark, Madelyn T., and Rohweder, Anne W.: Scientific principles applied to nursing, Philadelphia, 1959, J. B. Lippincott Co., pp. 199-206.
11. Thompson, La Verne R.: Evaluating disinfectants, American Journal of Nursing **62**:82-83, Jan. 1962.
12. Thompson, La Verne R.: Thermometer disinfection, American Journal of Nursing **63**:113-115, Feb. 1963.
13. Wilson, William J.: Heat injury, American Journal of Nursing **60**:1124-1125, Aug. 1960.

Chapter 12

Hygiene and comfort

The varied adaptations involved in the process of helping patients cope with problems encountered in meeting basic comfort needs, an understanding of what constitutes hygiene and comfort, and a correlation of this knowledge with the factors that complicate the maintenance of hygiene and comfort are areas of nursing care that are scientific and universal regardless of the patient's diagnosis. This particular aspect of nursing care is considered in this chapter, and it involves at least a beginning understanding of what constitutes the identification of the science and art of nursing. Actually this "comforting" aspect is a great part of what constitutes nursing.

CONCEPT OF HOMEOSTASIS

According to Webster, hygiene is defined as "a science of the establishment and maintenance of health."[*] It is well to recall that science is a word adapted from the Latin *scio*, meaning "to know"; therefore, science implies knowledge. Knowledge in the scientific sense indicates fact as it is perceived in the light of investigation that is planned, methodical, objective, complete, and conclusive. Thus, hygiene is concerned with the application of knowledge in the institution of practices designed to maintain and promote optimal health. Such practices are intended to support man's state of equilibrium in relation to his total environment and include both physical and mental aspects. Like many major factors in life, personal health is relative.

"Levels of wellness" as defined in the literature is a variable influenced by personal and social values, education, attitudes, and habits as much as it is altered by physiological changes. In the person "apparently free from disease," the level of health may fluctuate from day to day according to practices related to personal cleanliness, nutrition, exercise, rest, sleep, elimination, recreation, occupation, and emotional adjustment. These are the critical elements that science has identified as basic determinants in the

---

[*]By permission. From Webster's Seventh New Collegiate Dictionary, copyright 1963 by G. & C. Merriam Co., Publishers of the Merriam-Webster Dictionaries.

maintenance of homeostasis. In the well person, understanding of knowledge concerned with supplying these needs in proportion to the individual physical and mental demands is important not only in preventing disease but also in the achievement of the optimal level of health. In states of physiological stress, factors such as personal cleanliness, nutrition, exercise and rest, sleep, and elimination assume increased significance. Limitations imposed on patients by disease or injury frequently complicate the ability to ensure good hygiene and physical comfort.

HYGIENE AND COMFORT

As a nation, we attach a high degree of cultural value to comfort in all aspects of daily living, whether at work, at play, or at home. The ingenuity of scientific investigation on all levels and in every area of business and industry has resulted in an almost inexhaustible array of comfort-producing paraphernalia and settings. In this explosion of facilities, however, major emphasis has been focused on consumer conveniences to promote business. To understand the implications of comfort in relation to health, it is well to analyze certain concepts implied in its meaning.

Contrary to the popular "physical" frame of reference, the word "comfort" is defined in the dictionary as relating primarily to the provision of strength in alleviating mental or emotional distress. Because the physical and mental components of man are indissoluble in the life process, whatever affects one inevitably affects the other. Understanding of their functional interrelatedness, the factors that affect their integrity, and measures designed to alleviate discomfort are inherent in nursing. The classical concept of *"Mens sana in corpore sano"* has genuine significance in the concept of hygiene and health.

Causes of discomfort

During the course of illness and hospitalization, patients are subjected to situations and circumstances that cause discomfort. In fact, the incidence of disease and the necessity for hospital admission are the wellsprings of physiological and psychological distress. Fear, anxiety, and depression as responses to physical illness are as real a source of discomfort as the myriad patterns of pain that are the body's responses to pathological processes. In a similar vein, authoritarian, punitive, and insensitive nursing personnel are as much a source of discomfort as are neglect of personal hygiene, incompetent physical manipulation, or lack of adequate provision for individual problems related to nutrition and elimination. Comfort is literally endemic in every facet of patient care. For this reason, detailed discussion of its many aspects will be carried like a common thread into each area included in total hygiene.

In order to provide adequately for individual hygienic and comfort needs of patients, specific knowledge of scientific principles underlying methods and procedures must be applied. It is not sufficient that the nurse "knows how"; she must also "understand why."

Scientific principles related to hygiene and comfort

Personal hygiene. Bathing and care of the hair and nails are matters that become routines at a relatively early age in the American cultural pattern. Actually, the daily bath plus deodorant, the weekly shampoo, and the usual routine of fingernail and toenail care are habitual in our society. Although in many instances the operational basis of body care is related to social acceptance and approval, there is nevertheless a marked degree of national understanding of the scientific bases for such physical hygiene. The nurse must understand this if the needs of the knowledgeable patient and the needs of the unknowledgeable patient are to be met. The patient who knows requires assistance in maintaining personal hygiene. The patient who does not know requires assistance in promotion of personal hygiene. The nurse must understand the scientific bases on which the specific aspects of personal hygiene are structured in order to provide nursing care for all.

Physiological basis. The mechanical operation of friction employed in washing, rinsing, and drying the body surface stimulates peripheral circulation and so induces nutrition to the parts. This contributes to ensuring the integrity of skin and subcutaneous tissues and is of particular significance when body motion is impaired by physical limitations. Simple massage of areas that bear body weight also increases blood supply to parts, relieves local hemostasis, and aids relaxation of voluntary muscles. In massaging the body, the use of a pharmaceutical agent that is emollient-astringent serves to help maintain normal skin turgor. Of no less importance is the application of particular physiological knowledge to hygienic care of the body appendages. Removal of dead cells and debris from toenails and fingernails, as well as clipping and filing to ensure normal contour that prevents edges from becoming imbedded in tissues, enhances circulation and avoids infections due to impairment of cell nutrition. Brushing the teeth and massaging the gums promote local nutrition through increased blood supply.

Microbiological basis. There are two clear-cut aspects of nursing intervention related to total physical hygiene that are based on scientific principles concerning microorganisms as one cause of pathological processes. Because many types of pathogenic organisms are omnipresent in the environment and find favorable conditions for growth in certain media, measures that militate against their growth must be instituted if health is to be promoted. Washing secretions, excretions, and debris from body surfaces removes sources of infection. This is critical in care of the hands, face and external genitalia. It is critical in the care of hands because of their use in eating and drinking and in cleaning skin surfaces after elimination and because of the common habit of touching the face with the hands. It is critical in care of the face, because the nose and mouth are major "portals of entry" for disease-producing organisms. It is critical in care of the external genitalia because of the incipient danger of contamination from fecal material. Normally, stool contains organisms that are not harmful in the intestinal tract but become a threat in other systems of the body.

Still another aspect of care that applies the same principle relates to oral hygiene. Oral hygiene requires consideration of three areas of need: optimal nutrition, routine cleansing, and adequate professional dental care. Nursing must include provision for health teaching as it is indicated in each situation, as well as instituting mouth care directly. Brushing teeth and washing and rinsing the oral cavity removes food particles and mucus that provide favorable media for and harbor disease-producing organisms. Oral hygiene thus promotes total hygiene.

Psychological basis. In addition to the national cultural value referred to in the opening of this discussion, it is essential that the nurse be aware of the personal value that individuals attach to personal cleanliness. Patients as individuals may have either positive or negative feelings about body care. Understanding and acceptance of patients' attitudes will enable the nurse to meet patient needs and still maintain and promote good hygiene.

The foundation of positive attitudes is commonly centered in a "feeling of well-being" that is not entirely without physiological basis but that is most commonly associated mentally with "being at one's best." It would seem to have some root in the natural law of self-preservation. Nursing care designed to satisfy this need has a certain psychological basis. Negative attitudes are frequently associated with ignorance, poor habit training, or personality disorders. Not uncommonly, there are feelings of physical or mental discomfort or a rejection of society attached to responses of this type. However, identification of the problem and utilization of personal resources to ameliorate it without violating the individual's right to have and express feelings is an integral part of the nursing care plan.

Sociological basis. From what has already been said regarding the high degree of value that present-day society attaches to cleanliness as a primary adjunct to health as well as a goal of personal worth, it would seem evident that measures concerned with supporting the cause of physical hygiene have sociological implications. Of equal significance in the approach to understanding the patient's nursing problem is an awareness of the relatedness of good hygienic practices to total community health. A healthy community is a successful community intent on the full and happy life with all of resultant sociological implications.

NURSING INTERVENTION

In providing direct nursing care to meet physical hygiene needs of patients, certain generalizations must be used as guidelines to secure patient safety. The generalizations deal with time and method and are drawn from the basic sciences just discussed.

In accord with common social practices, patients are usually given a complete bath daily. Other than this, additional provision is made for partial bathing, i.e., for washing the face, neck, arms, hands, and back at least once. Current hospital routines provide for a complete bath in the morning and other physical care in the afternoon and/or evening. Mouth care is generally provided three times daily, most commonly in conjunction with the washing procedure. Brushing and/or combing hair are managed in the same fashion. Fingernails and toenails are generally cleaned at bath time and filed or trimmed whenever necessary. Such routines are adapted to general staffing patterns and should, in particular instances of patients' preferences or settings, be adjusted.

In the use of the term "method," it is not so much a matter of equipment or inflexible steps in routines but rather a reference to the combination of manual facility and patient safety and comfort. Within this framework, awareness of three factors is fundamental: (1) sensitivity to the effect of touch and stroke motion in the physical process of washing, massaging, and drying patients, (2) understanding of the scientific and esthetic aspects of the sequence of washing body parts, changing wash water, and keeping patients adequately covered during the bathing procedure, and (3) knowledge of measures to ensure effective and safe care of the oral cavity and the appendages.

As in all nursing procedures, modifications and adaptations are dictated by specific patients' needs or problems. From these facts evolve the following nursing generalizations or principles governing the "when," "what," and "how" of providing this aspect of patient care:

1. In so far as it is possible, all plans should be adapted to individual patient's preferences.
2. Acutely ill patients should be given this care at a time when physical capacity is optimal.
3. Acutely ill patients should receive minimal physical care in order to conserve energy needed for reparative processes.
4. Care should be organized to avoid physical and/or emotional distress in all patients.
5. Routine daily bathing of elderly (geriatric) patients should be avoided since the natural skin lubrication is reduced.
6. All patients who have increased secretions and uncontrolled excretions should be washed as often as necessary to maintain a total hygienic environment.
7. Emollient agents should be applied to skin areas regularly to counteract the effect of soap and water and degenerative processes resulting from disease and/or age.
8. Patients with long-term illnesses should be bathed totally and partially at regular intervals to counteract the deforming aspects of physical limitation and inactivity.
9. All patients should have their hair brushed and combed at regular intervals. Attention to styling is of significance in women.
10. Patients who have specific problems related to the hair and/or scalp should receive prescribed medical treatment.
11. Men patients should be afforded services and/or facilities for shaving.

12. All patients should receive mouth care at least three times daily, preferably after meals.
13. Patients who are acutely ill should receive special mouth care every two to three hours in accord with their need.
14. All patients should receive care related to fingernails and toenails daily at bath time.
15. Patients who have specific health problems involving the feet and toenails, i.e., calluses, corns, ingrown toe nails, and excessive dryness should receive special care involving soaking, cuticle care, lubrication, and square trimming. The toenails of patients who have diabetes mellitus should be managed under direct medical supervision.

Nursing care relative to securing patient comfort in the process of providing for cleanliness and freedom from physical and mental disturbances requires understanding of causative factors and knowledge of measures to alleviate or at least minimize their impact on the individual patient. The nurse must understand the psychosocial implications of the "invasion of privacy" when a person is forced to submit to being bathed by a stranger because he is unable to provide for this need. The nurse must understand the physical distress that results from disease and disability when physiological debilitation or anatomical impairment limits natural body activity. The nurse must understand that a physical being subjected to the destructive forces of any illness requiring confinement suffers a relatively sharply defined pattern of aches and pains associated with physiological dysfunction.

Nursing generalizations governing the "how" of protecting patients' comfort in this regard may be summarized as follows:

1. All patients must be positioned (in bed or in chair) so that dependent body parts are supported to avoid muscle strain.
2. All patients must be anatomically positioned so that all major movable body portions are in natural alignment to avoid muscle strain.
3. All patients' positions should be changed at regular intervals regardless of their health problems. Modification of this principle is essential in gross physical limitation, but it still must be provided for within a set range of motion.
4. Supportive devices such as pillows, pads, rings, and footboards should be employed specifically to maintain posture or to relieve pressure due to position or weight of bedclothes.
5. Mechanically adjustable beds should be raised and lowered, both head and foot, at regular intervals to support normal anatomical motion.
6. In accord with individual limitations, bathing, massaging (back care), change of clothes, and change of bed linen should be provided with regularity.
7. Provision of an environment that is physically and psychologically acceptable is essential to all patients. Temperature, ventilation, and serenity are key words in nursing responsibility in this regard. Spe-

cific acts in implementation of such are centered in the needs of the individual patient.

The nursing practices involved in meeting the needs of patients related to basic hygiene and comfort are much more complex than could possibly be summarized in a textbook. They are completely and critically individual, and on the understanding of this fact rests the foundation of what constitutes good nursing practice. Better patient care is dependent upon the application of scientific knowledge to specific patient problems; however, the effectiveness of such care is ultimately dependent on the patient's response to the care. When this is limited by nature, the results are frequently irreversible. In the area of "maintaining hygiene and comfort," the results are directly affected by the understanding and facility of nursing intervention.

BIBLIOGRAPHY

1. Fuerst, Elinor V., and Wolff, La Verne: Fundamentals of nursing, ed. 2, Philadelphia, 1959, J. B. Lippincott Co., pp. 215-227.
2. Harmer, Bertha, and Henderson, Virginia: Textbook of principles and practice of nursing, ed. 5, New York, 1955, The Macmillan Co., pp. 322-362.
3. Johnson, Dorothy E.: The significance of nursing care, American Journal of Nursing **61:**63-66, Nov. 1961.
4. McClain, M. Esther, and Gragg, Shirley H.: Scientific principles in nursing, ed. 4, St. Louis, 1962, The C. V. Mosby Co., pp. 119-159.
5. Nordmark, Madelyn T., and Rohweder, Anne W.: Scientific principles applied to nursing, Philadelphia, 1959, J. B. Lippincott Co., pp. 155-164, 171-180, 241-267.
6. Tassman, Gustav C., Zayon, Gilbert M., and Zafran, Jack N.: When patients cannot brush their teeth, American Journal of Nursing **63:**76, Feb. 1963.

Chapter 13

Posture, activity, and rest

Freedom from disease or injury alone is not sufficient to ensure an optimal "level of wellness." Adequate physiological function is directly affected by body posture, activity, and rest. As a functioning organism, the human body is maintained by two natural operations: innumerable mechanical motions that trigger muscular and circulatory responses essential to its efficiency and regular period of relative cessation necessary to restoration of power or energy. In this respect, as in many others, it is analogous to a machine that requires use to preserve function, but that must not be overused because parts will become worn rapidly. In the routine of daily living, actions involved in standing, sitting, walking, eating, washing, and the like maintain body mechanics and support physiological function on a minimal level.

All actions are totally dependent on the integrity of movable body parts. A person cannot stand unless knee joints and hip joints can be altered from a position of flexion or angulation to one of extension or straight line. Conversely, a person cannot sit unless the motions can be reversed. Walking is dependent upon ankle, toe, and knee joint function, and eating is dependent upon digital, wrist, elbow, and shoulder joint function, as is combing hair, brushing teeth, and blowing the nose. The almost prosaic business of taking a bath puts into action literally every movable part of the body. There are many other activities regularly engaged in that improve the level of function. The usual routines and chores of the homemaker and homeowner serve to supply a relatively fair amount of the kind of activity the body needs. Through various stages of growth in life the activity need tends to diminish. Although high in the early years of life, activity should lessen after a person reaches full physical maturity. In many instances, the amount of physical activity in which people can engage is fully a matter of personality makeup and habit patterns. However, there is an actual scientific basis for the natural "slowing down" in physical activity associated with middle years and later life. In the relative state of health, then, there exists throughout life a rather consistent picture of the body's need for varying amounts of activity and rest. Regardless of how widely the need varies, it never ceases to exist.

Regular periods of relative cessation from activity are procured by the body through normal rest and sleep. The term "relative" is employed here deliberately, because total physiological action never ceases. The skeletal and muscular systems of the body are capable of complete mechanical inactivity for short periods of time when the body is at rest. Physiological activity, however, while sharply reduced, never actually stops for any period. When and if it does, the result will depend on the vitality of the deficient activity. A nonfunctioning colon constitutes a serious health problem, but a nonfunctioning heart or nonfunctioning lungs constitute death. Although such facts are obviously elementary, understanding of them is fundamental for anyone concerned with health preservation or restoration. When a person is at rest, sitting in a chair, or lying in bed, cell metabolism is decreased and energy requirements are minimal. When a person sleeps, the reduction in these areas is even greater, because more energy is utilized during conscious activity. Although patterns of physical and mental activity during sleep are peculiar to individuals, there is universal acceptance of the fact that the levels of both kinds of activity are less during sleep than when awake. As has been stated in regard to activity, although the need for rest and sleep varies in individual life patterns and life stages, both are essential to health and life.

WHAT CAN GO WRONG

Patients' needs for maintenance of normal posture, activity, and rest are directly thwarted by disease and by injury, with associated physical limitations as well as the necessity for hospitalization. Pathological processes that are debilitating may render a patient incapable of even the most simple kind of self-directed or self-initiated physical or mental action.

A patient who is febrile, toxic, or dehydrated lacks the strength to bathe, eat, drink, turn in bed, or even make the decision that he would like to do so. Other health problems are of a nature that require a patient to refrain from ordinary activities of which he may feel capable in order to conserve energy in vital organs. A patient who has coronary heart disease is forced to remain at rest in bed and frequently to refrain from the routine procedures of bathing, eating, and the like in order to reduce the work load on the nutritionally deprived heart.

Primary diseases of any part of the central nervous system may cut off the innervating current to motor activity at its source. Paralysis renders a patient unable to move a part or all of his body. Depending upon the extent of nerve impairment, the patient is limited in motion. Traumatic conditions produce the same effect, even though in a different way. A patient with a fractured pelvis, femur, tibia and fibula, or radius and ulna is equally as limited in range of normal activities as the patient who is hemiplegic as a result of a cerebrovascular accident. Activity and motion are commonly further limited in a variety of health problems when pain is a constant factor or occurs when a part is used.

The physical and psychological trauma of hospitalization has been discussed previously but bears repetition. The ritualistic, compulsively "unfeeling," and totally unnecessary pattern of routine in the majority of hospitals places patients in a physical and psychological environment that is incompatible with any concept of rest or sleep except under chemical hypnosis or narcosis. Pain, positional and other physical discomforts, anxiety, environmental noise, and routines geared to personnel needs but ill-timed in relation to patients' needs make no contribution to the cause of rest and sleep. Although it is readily conceded that there are many situations in which vital treatment must take precedence in order of need, it must in honesty be admitted that patients' rights in regard to rest and sleep are often violated without justification by thoughtless personnel on all levels.

NURSING INTERVENTION

If the needs of patients for activity and rest are to be maintained, nursing care must be planned and implemented within the following six major areas of function:

1. Astute and critical observation of positional and motional limitations or deviations
2. Retention of normal body alignment
3. Provision of optimal hygienic activities fundamental to homeostasis
4. Consistent and regular alteration of posture as an adjunct to minimal activity and prevention of complications
5. Regular institution of active and/or passive exercises to include full range of joint motion to prevent ankylosis
6. Provision of optimal physical and psychological comfort as a prerequisite to rest and conducive to sleep

Occurring directly or indirectly as a result of a patient's health problem, limitations and deviations in position or motion are highly meaningful in terms of prognosis and rehabilitation. The fact that a patient who yesterday was unable to grasp a spoon but today can clasp your hand is a significant one. Similarly, the fact that a patient who yesterday had a cast applied to a lower extremity but today cannot move the toes is equally significant. Such examples of critical change, although somewhat dramatic, give direct indication to medical action in regard to therapy. Positional and motional limitations are sometimes obscured deliberately by patients in order to reduce or to prevent pain. The mechanism of "self-splinting" painful parts requires astute and continuous observation in order to detect and to prevent deformities that will permanently militate against normal activity.

Retention of normal body alignment is basic to rehabilitation when a patient is denied normal body motion to any extent. Patients who have long-term or chronic illnesses producing physical and physiological restrictions require positive nursing measures to maintain body alignment and to prevent or to correct deformities. Drop foot, wristdrop, and drop shoulder can result in permanent loss of function when major nerves die as a result of nutritional (circulatory) deprivation. Such tragedy is readily preventable by the strategic use of supportive measures and devices to sustain normal body alignment during a period of physiological stress. The rudimentary principles of competent preventive nursing care in this problem are summarized as follows:

1. Maintain normal posture of all body parts in any position or motion whether lying, sitting, walking, i.e., normal articulation of parts in any position.
2. Use specific methods and devices to correct bizarre positions or to support inert or weak body parts, i.e., footboards to prevent or to correct drop foot, pillows to maintain body posture or extremity alignment, and continuous evaluation of the efficiency of corrective devices such as traction and casts.
3. Apply supportive materials such as bandages, binders, and cravats so that they are functionally efficient, i.e., achieve purpose but do not impair circulation or unnecessarily limit motion.

The usual nursing routines of ordinary body hygiene provide a good margin of minimal physical activity for patients who are confined. In many instances, the procedures of bathing, massaging the back, giving oral hygiene, and lifting the patient on and off a bedpan provide activity basic to maintenance of any function for the totally helpless patient. Unfortunately, in most hospital settings, routine aspects of physical care are implemented on a time schedule, a method that results in long periods of time when patients have literally no activity. Regular administration of morning, afternoon, and evening care to provide basic hygiene must be supplemented by additional nursing measures when body mechanics are impaired.

Prolonged retention of any body posture interferes with circulation and is a direct cause of functional loss. When a patient cannot alter his position of his own volition, the nursing care must provide for regular and frequent alteration of posture as an adjunct to minimal activity. The physically dependent patient should be turned at least every hour from one side to the back to the other side in a regular rotation sequence. Whenever the patient's physical condition permits, without danger or gross discomfort, the rotation should include the prone position or lying on the abdomen. Each time the patient is repositioned, normal alignment and support of the body must be assured.

Besides constituting a threat to functional efficiency of movable body parts, prolonged retention of any position is a direct cause of decubitus ulcers or pressure sores. Undue pressure on any skin surface or area shuts off blood supply to the part. When this state persists for a period of time, the tissue cells become devitalized from lack of nutrition, and there is a dissolution of tissue. Regeneration of cells will take place if nutrition is provided by reestablishment of circulation. If it is not restored, the tissue cells become necrotic or die. Necrosis is the term used to describe death of tissue in a localized area. When the tissue death is massive, over a large area and involving deep-lying tissues, the condition is termed gangrene. There are several physical factors that predispose patients to decubitus ulcers. Nurses must be aware of the inherent danger when any of these conditions are present:

1. Immobilization due to any cause
2. Inability to contain excreta
3. Physical weakness, malaise, or debilitation associated with disease or senescence
4. Mental apathy or depression associated with disease or senescence
5. Senile regression (infantile dependency)
6. Physical malnutrition or cachexia
7. Obesity

Preventive aspects of nursing care are critical in any and all of these circumstances.

Certain areas of the body have a predilection for breakdown because circulation is limited or because body weight is greater as the center of gravity shifts with positional changes. This poses no problem in health, because normal activity involves continuously alternating rotation of rest and exercise of all body parts. When activity is limited, vulnerable areas include all

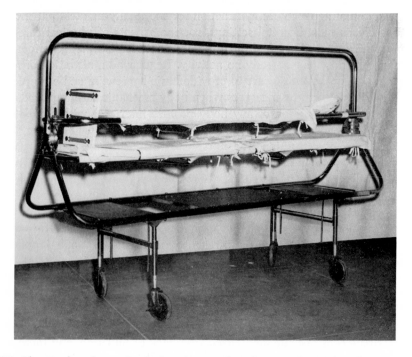

Fig. 21. The Stryker frame is designed to make change of position from supine to prone possible and easy for patients with limitation of motion, such as fractures or paralysis.

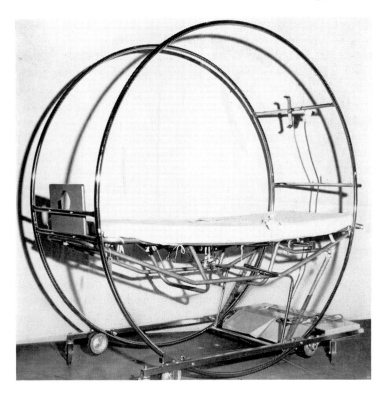

Fig. 22. The "circular" bed performs the same basic function as the Stryker frame. It can be manipulated by the patient and causes less apprehension than similar apparatus.

bony prominences and specific points at which pressure of weight is high. The coccygeal, scapular, elbow, and ankle areas are common sites of pressure sores involving sparsely circulated regions. The buttocks and heels are common site pressure sores involving high pressure due to weight. An additional factor in obesity is that the dissolution of adipose tissue inhibits wound healing. Summarily, these patients must be kept clean and dry, be repositioned frequently, be kept free of all undue pressure on any body area, be massaged frequently with emollient skin lotions, and be provided with and encouraged to take an adequate nutritional and fluid supply.

When decubitus ulcers exist, nursing measures must be directed toward removal or control of the cause and preservation of tissue integrity from infection. A patient who has a pressure sore should never be positioned so that there is direct weight on the area. When specific health problems prevent turning a patient to alternate postures, supportive devices must be strategically employed. Such equipment ranges widely from simple foam rubber rings that physically relieve pressure on given areas to the elaborate electrically driven alternating pressure mattress that continuously and regularly changes pressure exerted on all surfaces in contact with the mattress surface. Several specially designed beds are utilized in hospital settings to facilitate patient safety and comfort. The Stryker frame and CircOlectric bed are also adjuncts to prevention and correction of decubitus ulcers in patients with marked physical and mechanical limitation.

When a patient has bladder or bowel incontinence, control of the frequency of skin contact with excretions is primary. Body excreta excoriates skin, and moisture reduces skin turgor and tissue tension. Positive means of avoiding incidence to this include immediate meticulous skin care and change of linen whenever involuntary excretion occurs, providing the bedpan and the urinal at regular and frequent time intervals, inserting retention or indwelling catheters, and giving cleansing enemas every second or third day. Catheterization and rectal irrigation are both dependent nursing measures requiring legal medical prescription.

Decubitus ulcers are complex problems. Their complexity is compounded when bacterial invasion of tissues complicates the healing processes. Any dissolution in the continuity of skin predisposes subcutaneous tissue to infection. When tissues are devitalized, the process of infection is rapid. Efficient treatment of decubitus ulcers requires use of surgical aseptic techniques. Plans for specific treatment should be made in consultation with the medical team leader and the method of therapy carried out by medical prescription. As in the protection of any wound against superimposed infection after incidence, preventive measures are a nursing responsibility. The basis of surgical asepsis is physical cleanliness. Keeping surrounding body surfaces clean of contaminants with soap and water is the first line of defense against wound infection. Specifically prescribed medical therapy must be instituted by the nurse with full understanding of method and precautions involved. Sterile dressings, synthetic plastic coating agents, heat or light, open-air or surgical debridement, and skin grafting may all be employed in the treatment of pressure sores. The selection of method is individual to the patient's problem, the doctor, and the health institution.

The safety of the patient is dependent upon the nurse knowing what to do, how to do it, and what not to do. Nursing care of patients with decubitus ulcers poses one of the greatest challenges to the fundamental principles and practices of nursing as a unique service to patients. Although in some patients the correction of this complication is not physiologically possible, in many patients the processes of physical trauma can be reduced markedly by careful institution of measures to control infection and to promote regeneration of tissue.

An aspect of nursing function concerned with maintaining operational efficiency in movable body parts requires the provision of full range of motion for all physically limited joints. Exercises of this nature may be initiated by the patient when he is able or may be initiated by the nurse when the patient is incapable of self-mobilization. In relation to the moving force, they are classified as active (self-initiated) or passive (initiated by someone other than the patient). Full range of motion of movable body parts involves flexion, extension, and rotation in accord with normal physiological function. Routine exercises through full range of motion is essential to prevention of deformities and restoration of optimal function when body mechanics are impaired by disease and injury. Joint ankylosis or "frozen joint" is frequently an unnecessary complication of many diseases and injuries. In many patients, the state becomes irreversible and the resultant physical handicap permanent. It is a well-acknowledged fact that many patients have permanent physical handicaps because of ignorance and neglect on the part of members of a health team during the acute phases of illnesses. Team planning and medical consultation to identify areas of danger as well as knowledge of method of procedure are essential to patient safety. Body parts being exercised must be manually supported so that muscle action or circulation is not impaired. Exercises must not be so prolonged as to fatigue patients unnecessarily. Patients must be encouraged to work toward independent motion through full utilization of even the most minute degree of physical capacity in any part of the body.

Individual patient problems related to rest and sleep commonly result from physical and emotional disturbances caused by illness and hospitalization. Pain, nausea, vomiting, loss of body function and surgical disruption of the body are readily identifiable as experiences that interfere with a patient's achievement of a normal amount of rest and sleep. In many clinical settings, lack of administrative organization on any level results in a health service that makes more demands on the patient than it does on the health personnel. The end result of this is a picture of a patient in an average hospital setting that has a sixteen-hour period of wakefulness and an eight-hour period of sleep. In view of the fact that this is a norm recommended for healthy individuals, there is some reason to question the adequacy of what is provided for patients in a hospital. In many instances, the variety of diagnostic and therapeutic means required to rescue the body from illness may well justify the bombardment of a patient in acute illness at any time of day or night. Outside of this situation, much of the disturbance can be greatly reduced by a well-organized plan of patient care. The nurse must literally become a self-appointed custodian of patient rest and sleep. To paraphrase a quotation, the patient must be the center of nursing care, not the target. Direct nursing measures prerequisite to ensuring optimal rest and sleep for patients may be summarized as follows:

1. Adequate provision for total physical hygiene needs and comfort at all times
2. Control of temperature and ventilation in the environment
3. Planned rest periods during the day
4. Control of noise and personal interruptions of patients during rest periods
5. Administration of medications prescribed to support rest and sleep as prescribed
6. When preparing patients for sleep at night, particular emphasis placed on physical and emotional support that will alleviate anxiety that commonly results from fear and lonesomeness during stages of illness and enforced confinement in a strange environment

Like the area of nursing care related to prevention and treatment of decubitus ulcers, the area concerned with promotion of adequate rest and sleep is a challenge to the nurse practitioner. Rest and sleep are real needs in the day-by-day business of living. It is regrettable to observe that it is the one area of service about which a variety of patients in a variety of hospital settings complain most consistently and most bitterly. The total responsibility rests with many people. Efficient hospital, medical, and nursing service administrations can do a great deal to alleviate this problem. In the meantime, well-organized and effective nursing care gives optimal protection to the rights and the needs of patients for an adequate amount of rest and sleep.

BIBLIOGRAPHY

1. Fuerst, Elinor V., and Wolff, La Verne: Fundamentals of nursing, ed. 2, Philadelphia, 1959, J. B. Lippincott Co., pp. 107-116, 263-307.
2. Harmer, Bertha, and Henderson, Virginia: Textbook of principles and practice of nursing, ed. 5, New York, 1955, The Macmillan Co., pp. 467-506.
3. Larson, Carroll B., and Gould, Marjorie L.: Fractures of the hip and nursing care of the patient with a fractured hip, American Journal of Nursing 58:1558-1563, Nov. 1958.
4. Madden, Barbara W., and Affeldt, John E.: To prevent helplessness and deformities, American Journal of Nursing 62:59-61, Dec. 1962.
5. McLain, Esther M., and Gragg, Shirley H.: Scientific principles in nursing, ed. 4, St. Louis, 1962, The C. V. Mosby Co., pp. 119-135.
6. Mendelson, Janice A.: Sprains and strains, American Journal of Nursing 61:45-50, June 1961.
7. Nordmark, Madelyn T., and Rohweder, Anne W.: Scientific principles applied to nursing, Philadelphia, 1959, J. B. Lippincott Co., pp. 130-154.
8. Stilwell, Elizabeth J.: Pressure sores, American Journal of Nursing 61:109-110, Nov. 1961.

Chapter 14

Basic aspects of nutrition and elimination

The maintenance of health is dependent upon the maintenance of nutrition in all body cells and the elimination from the body of 'the waste products of digestion and of cell metabolism. Consideration of .these factors is essential to any study related to the provision of patient-centered nursing care. Therefore, this chapter will deal with specific aspects of food and fluid intake required for normal nutrition and with significant facts of the elimination of wastes through the urinary and intestinal tracts that are basic to general physical hygiene. At this point, there is no concern with nursing problems directly resulting from physiological disturbances of digestion, absorption, assimilation or excretion. The major emphasis is on the provision of essential nutrients and assurance of a physiological and psychological climate that will support their optimal utilization and facilitate the natural disposition of the resulting waste products when no specific pathological processes are existent.

NUTRITION
Physiological aspects of nutrition

The body requires specific elements or nutrients in order to function. These elements are identified broadly as proteins, carbohydrates, fats, vitamins, minerals, water, and cellulose. From these nutrients, the body derives the factors necessary to produce heat and energy, to build and repair tissues, and to regulate the body processes. Adequate nutrition is dependent upon a minimal supply of each of these nutrients. Actually, the body should be supplied with optimal amounts in order to provide a margin of safety during physiological stress. During the various periods of growth and development in the life cycle, the quantity and quality of food must be adapted to the particular needs of the body. For example, the caloric energy requirements of the body gradually decrease from the period of infancy to the period of full physical maturation and continue to decrease throughout the life cycle with the normal reduction of physical activity. Similarly, when the body is subjected to disease, the quantity and quality of food must be adapted to support the regulatory functions involved in reparative processes. In febrile states, patients require increased water intake to support the regulation of body temperature and increased carbohydrate intake to replenish energy dissipated through increased metabolism.

The achievement of good nutrition is ultimately dependent upon a pattern of dietary habits that regularly ensures the intake of the quality and quantity of foods essential to physiological homeostasis.

Sociological aspects of nutrition

Food and its intake constitute a significant and emotionally charged aspect of life, because eating is very closely related to cultural value systems. What one eats, how one eats, with whom one eats, and how one disposes of garbage may reflect and indicate one's nationality, religion, and social status. Foods that are considered a delicacy in one culture may be considered repulsive in another. Taboos in regard to acceptable foods are as numerous as the sub-groups in any society. In the South grits are served with breakfast, on the West Coast fried potatoes are served with breakfast, and in the Northeast neither of these are served with breakfast. Snails are a delicacy in France, but many Americans gag at the very idea of eating a snail. The eating of pork is forbidden by certain religions. Foods that are served with pleasure in one social group may be prohibited in another social group.

Whether one eats with a knife and fork or with one's fingers depends, to a great extent, on where the individual was born and reared. Even more sensitive is the subject of with whom one eats. We are fully aware of the obvious segregation that exists in the United States, but the not-so-obvious segregation in regard to "eating together" is even more widespread. We may invite a pretty narrow range of people to eat in our homes, comprising a limited ingroup. There are people with whom we will eat in a restaurant but will not invite into our homes. We would not eat at all with many more people. If the people with whom we eat have table manners that differ markedly from our own, we are very likely to have strong negative feelings about them.

The social implications of what and how we eat have their own influence on the adequacy of the maintenance of nutrition for any given individual.

Psychological aspects of nutrition

Another aspect of food and its intake that is significant is the individual personality as reflected in dietary habits or patterns. The intake of food, in addition to alleviating the "pain" of hunger, also satifies the pleasure instinct in man. In the healthy, well-adjusted person, eating is a "pleasurable experience." As a result of varied experiences with foods during the stages of growth, the average person eventually achieves a capacity to eat a well-balanced, varied diet regularly and in proportion to bodily needs.

However, this capacity is frequently hampered by emotional disturbances that occur as a result of previous life experienes. The child who learns that refusal to eat arouses a response in parents may eventually learn to use this as an "attention-seeking" device. Continuous behavior of this kind may eventually lead to the development of dietary habits exemplified by the "poor or picky" eater or the "food fadist" with strong aversions for some foods or a predilection for others. Another type of personality may exaggerate the "pleasure instinct" of eating to satisfy encountered frustrations. People who meet situations of stress with compulsive eating are not at all unusual. Sustained behavior of this kind may eventually lead to the development of dietary habits exemplified by the gourmand, or greedy eater, who tends to luxuriate in the business of eating any kind of food. In between these two extremes are numerous aspects of the individual personality that have strong influence on food intake. The presence of a disturbed emotional state impairs normal appetite or desire for food. Although this is directly caused by the physiological changes produced by emotions, the ultimate effect is nutritional deficiency. Anxiety, anger, or depression may not only destroy appetite or increase it beyond reason, but may also interfere with digestive processes essential to absorption and utilization of essential nutrients.

In the maintenance of good nutrition, individual psychological needs must be considered. Deficiencies or excesses in quantity or quality of foods stem from emotional disturbances and result in nutritional problems.

Normal nutrition and health

The interrelatedness of normal nutrition and health is obvious. The vital capacity of the individual is centered in adequate physiological function, optimal physical and mental energy, the capacity to enjoy life, and the resources to solve problems in the life situation. *Malnutrition* militates against the individual's achievement of his optimum potential. Poor dietary habits or indiscriminate dieting frequently means an inadequate intake of food and a decrease in total mental and physical energy, resulting in an "underachiever" at work or play in addition to a body predisposed to infections. Poor dietary habits that exclude essential nutrients directly contribute to physiological dysfunction. Poor dietary habits that are characterized by excesses of quantity or quality are responsible for the complex and universal health problem of obesity, as well as many specific health problems believed to be associated with excessive intake of food.

What is true of the individual is no less true of the optimum potential of a total population. Economic depression along with political and social abuses results in poverty, hunger, and disease in "backward" nations as well as among the underprivileged people of the "privileged" nations. The sociological and psychological aspects of eating dictate that not only must food be available but also that understanding of the significance of food and the emotional stability to use it effectively are positive factors in relation to health.

Nursing intervention and nutrition

Nursing intervention in regard to nutrition may be divided into two broad areas:

1. Knowledge and understanding required to provide for nutritional needs of patients
   (a) Relatedness of physiology and nutrition
   (b) Function and sources of essential nutrients
   (c) Social, cultural, economic, and psychological factors affecting dietary habits
   (d) Limitations and adjustments indicated in sickness and injury
2. Nursing functions related to providing these needs

The nurse must have a knowledge of the importance of the essential value of proteins as fundamental structural elements of all body cells, the functions of fats as assistants in regulating body heat and as carriers of fat-soluble vitamins (A, D, E, and K) and specific sources of fatty acids essential for growth and survival, and an understanding of carbohydrates as chief sources of energy and cellulose and, consequently, as a prerequisite to metabolism of other nutrients.

The best source of essential nutrients must be approached from the standpoint of the foods that contain the greatest amount, with consideration for the economic availability and cultural and individual acceptability of sources. Reference to limitations and adjustments imposed by sickness or injury includes a broad knowledge of physical conditions that interfere with adequate intake of food or fluid. Understanding of the implications of symptoms that threaten good nutrition, such as nausea, vomiting, pain, change in skin color or turgor, anorexia, inability to masticate, and dysphagia, is basic in nursing.

Although the nurse is frequently limited in helping patients to meet nutritional needs because of the circumstances of hospital dietary services, there are several critical aspects of nursing that can be controlled.

An environment that is physically, socially, and psychologically acceptable to patients is a positive force in fostering adequate intake and digestion of food. Sights, sounds, odors, and experiences that are unpleasant should be eliminated from the patient setting at mealtime or whenever nourishment or fluid is presented. Physical comfort, emotional ease, and social and psychological security are essentials that depend on nursing function to a great extent. An uncomfortable bed, strained interpersonal relationships, provision of food in an unpalatable or unmanageable way do nothing toward providing a desirable setting at mealtime.

Observation of eating problems related to difficulties with mastication, difficulties in swallowing, or emphatic food preferences and aversions should not only be made and reported by the nurse but, in addition, require positive action to correct the degree to which they interfere with nutrition. The provision of foods that are readily ingestible is as important as the provision of foods rich in essential nutrients. In the nursing care of patients who have problems of ingestion for any reason, the consistency, form, and type of

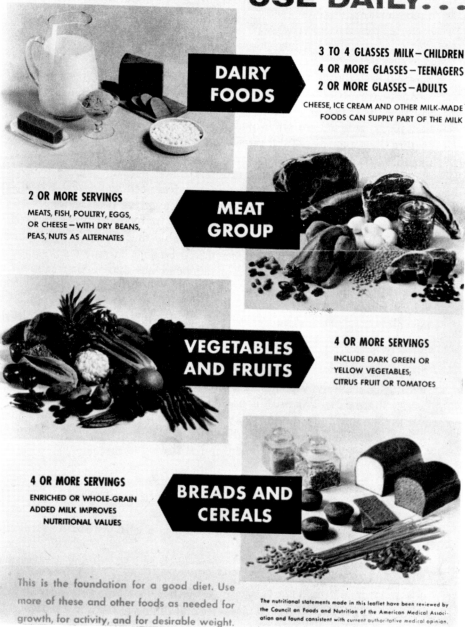

A Guide To Good Eating

USE DAILY...

DAIRY FOODS

3 TO 4 GLASSES MILK—CHILDREN
4 OR MORE GLASSES—TEENAGERS
2 OR MORE GLASSES—ADULTS

CHEESE, ICE CREAM AND OTHER MILK-MADE FOODS CAN SUPPLY PART OF THE MILK

2 OR MORE SERVINGS

MEATS, FISH, POULTRY, EGGS, OR CHEESE — WITH DRY BEANS, PEAS, NUTS AS ALTERNATES

MEAT GROUP

VEGETABLES AND FRUITS

4 OR MORE SERVINGS

INCLUDE DARK GREEN OR YELLOW VEGETABLES; CITRUS FRUIT OR TOMATOES

4 OR MORE SERVINGS

ENRICHED OR WHOLE-GRAIN ADDED MILK IMPROVES NUTRITIONAL VALUES

BREADS AND CEREALS

This is the foundation for a good diet. Use more of these and other foods as needed for growth, for activity, and for desirable weight.

The nutritional statements made in this leaflet have been reviewed by the Council on Foods and Nutrition of the American Medical Association and found consistent with current authoritative medical opinion.

Fig. 23. The basic four groups of food constitute the foundation for an adequate balanced diet. (Courtesy the National Dairy Council, Chicago, Ill.)

food provided is of major importance in any attempt to provide adequate nutrition.

In the presence of anorexia, meals should be planned to be small, frequent, and selective as to personal food preferences while still including minimal quantities of essential nutrients. In attempting to encourage adequate nutrition, the nurse never should insist that patients eat certain foods because "they are good for you." This approach invariably produces negative responses. During any phase of physiological or psychological stress, any aspect of nursing care designed to maintain nutrition must consider the personal preferences of patients.

Another aspect of nursing care concerned with maintaining nutrition is assisting patients to eat or feeding them. Because of a variety of physical limitations, patients are often unable to partake of food independently and require the direct services of nursing personnel to get food or fluid into the mouth.

Feeding is probably the first essential function that man learns to perform for himself. Strongly motivated by physical need and psychological satisfaction, the baby learns quickly to outmaneuver the problem of spooning food from plate to mouth or transferring liquid from cup to lips. The rewards are great. It is therefore readily understandable that the loss of the ability to provide such basic wants arouses mixed feelings in patients. Generally, such feelings are centered in loss of independence and "embarrassment at being forced into the role of a baby." In feeding patients, genuine consideration of these feelings will guide the nurse in action. In addition, specific aspects of physical safety, aspiration, and asphyxiation must be clearly understood when patients are handicapped by positional limitations or functional or organic dysphagias.

Crucial aspects of feeding patients may be summarized as follows:

1. See that food is palatable and ingestible.
2. Place patient in a sitting or side-lying position.
3. The nurse assumes a position that is comfortable for the mechanics of feeding, sitting, or standing.
4. Present food in the amount and at the rate that is "natural" for the individual patient.
5. Vary types of food served at the same time in a "natural sequence."
6. Provide social atmosphere amenable to the individual patient, i.e., conversation, radio, television, or silence.
7. Use drinking tube, spoon, fork, etc., in accord with patient's limitations and preferences.
8. Test food and beverages for heat and cold by offering a very small amount first.
9. Encourage but never force any patient to ingest any form of food.
10. Use extreme caution in quantity and timing in feeding a patient with dysphagia, and discontinue oral feeding of food or fluid whenever the patient gags, coughs, or chokes.
11. Observe, report, and record all significant facts concerning quan-

tity, quality, facility, and tolerance in regard to food intake, especially if adequate nutrition is critical to patient welfare.

Finally, in the area of health teaching, the nurse in fulfilling her responsibilities must be aware of her own limitations. Teaching, to be effective, must be based upon the social, cultural, and individual capacity of the patient to accept relevant knowledge. Limitations imposed by personal and emotional experiences may negate learning in any area. Therefore, in her projection of knowledge, the nurse must avoid imposing her own personal food preferences, accept the limitations of the patient in any adjustment required, and project positive knowledge in a simple, understandable way. Acceptance of our own limitations to effect change is as true in nutritional areas of patient need as it is in any other. It is not easy to change dietary habits of long standing. Helping patients make such changes is often complicated by the nurse's own cultural and personal attitudes toward food. Improved nutrition in patients is largely dependent upon the ability to change dietary patterns. We cannot always help patients to reverse eating habits, but we can help them to alter scope and breadth in the majority of situations.

ELIMINATION
Output of body wastes

Substances that cannot be utilized by the body to maintain physiological function are regularly eliminated as waste products through the respiratory, urinary, and intestinal systems. (Although the majority of textbooks generally name the skin as an organ of excretion, its function is relatively limited in comparison with the other systems. For this reason it will not be included in this discussion.) Failure of the body to excrete waste materials with a relative degree of regularity impairs normal body function. The degree of failure and the system involved determine the severity of the patient's problem. When any of the major organs of elimination (the kidneys, the intestines, and the lungs) fail, the patient faces a major health problem. Consideration of primary pathological processes involving major systems of elimination will be found in a subsequent chapter. Discussion of problems of elimination in this section will be confined to those which result from limitations imposed by clinical conditions of other systems of the body, and problems of elimination through the alimentary and urinary tracts will be further delineated.

Physiological aspects of urinary elimination

Urine is manufactured by the kidneys and passes through the ureters into the bladder. When a sufficient amount of secretion accumulates, pressure on the sphincter muscle of the bladder stimulates the patient to feel a need to void, and urine passes through the urethra to the external surface of the body. The amount of urine that can be retained before expulsion is necessary or the frequency of micturition is affected by habit training patterns, total fluid intake, and the emotional status of an individual. Additionally,

Table 7. *General properties of a normal pattern of urinary elimination*

Properties	Normal findings
Amount	1000-2000 ml. daily (24 hr.)
Frequency	6-8 times (approximately 200-250 ml. each time)
Color	Amber
Consistency	Clear

total urinary output in any given period as well as the color of urine will be influenced by fluid consumption, because urine largely consists of the nitrogenous waste products of protein metabolism and water. The amount of solid substances present in the urine is known as the specific gravity. This factor, too, varies sharply in individuals, because it is dependent upon the amount of sodium chloride and protein consumed. Within a structured framework, however, it is possible to assume that the amount, frequency, color, and consistency of urinary excretion has some degree of constancy. A normal pattern of urinary elimination is shown in Table 7.

Physiological aspects of intestinal elimination

The bulk of residue of digestion is eliminated from the body through the large intestine. Major absorption of food nutrients occurs in the small intestine. When digested substances reach the cecum, they mainly consist of cellulose and water. The function of the large intestine then is threefold: (1) absorption of water, (2) breakdown of cellulose (which requires the action of bacteria present in the colon), and (3) elimination of the bulk which is referred to as feces or stool. The gross bulk eliminated from the body is directly dependent upon the amount of cellulose ingested. However, within a norm, the average adult person with regular dietary habits evacuates once or twice daily. Actually, the number of times or frequency with which evacuation of the bowel occurs is a distinctly individual function influenced by the following variables:

1. Individual physiological capacity in the digestion and absorption of nutrients and water as well as peristaltic action
2. Dietary habits which provide adequate amounts of nutrients, cellulose, and water
3. Exercise or physical activity appropriate to physiological needs
4. Regular habit patterns in planning sufficient time for evacuation in a regular daily schedule and reasonably immediate response to physiological stimuli indicating the body's readiness to evacuate at any time —planned or unplanned.

The rate of total digestive processes is not constant in all people. For this reason it is not considered abnormal for healthy individuals to eliminate less frequently than daily. Normalcy in relation to frequency can only be evaluated in terms of what is usual for the individual. The consistency, color, and facility of disposal of the stool gives relatively constant indication of normal elimination. Throughout the whole digestive process the action of multiple juices, enzymes, and bacteria, plus absorption of elements and water, produces residue that is characteristic in consistency, color, and relative ease with which it is expelled from the rectum. Although these qualities can deviate mildly and transiently in relation to occasional dietary digressions, they are still relatively stable within individual patterns. Normal stool is expelled easily from the rectum without undue strain or pain and appears generally as a brown mass softly formed to the contour of the rectal canal.

Common deviations in elimination

Any gross deviation in a pattern of elimination through the urinary or intestinal systems is indicative of a disturbance in homeostasis. Deviations are fundamentally manifested by (1) excesses, (2) deficiencies, and (3) failure to control the functions.

The terms "excesses" and "deficiencies" are used here to include gross changes in quantity, quality, and color of waste products as three prime indicators of homeostatic disturbances. Excesses in elimination may be "normal" or nonpathological, resulting from fluid and food intake or emotional disturbance. Frequency in voiding, polyuria (increased urinary output), and diarrhea are not unusual when directly attributable to increased fluid consumption, ingestion of foods that are incompatible with personal dietary patterns, or individual experiences that arouse anxiety or excitement.

In a similar vein, deficiences in elimination may result directly from the same factors. Oliguria (diminished urinary output) and constipation are not unusual when related to inadequate fluid intake, a diet deficient in nutrients and cellulose, or individual experiences that arouse anxiety or depression.

Inevitably, the usual response of excess or deficiency in otherwise "healthy" individuals is an entirely individual one. However, in terms of nursing problems in maintenance of elimination, specific disturbances are significant. Understanding basic causes is essential to effective nursing care. The physiological process of elimination can be affected by six causes:

1. Pathological changes within the organs involved
2. Mechanical obstruction of any of the organs involved
3. Systemic changes
4. Pathological changes in the central nervous system
5. Drugs that directly or indirectly affect elimination
6. Emotional disturbances

At this point in the discussion, the concern is not with the disease processes that directly or indirectly affect elimination but rather with understanding the effects produced in terms of changes in patterns.

Deficiencies are manifested by oliguria, suppression, and retention in relation to urinary output. Suppression (kidney failure) is caused by renal pathology. The term "anuria" is generally related to suppression. Oliguria, however, may occur in conjunction with other conditions. In febrile states, dehydration occurs when body water is depleted, total urinary output is diminished, the color of the urine is dark, and the product appears concentrated. Generally, it is practical to conclude that in any situation in which there is restriction or limitation of fluid intake or a gross loss of body fluid, as in major surgery or hemorrhage, these changes in urinary excretion will occur. Retention or inability of the ureters, bladder, or urethra to allow urine to flow may be caused by mechanical factors internally obstructing or externally impinging on the channel, central nervous system diseases, or emotional states affecting enervation of sphincter muscles.

Deficiencies related to output of waste through the intestinal tract are indicated by constipation or obstipation (no stool). Constipation is a relatively common problem among hospitalized patients, and, judging by the amount of advertising spent on laxatives and cathartics, it is a national problem. Constipation is mainly attributable to altered routines in dietary and activity patterns, functional impairment due to surgery, and the psychological aspects of restricted use of toilet facilities. Obvious manifestations of constipation include changes in color, consistency, and facility of expulsion. Because the stool has been retained abnormally long in the intestine, it becomes darker, hard, and difficult and/or painful to pass.

Excesses in urinary output are demonstrated in polyuria (frequency) or changes in color and consistency. When polyuria is not associated with massive fluid intake to offset dehydration, it is suggestive of endocrine or metabolic disturbance. Voiding small amounts at frequent intervals may be due to pressure on the bladder or the urethra exerted by surrounding structures. Patients who develop enlargement of the prostate gland or uterine tumor or prolapse are commonly troubled with frequency. Changes in color and consistency of urine are caused by the presence of abnormal constituents such as blood, bile, mucus, or pus.

The excess pattern in terms of the intestinal tract is similar. Diarrhea is not technically characterized by an increased number of stools but rather by the consistency, i.e., loose and watery. However, when this factor is related to causes such as infection and inflammation, there usually is a common picture of loose, watery stools at frequent intervals. Color changes in stool are produced by the gross presence of abnormal constituents. The presence of blood that originates in the upper intestinal tract produces a stool that is "tarry" in color, for the blood has been digested. Frank blood in the stool is characteristic in color and is obviously due to hemorrhage in the rectal or anal regions. A dark green color is indicative of excessive bile. In addition to these classical and rather critical color changes, there are others that can be related to dietary excesses and the presence of microbiological agents within the intestinal tract.

The third major area of gross deviation in physiological function is exhibited in patients who are unable to control elimination through the urinary or intestinal systems. A problem of loss of control is often a complex and irreversible one, but, in many instances it may be a temporary or transitory condition. Such widely divergent conditions as neurogenic or cerebrovascular diseases or pathology and/or surgery of urological, gynecological, or alimentary tracts may be directly responsible for problems related to the control of output.

Postoperatively, incontinence is often temporary; at other times, it is irreversible. Postoperative patients may be subjected to enforced loss of urinary control because of insertion of a catheter prior to surgery. This is done in order to prevent distention during surgery and retention following surgery and to provide a clinical indication of fluid and electrolyte balance in the early postoperative period. The serious problem related to loss of continence involves patients whose problems are directly caused by pathological processes of the total system or the central nervous system. Patients who have a high fever, dehydration, or acidosis are equally as prone to loose bowel and bladder control as patients with brain tumors, cerebral arteriosclerosis, or spinal nerve destruction. Regardless of the cause, the manifestations are consistent. The patient is unable to control and personally direct elimination of waste from the bladder and/or the intestinal tract.

Psychological aspects of elimination

A patient's response to any interference with normal elimination, although strongly individual, is still characterized by common elements despite cultural or national differences in patients. Such elements are intrinsically concerned with privacy, comfort, freedom from pressure, and normalcy of characteristics of body excretions. Any experience that militates against these aspects of cultural patterns constitutes a source of psychological discomfort. Conversely, psychological discomfort constitutes a threat to normal elimination.

When considered from the aspect of what can go wrong, these facts become significant. It is not unusual for patients who are confined to bed to develop constipation because of inadequate privacy, the discomfort associated with using a bedpan, and being forced to evacuate in an abnormal anatomical position. It is also generally conceded that patients who are emotionally disturbed by anxiety instigated by hospitalization or medical treatment are suddenly unable to void despite the absence of physical cause. Like feeding oneself, control and direction relative to elimination of wastes from the body is an early developmental task. Loss of such control constitutes a threat to independence and may distort the patient's self-image. In addition, the general appearance of the products of elimination that deviate from accepted normal standards are anxiety-provoking factors. Although in many instances in patient care it may be a matter of the proverbial "chicken or egg," it is essentially undebatable that emotional problems related to elimination genuinely result from attitudes and feelings developed through life experiences. The problem becomes overt when such patterns are disturbed.

Nursing intervention and elimination

Nursing care directed toward the maintenance of elimination must essentially be concerned with what has gone wrong. Regardless of whether the nursing function is dependent or independent, efforts are directed toward three central objectives:

1. Maintaining optimal function
2. Restoring optimal function
3. Rehabilitating the patient

Nursing measures involved in maintenance of function are supportive and preventive. Because hospitalization and enforced bed rest constitute an invasion of privacy as well as a major change in physical habits and eating habits, steps must be taken to prevent deficiencies in elimination. Privacy, comfort, and adequate services are fundamental to patients' needs in this regard. Screening the patient from public view during elimination preserves his sense of personal dignity, thereby avoiding emotional disturbances that inhibit normal function.

The patient's need for physical comfort is provided mainly by correct positioning. The normal anatomical position for bowel evacuation is the normal sitting position. When patients are confined to bed, it is sometimes necessary to modify this in view of physical limitations. The nurse must learn how to secure optimal comfort in light of all limitations. This requires knowledge and judgment. Many variations of normal position may be adapted when patients cannot ambulate to the toilet. The method selected depends on the physical capacity of the patient. When a patient is unable to get out of bed, support of the back, shoulders, and head on a line with or above the level of the hips (on the bedpan) will afford maximum comfort. The degree of the angle of elevation must be related to the patient's limitation. The head of the bed should be "gatched" to a height that is comfortable for the patient. The correct position of the patient on the bedpan facilitates normal relaxation of the anal sphincters. Placing a bedpan on a chair or providing a commode for a patient whose activity is confined to sitting out of bed simulates natural circumstances of elimination effectively.

Normal anatomical position for bladder evacuation in women is identical with bowel evacuation. Nursing measures to provide for patients' needs in this area are essentially the same. However, because of anatomical structure, men naturally void in a standing position; male patients confined to bed frequently encounter difficulty in using a urinal. Whenever it is possible, provisions should be made to allow the patient to attain as closely as possible the normal voiding posture. If a patient has difficulty in voiding because of position, consultation with the physician is indicated to determine activity adjustments that can be made safely to alleviate the problem.

Additional aspects of providing comfort in elimination include room temperature and the collecting receptacles, i.e., bedpan and urinal. Although it would hardly seem necessary to elaborate on the significance of room temperature to comfort, one point needs to be emphasized here. When a body is chilled, muscles and blood vessels constrict. Such physiological action is opposed to the relaxation of muscles required for evacuation. A cold bedpan or urinal in contact with a warm body produces the same effect and is a most unpleasant feeling. It is a relatively easy matter to warm these utensils to approximate body temperature before use. From the standpoint of safety, however, caution must be taken that they do not burn the patient.

Adequate service to maintain optimal function in elimination requires provision of necessary facilities as often as needed and allowance of a sufficient time for their use. In planning patient care, provision for elimination should be made routinely in the usual pattern of function, i.e., early morning, before and after meals, and at bedtime. It is readily understandable that such plans will not completely coincide with patients' needs in general. In this regard, it is important to remember that nursing plans must be adjusted to patients, and not vice versa.

When excesses in elimination are present, specific supportive nursing measures are related to comfort and safety. Diarrhea and polyuria are distressing to patients, and every effort should be made to provide the facilities required, rapidly and frequently. Because diarrhea may be infectious, meticulous attention to the patient's body and hand hygiene is important. Skin areas surrounding the excretory orifices may become excoriated. The use of emollient agents or talcum powder is effective in counteracting this condition. It is also necessary to be sure that bed linen is clean and dry to control spread of infection and to promote comfort.

In general, these same practices are applicable to nursing care of patients who are incontinent and involuntary, with emphasis on the predisposition to skin breakdown and reenforcement of measures to prevent this.

Preventive nursing measures directed toward maintaining elimination are essentially related to food and fluid intake. The specific point made here is in direct relation to the role of nutrients and water in preventing constipation. It is the responsibility of the nurse to bring about any adjustments required to meet this need. Planning a regimen of fluids to be taken at regular intervals and arranging for the exclusion of foods that are not liked are the kinds of things the nurse must do to ward off elimination deficiencies.

Nursing measures to facilitate restoration of optimal function in elimination include, among others, catheterization, irrigation, administration of medications, and regulation of diet and fluid intake. Catheters are inserted for a variety of reasons. The concern here is not with the procedure per se or the reasons why it is instituted, but with maintaining the patency of the tube once it is inserted. The lumen of a catheter may become occluded by constituents from the bladder, such as mucus, pus, or urate crystals. This may be prevented or corrected by periodic irrigation with an isotonic saline solution. In some situations this procedure is standard, while in others it is carried out only on specific medical order. Regardless of policy in relation to irrigation, the major nursing responsibility is to know whether or note the tube is patent and to do something about it immediaely and directly if it is not.

Rectal irrigations or enemas are frequently prescribed. There are several types of enemas given for specific purposes. The procedure used to stimulate bowel evacuation and to relieve constipation is classified as a cleansing enema and commonly consists of the rectal injection of solutions of tap

Table 8. *Scientific knowledge related to the safe and effective administration of rectal irrigations*

Science	Fact	Safe practice
Physiology	Body temperature 99.6°F. Mucous membrane is delicate structure Moderate heat increases circulation and stimulates involuntary muscles	Administer solution at approximately 105°F.
Anatomy	Rectum in adults approximately 6 inches long	Insert rectal tube approximately 4 inches
Anatomy	Anal sphincter and mucous membrane are delicate structures	Lubricate rectal tube to facilitate insertion to avoid trauma
Physics	Height of a column of fluid determines amount of force exerted at point of application	Suspend fluid approximately 12-16 inches above level of rectum to prevent trauma and to reduce muscle spasm
Physiology	Distention of wall of rectum stimulates peristaltic action in intestines	If patient complains of "cramplike" pains, shut off inflow until spasms subside If pain is *acute*, siphon out solution and discontinue treatment

water, soapsuds, or saline solution to stimulate peristaltic action. The solution should be specified by the doctor in a legally written order. Safe and effective administration of the treatment requires application of scientific knowledge. The critical facts and implications for appropriate action are summarized in Table 8.

The precise amount of solution that can be retained without unduly taxing the capacity of the rectum and still be effectual is an individual matter. It is directly affected by physical constitution, bowel hygiene, and previous experience with enemas. Many patients can retain only 500 ml. and achieve satisfactory results. Still others may require 1000 ml. or 1500 ml. to procure the desired effect. To quote an average is idle, but in order to provide a guideline, it is generally accepted that the average adult requires approximately 1000 ml. of solution in order to evacuate constipated stool completely.

A variation on the traditional type of enema is the commercially prepared compact disposable unit. The pinciple involved is the use of a relatively small amount of a hypertonic solution. The solution draws fluids from surounding tissues into the rectum and produces an effect similar to the routine procedure. This method is convenient, practical, and in many instances satisfactory. However, in certain situations the effectiveness of the treatment is not adequate. Like all treatments, such type of enema must be ordered specifically by name by the physician.

Medications employed to restore simple disturbances include drugs that produce evacuation and those that control diarrhea. When and how laxatives or cathartics are administered are dictated by their nature. Some are given at bedtime; others are given in the early morning. Reverting to a statement made previously, in view of the importance of water in elimination, patients who require catharsis should be encouraged to take fluids (especially water) freely. Catharsis may also be induced by the use of suppositories. To be effectual, a suppository must be inserted approximately three inches and remain in place for the recommended period of time. Antidiarrheic agents commonly contain drugs that are antispasmotic in action, i.e., they reduce muscle spasms. Some agents are prescribed at regular intervals; others are ordered in relation to the frequency of bowel movements. Fluid replacement is of paramount importance in diarrhea, because of the large quantity of fluid lost through the excreta. A nursing plan designed to provide small amounts of clear fluids at frequent intervals will replenish losses without overtaxing the upper digestive tract. Fluids that have residue, such as eggnog or creamed soups, are contraindicated in order to allow the colon to rest.

Consideration of the rehabilitation of patients who have uncomplicated problems related to elimination is confined here to the explanation and clarification of hygienic practices to promote optimal function and prevent recurrence. Within this frame of reference, the most prevalent problem of constipation takes priority. Helping the patient to accept and to understand the effectiveness of simple practices related to nutrition and regular habits is paramount. Patients should be made aware of the dangers inherent in the indiscriminate use of cathartics and laxatives. The vital importance of seeking medical advice when constipation persists cannot be overemphasized, because chronic constipation may well be considered as predisposing to many more serious health problems.

Summary

The ability of the body to eliminate waste products through the urinary and intestinal systems is an intrinsic factor in maintaining and/or restoring homeostasis to optimal levels. Nursing intervention may be concerned with providing a variety of patient needs through institution of preventive and supportive measures. As in all areas of patient care, the ability to make critical observation of significant symptoms is a serious responsibility. In the care of patients with problems in relation to elimination, any deviation from normal must be carefully reported and recorded in accurate and descriptive terms.

BIBLIOGRAPHY

1. Burton, Benjamin, executive editor: Heinz handbook of nutrition, New York, 1959, McGraw-Hill Book Co., Inc., pp. 3-106, 129-203.
2. Cooper, Lenna F., Barber, Edith M., Mitchell, Helen S., and Rynbergen, Henderika J.: Nutrition in health and disease, ed. 13, Philadelphia, 1958, J. B. Lippincott Co., pp. 3-18.
3. Fuerst, Elinor V., and Wolff, La Verne: Fundamentals of nursing, ed. 2, Philadelphia, 1959, J. B. Lippincott Co., pp. 153-163, 167-190, 335-397.
4. Gray, Florence, and Little, Dolores: It's not just a matter of will power, American Journal of Nursing 60:101-103, Nov. 1960.

5. Harmer, Bertha, and Henderson, Virginia: Textbook of the principles and practice of nursing, ed. 5, New York, 1955, The Macmillan Co., pp. 407-423, 429-464.
6. Kaufman, Margaret A., and Brown, Dorothy E.: Pain wears many faces, American Journal of Nursing 61:48-51, Jan. 1961.
7. Kelly, Cordelia W.: Nurses, nutrition and the general public, American Journal of Nursing 58:217-218, Feb. 1958.
8. Krause, Marie V.: Food, nutrition and diet therapy, ed. 3, Philadelphia, 1961, W. B. Saunders Co., pp. 115-180.
9. MacGregor, Frances C.: Social sciences in nursing, New York, 1960, Russell Sage Foundation, pp. 181-202.
10. McHenry, Earl W.: Basic nutrition, Philadelphia, 1957, J. B. Lippincott Co., pp. 234-257, 290-330.
11. McClain, Esther M., and Gragg, Shirley H.: Scientific principles in nursing, ed. 4, St. Louis, 1962, The C. V. Mosby Co., pp. 160-188.
12. Monge, Bertha, and Throssell, Dorothy: Good nutrition on a low income, American Journal of Nursing 60:1290-1292, Sept. 1960.
13. Mowry, Lillian: Basic nutrition and diet therapy for nurses, ed. 2, St. Louis, 1962, The C. V. Mosby Co., pp. 1-82.
14. Newton, Marjorie E.: Nutrition in an associate degree program, Nursing Outlook 9:678-679, Nov. 1961.
15. Nordmark, Madelyn T., and Rohweder, Anne W.: Science principles applied to nursing, Philadelphia, 1959, J. B. Lippincott Co., pp. 71-85, 124-129, 234-276.

Chapter 15

Administration of medications

A fantastic increase in the use and the diversity of chemotherapeutic agents has come with the explosion of scientific knowledge. Almost every patient receives medication of some type. The time when any one nurse could know all there was to know about every medication commonly given has long passed. In addition to the increase in the number of medications, the names by which they are known may vary widely, for most drug companies do not use the generic names of drugs but market them under trade names. For example, norepinephrine or levarterenol is marketed under the trade name of Levophed; a similar preparation, used for the same purposes, is Aramine bitartrate. The administration of medications, a dependent nursing function that involves carrying out medical directives, occupies a considerable portion of nursing time. Because medications represent an almost universal experience for patients, the basic guidelines for their use is included in the unit on basic needs of patients.

The administration of medications is an area of nursing responsibility in which legal implications are relatively easy to pinpoint. The nurse who administers a medication is legally responsible; if the wrong medication, or the wrong dosage is given, the nurse may well be held liable. This means that the administration of medications can never be a routine performance, perfunctorily carried out.

In general, medications are used for three purposes: (1) preventive, (2) palliative, and (3) restorative. Some drugs, such as vitamins, may also be used for all three purposes. Preventive medications include those used to prevent disease or to promote health and include such agents as vitamin preparations, vaccine to prevent smallpox, diphtheria toxoid to prevent diphtheria, typhoid vaccine to prevent typhoid fever, and similar preparations. Other diseases that can be prevented by vaccine include cholera, pertussis, Rocky Mountain spotted fever, and yellow fever. Perhaps the most dramatic development in this area is the discovery of a poliomyelitis vaccine which represents the first great breakthrough in preventing viral infections.

Chemotherapeutic agents, when used for palliative reasons, serve to control symptoms while not directly modifying the disease process. Morphine, the classic narcotic, is often used for its ability to relieve pain. The morphine does not reduce the *cause* of pain, but it does reduce the sensation of pain and is thus valuable for the control of this particular symptom. Some medications, however, are used for restorative purposes because they directly affect the pathological processes. Digitalis, used to improve and strengthen the contraction of failing heart muscle, is an example. Vitamin C, administered to remove the symptoms of scurvy, is another example. Antibiotics also are specific, for they inhibit the growth of microorganisms, and varying agents are usually effective against specific microorganisms. Penicillin, for example, is effective against pneumococcus, *Streptococcus viridans*, *Treponema pallidum*, and other organisms. Streptomycin is effective against *Bacterium coli*, Friedländer's bacillus, and tubercule bacillus, among others. Certain antibiotics are classified as "broad spectrum," because they are effective against many kinds of microorganisms. With few exceptions (psittacosis, trachoma, and lymphogranuloma), antibiotics are ineffectual against viral diseases. However, in clinical medical practice, antibiotics are prescribed in viral infections to prevent complications due to secondary bacterial infections. The evaluation of the effectiveness of any medication must be made in the light of the purpose for which it is administered.

Medications are usually classified according to their physiological action or the purpose for which they are used. Because useful knowledge is organized knowledge, it is wise to learn about medications by grouping them as they are met and used in the clinical area or studies in relation to patient nursing care. For example, tranquilizing drugs are used to relieve anxiety or uncomfortable emotional states. Included in this grouping are such drugs as chlorpromazine (trade name, Thorazine), perphenazine (trade name, Trilafon), and thioridazine (trade name, Mellaril). Anticoagulant drugs, used to increase the clotting time of the blood, include such drugs as bishydroxycoumarin (trade name, Dicumarol) and phenindione (trade names, Danilone and Hedulin). Learning about medications by grouping should include learning the following about each drug: generic name, trade name(s), route of administration, range of and usual dosage, physiological action, contraindications, and signs of untoward or toxic effects. If untoward or toxic effects do occur, the specific measures to be taken should also be determined. For example, if the patient's pulse drops below 60, digitalis is withheld; or if a patient taking antibiotics develops a rash, the medication is withheld until the physician reviews the matter. In addition, wherever a medication has a narrow safety margin, such as morphine or digitalis, the range of dosage and the signs of untoward or toxic reactions should be thoroughly learned.

Before learning to administer medications, a knowledge of some of the standard abbreviations and symbols commonly used in ordering drugs must be mastered. The only way to learn these terms is through memorization. The most commonly used abbreviations are given in Table 9.

Table 9. *Standard abbreviations and symbols used in ordering drugs*

Abbreviation	Latin	English translation
āā	*Ana*	Of each
a.c.	*Ante cibum*	Before meals
ad lib.	*Ad libitum*	At pleasure
b.i.d.	*Bis in die*	Twice daily
c̄	*Cum*	With
elix.	*Elixir*	Elixir
ext.	*Extractum*	Extract; external
Gm.	*Gramma*	Gram
gr.	*Granum*	Grain
gtt.	*Gutta*	Drop
h.s.	*Hara somni*	At bedtime
I.M.		Intramuscular
I.V.		Intravenous
Pil.	*Pilula*	Pills
p.c.	*Post ciba*	After eating
P.O.	*Per os*	By mouth
p.r.n.	*Pro re nata*	According to circumstances
q.d.	*Quaque die*	Every day
q.i.d.	*Quarter in die*	Four times a day
q. 1(2,3,4)h.	*Quaque un* (etc.) *hora*	Every 1,2,3,4 hours
q.s.	*Quartum satis*	A sufficient quantity
Rx	*Recipe*	Take
s̄	*Sine*	Without
S.O.S.	*Si opus sit*	If it is needed
ss	*Semis*	A half
Sol.	*Solutio*	Solution
Stat.	*Station*	At once
sub. q.		Subcutaneous
t.i.d.	*Ter in die*	Three times a day
tab.	*Tabella*	Tablet
tr., tinct.	*Tinctura*	Tincture

There are three common sources of information concerning medication ordered for patients: one primary and two secondary. The primary source is the doctor's order sheet; the secondary sources, and therefore not completely reliable, are the Kardex and the medication tickets. It is helpful, of course, if all three are legible.

The doctor's order sheet contains, in addition to identification data concerning the patient, the date of order, the medication, the dosage, the time or times of administration (i.e., h.s., b.i.d., etc.), and, if other than the usual, the route of administration. Some medications are given usually by mouth and some usually by injection. In such instances, it is common for the physician who writes the order to assume that the nurse knows this. The one unfailing law is—when in doubt, ask questions. If the handwriting is not legible, if the dose is not clear, if the route of administration is uncertain, if the dose seems too large or too small, ask questions. It is easier to ask *a priori* than to have to explain *post facto*.

The Kardex contains (or should contain) the patient's name, age, diag-

| | | | THE COMMUNITY HOSPITAL AT GLEN COVE / GLEN COVE, N. Y. / PHYSICIAN'S ORDERS | | | |

O. S.
130-16 Atlantic Ave.
Freeport, L. I.
Adm. 6/1/63   3621458
Dr. Q. B. J.
↑ Prot. - 45 yrs.
Single   Room 107

Date	Time	Ordered by		How often	Date effective
6/1/63	4 pm	R. B. J.	1) Oxygen tent Stat		6/1/63
			2) Demerol 100 mg. Stat		
			then 75 mg.	q. 4. h.	
			3) Coronary precautions		
			4) N. P. O.		
			5) E. K. G. at bedside Stat		
			6) Sed. rate		
			7) Blood Cholesteral		

Fig. 24. The physician's order sheet is a primary source of information on the patient's therapy.

nosis, treatments, and medications. Sometimes it may also include specific approaches to nursing care or specific patient nursing problems. The Kardex is, however, a brief summary of some of the material in the patient's chart and is of value only if kept up to date. Otherwise, it can represent a certain potential danger through carrying directions for medications or treatments that have been discontinued. The Kardex should therefore be handled with the caution it deserves.

The medication ticket contains the patient's name, location, medication, dosage, route of administration, time for administration, and date ordered. It may or may not indicate when the medication is to be terminated or under what conditions to terminate. The medication ticket, like the Kardex, is a secondary source, and it, too, must be kept up to date in the interest of patient safety. In using secondary sources, as with primary, the law remains the same—when in doubt, ask questions.

Since the ordering and administration of medications follows certain routines established by, and all too often unique to, the particular agency, the nurse responsible for administering medications should have a knowledge of the following:

1. The system for noting new doctor's orders
2. How medication tickets are identified for differing hours of administration

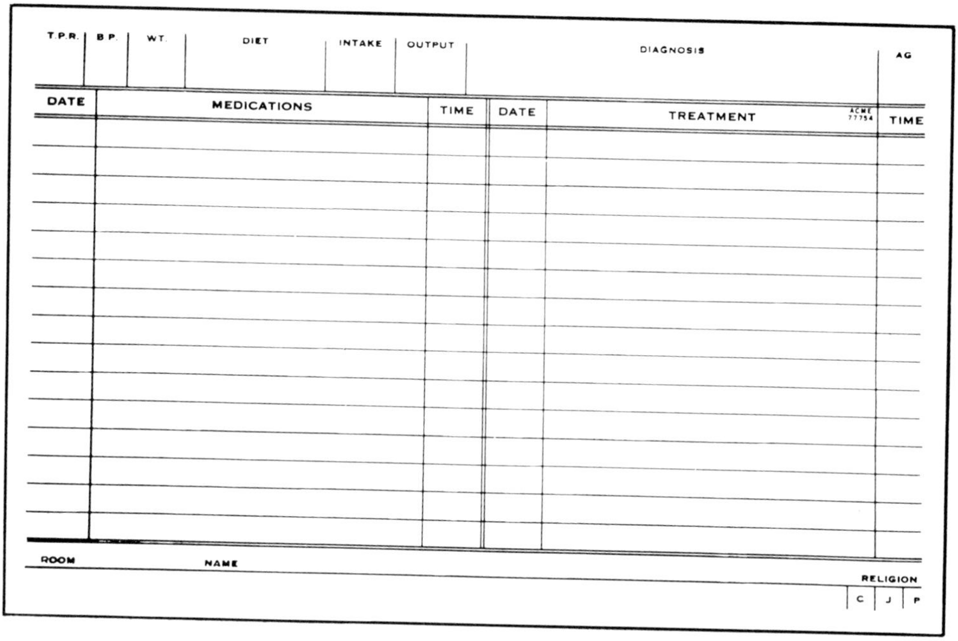

T.P.R.	B.P.	WT.	DIET	INTAKE	OUTPUT	DIAGNOSIS	AG

DATE	MEDICATIONS	TIME	DATE	TREATMENT	TIME

ROOM NAME RELIGION C J P

ACME 77754

A

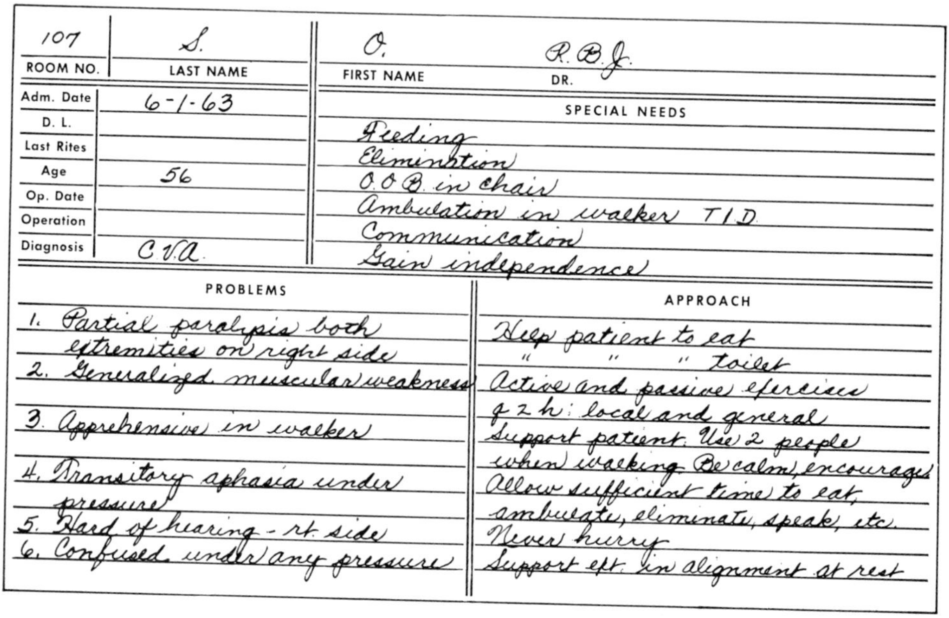

ROOM NO.	LAST NAME	FIRST NAME	DR.
107	S.	O.	R.B.J.

		SPECIAL NEEDS
Adm. Date	6-1-63	Feeding
D. L.		Elimination
Last Rites		O.O.B. in chair
Age	56	Ambulation in walker T.I.D.
Op. Date		Communication
Operation		Gain independence
Diagnosis	C.V.A.	

PROBLEMS	APPROACH
1. Partial paralysis both extremities on right side	Help patient to eat
	" " " toilet
2. Generalized muscular weakness	Active and passive exercises q 2 h: local and general
3. Apprehensive in walker	Support patient. Use 2 people when walking. Be calm, encourage.
4. Transitory aphasia under pressure	Allow sufficient time to eat, ambulate, eliminate, speak, etc.
5. Hard of hearing - rt. side	Never hurry
6. Confused under any pressure	Support ext. in alignment at rest

B

Fig. 25. A, The Kardex provides a space for a summary of treatments and medications. **B,** The Kardex may provide one original source of information: specific points in nursing care.

Southern Missionary College
Division Of Nursing, Library
711 Lake Estelle Drive
Orlando, Florida 32803

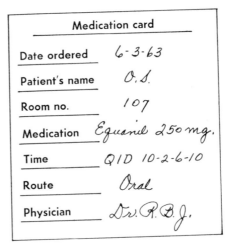

Fig. 26. Medication cards must carry specific information. They are dangerous unless accurate, up to date, and legible.

3. The usual hours for the administration of medications
4. How and when medication tickets and the Kardex are checked against doctor's orders
5. How medications are discontinued
6. Where information concerning new drugs is kept
7. What system is used for the identification of patients
8. What the system of organization is for the placement of drugs in the medicine cabinet
9. The formulary system used in the particular setting

In the administration of medications, there are certain critical factors that need special emphasis for patient safety: identification of the right patient, the right medication, the right dosage, the right route of administration, the right technique, and, when it is significant, the right time.

Any method that assures that the right patient receives a medication ordered for him is the right method. This is best accomplished by knowing patients, and while learning to know patients by their correct names is not usually considered part of the functional assignment to medications, it should be. Checking name bands, names on beds, asking the patient his name, and asking other patients or personnel who know the patient are helpful. Knowing when patients are disoriented, knowing those patients who have a wicked sense of humor, or knowing patients who have real personality problems can also help in avoiding mistakes. There is, however, no substitute for knowing individual patients to ensure that the right patient receives his medication.

Being certain that the right medication is given involves being sure what the right medication is and that the medication poured or prepared is the medication ordered. If there is any doubt about what the medication in question is, the doctor's order sheet should be checked. If this leaves any doubt, the physician should be consulted. It is this need to have a solid written reference that underlies the general practice of refusing to carry out verbal orders from a physician except in emergencies. The margin for error is much greater when verbal orders are accepted.

Having identified the correct medication to be given, the next step is to be certain that this is the medication that is prepared for administration. If a label is not clear, remove the container from circulation. The keynote here is alertness. Leaning upon a perfunctory habit is no substitute. Reading the bottle label when picking up the medication, reading it again when pouring or just before or after, and reading the label again when returning the bottle to the medicine cabinet protects no one if it is a routine habit carried out without thinking. Under such circumstances, a label read incorrectly the first time will probably be read incorrectly the second and third times as well. Whatever system is used (for example, checking the medicine ticket against the label), is effective only when the eyes and the mind are both focused on the medicine ticket and the label.

The next step requires the right dosage, and it is this step, perhaps, that is the commonest area of error. The sources of error are inaccurate computation, inaccurate transposition from apothecary to metric system or vice versa, and lack of knowledge concerning the usual dosage of the medication. Therefore, a nursing responsibility of considerable significance is to know how to add, subtract, multiply, and divide, and also to know how to handle fractions, ratios, and decimal points. The transposition of dosages from apothecary to metric or metric to apothecary is made simple by the numerous devices for this purpose that are available from many sources. Any doubt about usual dosages should be resolved by seeking accurate information.

The right route of administration and the right technique are interrelated. Medications that are injected (subcutaneous, intramuscular, or intravenous) require sterile technique. Medications given orally require cleanliness. There are a number of frequently used ways of administering drugs: orally, hypodermically, intramuscularly, intravenously, rectally, topically (on the surface, such as on the skin or in the eyes). Less commonly used routes of administration are intrathecal (via spinal canal), sublingual, and intradermal. Nurses are responsible for administering medications orally, hypodermically, intramuscularly, rectally, topically, sublingually, and by inhalation. Intravenous, intradermal, and intrathecal medications are given by physicians, although nurses may add medications to an intravenous infusion initiated by a physician or by technicians trained to do intravenous work. Sterile technique is routinely indicated in hypodermic, intramuscular, intravenous, intradermal, and intrathecal mode. The technique—medical or surgical asepsis—is adapted to the route of administration.

In addition to the other "rights" that ensure patient safety, the right time of administration may be important. Although all medications t.i.d. may be listed for 10 A.M., 2 P.M., 6 P.M., or 9 A.M., 1 P.M., 5 P.M., it is not usually necessary that they be given at the exact time. As a matter of fact, it would be impossible to do so unless there were one nurse for every medication. From the point of view of time, the time *interval* here is significant. The specific time is a factor in some instances, however. Examples are medications ordered for severe pain when a half hour's to an hour's delay could cause unnecessary discomfort, medications ordered before or after a meal when the relationship to the time of the meal is important, medications ordered to induce sleep, insulin ordered at specified times, or preoperative medications. Such orders should be noted and receive priority in administration.

The administration of oral medications is relatively simple provided the right patient is identified and the right medication in the right dosage

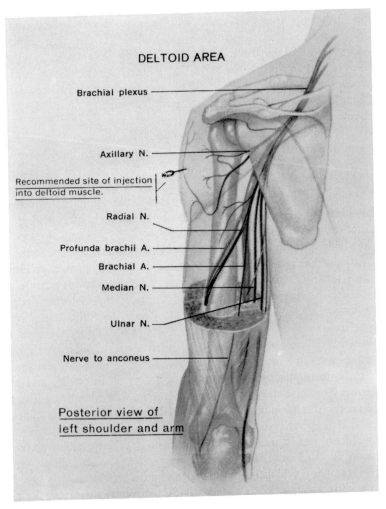

Fig. 27. The deltoid muscle is commonly used for hypodermic injection and may also be used for intramuscular injection. (From Spectrum; courtesy Charles Pfizer & Co., Inc., New York, N. Y.)

is given. Special precautions relate to the extent to which the patient is able and willing to accept his therapy and to the nature of the drug given. If the patient is unable to assume responsibility for his own behavior, then the nurse must remain with the patient and administer the medication. If the drug is an irritating one, it should be given after meals or be diluted with fruit juice or milk, if permitted, to provide protection to the stomach or intestinal mucosa. If the medication is given for cough and if part of its effect results from coating of the mucous membrane of the pharynx, it should not be followed by water.

The administration of medication by hypodermic injection (subcutaneously) requires the use of sterile technique. The skin at the site of injection is briskly prepared with alcohol or Zephiran. The most common site of injection is the outer aspect of the upper arm, although the anterior aspect of the thigh and the abdomen may also be used.

The needle, which may range from ½ inch to 1 inch in length and from 24 to 26 in gauge, is inserted at a 45° to 60° angle. The plunger of the syringe should be pulled back to check for accidental needle point insertion into a blood vessel. If blood appears in the syringe, the needle should be withdrawn, discarded, and another sterile needle reinserted. The medication

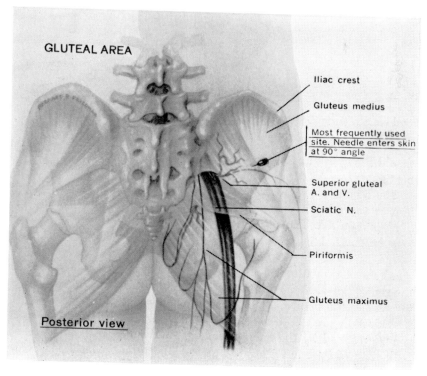

GLUTEAL AREA

Iliac crest

Gluteus medius

Most frequently used site. Needle enters skin at 90° angle

Superior gluteal A. and V.

Sciatic N.

Piriformis

Gluteus maximus

Posterior view

Fig. 28. The upper outer quadrant of the buttocks is one of the most common sites of intramuscular injections. The relation of this site to major nerves and vessels is shown. (From Spectrum; courtesy Charles Pfizer & Co., Inc., New York, N. Y.)

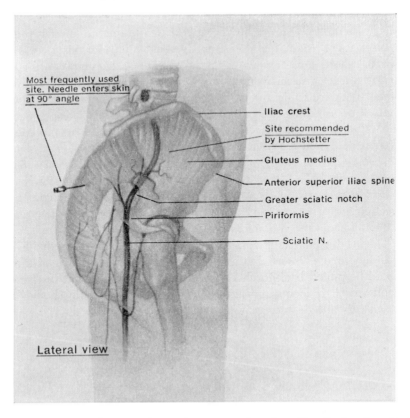

Fig. 29. Lateral view of commonly used intramuscular sites. The Hockstetter site is the most recent one and is recommended because there is less chance of damaging nerves and blood vessels. (From Spectrum; courtesy Charles Pfizer & Co., Inc., New York, N. Y.)

should be injected with smooth, steady pressure in order not to traumatize the tissues.

The administration of an intramuscular injection follows the same pattern as any other injection (i.e., sterile technique, including skin preparation) is required. The site of injection is into the muscle, and therefore, a longer needle, 1 inch to 2 inches in length and usually from 21 to 23 in gauge, is used. The most common site of injection is the upper outer quadrant of the buttocks, although a new site is currently being utilized— the ventrogluteal site. With the patient lying on his back, the area is located by placing the hand on the iliac crest, stretching the middle finger sidewise dorsally, and keeping the iliac crest palpable, pressing below it. The triangle formed by the iliac crest, the index finger, and the middle finger is the site of injection. The new site of injection is considered safer since there is less chance of damaging major blood vessels or nerves. Aspiration to ensure that the needle is not inserted intravascularly before injecting the medication is of major importance in intramuscular injections. Because many preparations administered via this route are not physiologically compatible with body fluids, they are a threat to patient safety. Damage to the sciatic nerve is not generally associated with the nature of particular medications. All medications may damage this nerve by increasing pressure in closely adjacent areas. Therefore, the site of injection is relatively circumscribed if trauma to nerves and major blood vessels is to be avoided.

In all uses of injection as a means of administering medications, the length of the needle used is affected by the size and condition of the patient, and the gauge of the needle is determined by the consistency of the fluid to be given. A thin, emaciated patient is protected by the use of a shorter needle, and an obese patient is protected by the use of a longer needle. Thicker solutions require a needle with a large lumen, whereas a needle with a small lumen can be used to administer free-flowing solutions. When in-

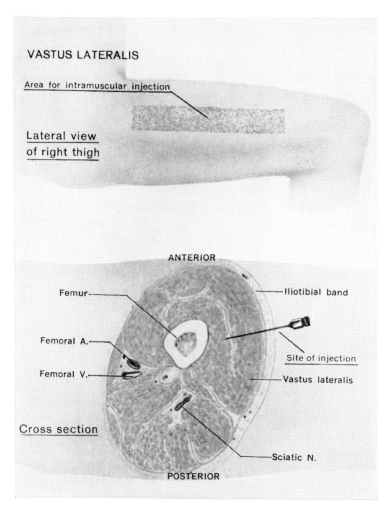

Fig. 30. The recommended site for intramuscular injection in the thigh. (From Spectrum; courtesy Charles Pfizer & Co., Inc., New York, N. Y.)

jections will be repeated or given frequently, the site of injection should be rotated to prevent permanent tissue damage at the site.

Medications may be administered by inhalation for either local or systemic effect. The two major types of inhalants utilized are (1) moist steam containing the prescribed drug and (2) nebulized drugs, i.e., drugs divided into very fine particles by the pressure of a gas (air or oxygen). Both methods bring the medication in contact with the mucous membrane of the respiratory tract where the rich blood supply makes absorption comparatively easy.

Other methods of drug administration that rely upon contact with mucous membrane include the sublingual (under the tongue) and rectal routes. Neither method is extensively used today. Exceptions include drugs used specifically, such as nitroglycerine tablets (sublingually) for angina pectoris, aminophylline suppositories for pulmonary edema, analgesic suppositories for rectal conditions, and certain hypnotic agents inserted rectally when oral administration is contraindicated.

The recording of medications on the patient's chart should be *accurate* and should include clearly the medication, dosage, time given, by whom given, and the patient's reaction, whether toward or untoward.

Part of the nurse's responsibility is observation for evaluation of the effectiveness of the chemotherapeutic regimen. In addition to knowing the purpose for which medications are given and possible untoward or toxic signs, the nurse must also give consideration to other factors that may influence the patient's response. Supportive measures may enhance or interfere with the intended drug action. Medications administered to promote sleep can be enhanced by environmental quiet and patient comfort and can be nullified by anxiety, noise, and physical discomfort. Patients may have idiosyncrasies to certain drugs and be unable to tolerate them. Allergic reactions are particularly important, and if any patient is known to have an allergy to any type of medication, this information should be clearly indicated in a place where personnel can see it. This may be on the patient's chart or bed, but always where it may be clearly seen.

In some institutions, new approaches to the administration of medications are being tried. In general, the new approaches rest upon placing responsibility for the preparation of medications with the pharmacy and placing responsibility for participating in taking medications as ordered with the patient. Medications are prepared for individual patients and sent to the patient care unit from the pharmacy ready to administer. In some instances, patients are responsible for taking the medications as ordered without the immediate supervision of nursing personnel. Both approaches have been favorably reported.

In summary, patient safety is maintained by adhering to the following guidelines designed to prevent error:

1. Be certain the patient is the "right" patient.
2. Be certain the medication is the "right" medication.
3. Be certain the dosage of the medication is the "right" dosage.

4. Be certain the route of administration is the "right" route, i.e., oral medication by mouth and injections by the appropriate route.
5. Be certain that the time of administration is "right," i.e., at spaced intervals if ordered every four hours or before meals if ordered thus.
6. Don't give medications if you have not prepared them.
7. Don't chart medications if you have not given them.
8. Use sterile technique for all injections.
9. Be sure equipment used is in good condition, for example, that needles are sharp.
10. If medications are not labeled or clearly labeled, do not use them.
11. Do not administer new or experimental drugs without finding out what is known about them.
12. Do not accept verbal orders except in emergencies.
13. Do not treat medication tickets and Kardex as though they were doctor's order sheets.
14. Do not assume that the doctor's order sheet is always completely correct.
15. *Know* the drugs administered—physiological action, dosage, toxic signs, contraindications, and indications for withholding or termination.
16. If a drug or medication has a narrow safety range, learn thoroughly all there is to know about it.
17. Be certain drugs are properly stored; i.e., refrigerate those that need it, place with proper category in medicine cabinet, and keep narcotics in narcotic cabinet.
18. If there is any doubt—don't! Ask questions first.

BIBLIOGRAPHY

1. Cohen, Lawrence S., and Cluff, Leighton E.: The sulfonamides, American Journal of Nursing **61**:54-58, June 1961.
2. Edwards, Lillian G., and Barker, Kenneth N.: Pharmacy notes for nurses, American Journal of Nursing **62**:68-69, Oct. 1962.
3. Ellison, Rose Ruth: Treating cancer with antimetabolites, American Journal of Nursing **62**:79-82, Nov. 1962.
4. Garb, Solomon, and Crim, Betty Jean: Pharmacology and patient care, New York, 1962, Springer Publishing Co., pp. 4-66.
5. Hall, James Whitney, III: Drug therapy in infectious diseases, American Journal of Nursing **61**:56-60, Feb. 1961.
6. Hansen, Daniel J.: Intramuscular injection injuries and complications, American Journal of Nursing **63**:99-101, April 1963.
7. Hershey, Nathan: Question that drug order, American Journal of Nursing **63**:96-97, Jan. 1963.
8. McClain, M. Esther, and Gragg, Shirley H.: Scientific principles in nursing, ed. 4, St. Louis, 1962, The C. V. Mosby, pp. 247-274.
9. Slomaker, Marian Ruth: Administering drugs from a central drug room, American Journal of Nursing **62**:108-110, Dec. 1962.
10. Unger, Donald L.: Nonallergic drug reactions, American Journal of Nursing, **63**:64-65, Jan. 1963.
11. Wempe, Bertha M.: The new and the old intramuscular injection sites, American Journal of Nursing **61**:56-57, Sept. 1961.

Overt nursing problems

Chapter 16

Reactions of the patient to disease processes

"The health of the cell depends on the state of its fluid environment, and, for the maintenance of the good health of the cells, this fluid must be kept fairly constant as regards its temperature, osmotic pressure and chemical composition."* When anything happens to disturb the health of the cells, the body reacts to restore this constant. "Thus we see that the body's efforts to re-establish equilibrium result in a series of positive activities of which the patient becomes aware. These are the symptoms of . . . disease."*

BASIC PATHOLOGICAL PROCESSES†

Cell health can be threatened from the external or internal environment, by physicial or chemical means or by living organisms such as pathogenic bacteria. Trauma as the result of an accident is an example of the physical source of cell damage; the inhalation of carbon monoxide, which displaces oxygen in association with hemoglobin in the red blood cell, is an example of the chemical source of danger. The invasion of the lungs by the tubercle bacillus is an example of the danger from living organisms. The human body reacts by passive changes at the site of the damage and by compensatory changes designed to restore equilibrium. When, for example, hemorrhage occurs, the body reacts to restore blood volume and replace lost red blood cells by constriction of small arterioles, contraction of the spleen, increased pulse rate, and decreased blood coagulation time. The passive changes that occur in disease include physical injuries, degeneration or necrosis of body cells, and hypofunction of the affected part or parts. The reactive changes include inflammation, a general response of hyperfunction of unaffected tissue in an effort to restore equilibrium, and the patient's emotional reaction to his illness. In general, the nurse's function relates to carrying out

---

*Apperly, Frank L.: Patterns of disease, Philadelphia, 1951, J. B. Lippincott Co., p. 1.
†This discussion on basic pathological processes is based on the approach used by Apperly, Frank L.: Patterns of disease, Philadelphia, 1951, J. B. Lippincott Co.

ordered therapy designed to remove or to neutralize the cause of disease, supporting the patient's compensatory reactions, providing rest for the diseased area, and providing supportive care for the patient's emotional response to his problem.

For the individual cell to remain healthy, it must have a continuous supply of food, oxygen, minerals, enzymes, and other substances necessary for the maintenance of life. The cell must also be able to utilize, i.e., metabolize, such ingredients. It must have the hormonal and nervous regulation that makes the metabolic process possible, and, finally, waste products must be removed from the cell. Passive changes in the cell will occur if deficiencies exist in any of the four essentials for health.

Atrophy, or the wasting away of mature cells, occurs when the cell remains healthy, but the supply of necessary materials is inadequate. This can happen as a result of disease, as a result of anything that interferes with adequate circulation, or as a result of inadequate innervation.

If there is any interference with the metabolic process in the cell, food materials may accumulate within the cell wall. The first materials to accumulate are carbohydrates and proteins; the cell increases its fluid content to dilute the accumulation, and the stage of cloudy swelling is reached. If the process continues, droplets of fat appear in the cell, and the stage of fatty degeneration is reached. Degeneration, in this sense, means deterioration in which the cell's vitality is diminished. The process can terminate in cell death.

If the area involved in cell death is a small localized one, it is identified as an area of necrosis; if the area involved is extensive, it is identified as gangrene. A necrosed area may liquefy and be absorbed, or it may coagulate. If the necrosed area does coagulate, immediately adjacent cells may digest it, or cells (i.e., macrophages) from other parts of the body may digest it, or the area may become encapsulated.

One of the body's most important reactive changes, one that serves as a major defense against bacteria and foreign bodies, is inflammation, with its cardinal signs of pain, heat, redness, and swelling. The symptoms result from vascular changes designed to localize and to neutralize or to destroy the invader. When the invading bacteria or foreign body comes in contact with a cell or cells, an increased blood supply immediately surrounds and infiltrates the affected portion. The local macrophagic cells, or histiocytes of the reticuloendothelial system, are reinforced by a greatly increased number of microcytes, neutrophilic polymorphonuclear leukocytes, hastily discharged from the bone marrow. Both histiocytic and microcytic cells are capable of phagocytosis, i.e., they engulf, destroy, and digest bacteria and foreign particles.

The attraction of cells capable of phagocytosis to the invaded area has a name, positive chemotaxis, but the mechanism of the operation is not understood. Because the invaded area has a marked increase in blood supply, and because more fluid is taken from the blood stream than is returned to it, the swelling, heat, and redness result from the hyperemia, or increased supply of oxygenated blood. Pain results from increased pressure upon nerve endings that are sensitive to pain stimulus. If the bacteria or foreign bodies are controlled at this point, the process ends and the body part affected returns to normal. If not, the blood flow slows down and the emigration of leukocytes from the blood stream to the affected part accelerates.

The next step is a slowing of the blood stream until it moves only with the pulse beat, and then finally cessation of the blood flow. When this occurs, the blood in the affected area coagulates and the part dies (necrosis). As the leukocytes in the area decompose, they liberate free enzymes that digest or dissolve the necrosed part, and pus is formed, leading to abscess development. The abscess ruptures, either spontaneously or by inducement, and granulation and healing occur. Granulation tissue is later converted to a fibrous scar.

Inflammation can be acute or chronic, localized or general. The process just described is an acute inflammation, local in type. Chronic inflammation can occur when the source of difficulty is mild but persistent or when an acute inflammation is not resolved. When the inflammation is not controlled at the local level, the bacteria and/or their toxins overwhelm local defenses and move through the circulatory system to invade the entire body. Septicemia (blood poisoning) or pyemia (a condition in which the body is infected with multiple local abscesses) may result.

The classic symptoms of inflammation are added to by interference with the function of the affected part. Inflammation occurring in the lungs, the eye, or the knee will present additional symptoms beyond those of inflammation, based upon the function of the part. Inflammation of the lungs will present problems in the exchange of oxygen and carbon dioxide between the blood stream and the alveoli. Inflammation of the eye will cause visual problems. Inflammation of the knee will present problems of locomotion. The combination of the character of the basic pathology, the function of the affected area of the body, and the patient's reaction to both of these constitute the pattern of any specific disease.

On occasions when there is an increased demand for function on the part of an organ or tissue, the part reacts with an increase in size to support the increased function. This may be hypertrophy (an increase in the actual size of the cells) or hyperplasia (an increase in the number of cells). Along with the increase in size and function must go an increased blood supply. The causes of hypertrophy and hyperplasia are adaptive, compensatory, and hormonal. The enlarged leg muscles of the ballet dancer are an example of adaptive hypertrophy, for the dancer uses leg muscles a great deal more than the average person. When the blood vessels narrow and offer greater resistance to the flow of blood, the heart increases in size to carry the additional work load, and this also is adaptive hypertrophy. Because many organs respond to the stimulation of hormones, excessive stimulation can lead to hypertrophy. On the other hand, a deficiency in iodine, a constituent of thyroxin secreted by the thyroid gland, can lead to the familiar hypertrophy known as goiter, because the thyroid must work harder to meet body demand for thyroxin. Although hypertrophy and hyperplasia can adapt organs and tissues to carry increased functions, it must be remembered that excessive and long-continued overuse can lead to exhaustion, atrophy, and tissue death.

There is a type of hyperplasia, or increase in cells, that is uncontrolled, serves no real physiological purpose, and represents what appears to be a disturbance of the normal growth process. Such new cell masses are called tumors, and they may be benign or malignant. When the tumor grows slowly, the cells resemble normal cells, and the growth is encapsulated by fibrous tissue, the tumor is benign. Benign tumors usually cause difficulties only for mechanical reasons—their pressure on surrounding tissue produces symptoms. Malignant tumors, on the other hand, grow rapidly and the cells produced have little resemblance to normal cells. Malignant tumors, usually referred to as cancer, invade the surrounding tissue rapidly and spread directly as well as indirectly via the circulatory and lymph systems. Secondary colonies of new cells that spread to other parts of the body are called metastases. Malignant tumors frequently result in death unless early diagnosis and treatment intervene. Death results from destruction of vital organs, destruction of blood vessels, causing hemorrhage, systemic debilitation that increases the patient's susceptibility to infection, systemic reaction to the absorption of the products of cell breakdown and necrosis, or to starvation or dehydration as a result of lowered intake.

The exact mechanism of the development of cancer is not yet clear, although recent discoveries about the structure of genes seems to promise much in terms of understanding. A number of predisposing causes, such as chronic irritation and exposure to carcinogens such as coal tar products, have been identified. The technical terms used to describe tumors are based upon the tissue from which they arise. The commonest forms of cancer are carcinoma, derived from epithelial tissue, and sarcoma, derived from connective tissue. Examples of benign tumors include fibroma (from fibrous or connective tissue), lipoma (from fatty tissue), myoma (from muscle tissue), and osteoma (from bone tissue).

PATIENT PERCEPTIONS OF DISEASE PROCESS

The patient's perception of his illness is most often experienced through the signs and symptoms produced by the basic pathological process rather than by direct perception of the process itself. This is not to deny that many patients can often diagnose their illnesses quite accurately. But the patient's awareness is triggered by pain, fever, weakness and malaise, nausea and vomiting, diarrhea, and similar occurrences. The physiological responses of the body to disease, the signs and symptoms produced, is most likely to be the signal that alerts the patient to seek help.

Pain

Pain is a complex phenomenon, only partially understood. Although theoretically the sensation of pain should be felt only in those areas of the body that are innervated with pain receptors, there seems to be sufficient evidence to indicate that pain can be felt on a purely psychological basis. Physically determined pain, however, is dependent upon the adequate functioning of nerve endings and pathways. The innervation of areas of the body by pain receptors varies widely in extent. The skin, for example, is liberally supplied, whereas the viscera and the brain are not. In fact, complete agreement on the mechanism of the production of visceral pain has not been reached. The periosteum that surrounds bone is also liberally supplied with pain receptors, while compact bone is not. Pain receptors do not respond selectively to type of stimulus but rather to intensity, regardless of whether the stimulus is thermal, chemical, or mechanical.

Pain initiates a response that is protective in character, designed to alert and to remove, if possible, injurious stimuli. Reflex actions to pain are withdrawal, the subordination of other reflexes, and the overriding of voluntary control. Pain is thus protective in nature, causing withdrawal from the painful stimuli, such as the reflex removal of a hand from a hot stove, or sounding a danger signal of threat or injury, such as the pain that accompanies a duodenal ulcer.

Pain itself also varies widely in type. Injury to the body surface tends to produce an initial sharp, pricking type of pain, followed by a slower, burning type of pain. Pain either can be felt at the area affected or can be referred to other parts of the body. A good example of the latter is the chest pain that radiates down the left arm when the heart suffers damage. Pain can be sharp or dull, constant or intermittent, mild or severe, local or diffuse, or cramping or steady.

People react differently to the experience of pain, and the response is influenced by the past experience and personality makeup as well as the so-called "pain threshold" of the individual and the prevailing cultural attitudes. Actually, the pain threshold, or the point at which the person perceives pain, is remarkably the same in any individual, although it varies widely from individual to individual. Patients responding to the same painful stimuli may differ sharply on the degree of intensity of the stimulus at which they become aware of pain.

Cultural attitudes in regard to the ability to tolerate pain and the freedom to express it also vary widely. Many puberty rites in some of the older civilizations feature a test of the ability of the adolescent boy to tolerate pain without overt response as evidence of having achieved mature manhood. "To bear it like a man" illustrates a fairly common cultural behavior norm expected of the male of the species. On the other hand, other cultural patterns (for example, some of those in the Southern Mediterranean area) encourage the expression and dramatization of pain.

The final factor that determines individual response to an expression of pain relates to the kind of person who experiences it. Some people complain bitterly; some people "grin and bear it." Some people are frightened by pain; some people are not. Some people acknowledge pain; some people deny it. At one time or another in her career, the nurse will see almost every possible response there is to pain. This individual variation in response occurs even in the presence of intractable pain, found sometimes in patients with central nervous system disease or in patients with terminal cancer.

Perhaps the most difficult type of pain to evaluate is pain that results from emotional conflict and cannot be identified with any specific injurious stimuli. Pain of such origin can involve any part of the body and can be of any character.

Pain, then, is a response to an injurious stimulus, physical or psychological in origin, varies greatly in type, character, and duration, may be direct or referred, and may elicit a widely varied kind of response from the persons who experience it.

The symptoms of pain, or clues to its existence, include subjective complaint, restlessness, irritability, withdrawal, tense facial expression, pallor, cold and clammy skin, anorexia, nausea and vomiting, muscle tension, spasm, guarding or limitation of movement, splinting a part, refusal to move, and increase in pulse rate and in respiratory rate.

Nursing responsibilities in relation to patients who suffer pain include the following broad areas:

1. The observation, assessment, and description of pain
2. Independent nursing measures to provide relief and reduction of pain
3. The administration of medical orders for the relief of pain
4. The prevention of pain

Pain may be detected by objective or subjective evidence. Keeping firmly in mind that patient reactions to pain may vary from Spartan endurance to exquisite agony at the slightest twinge and that the patient's personal reaction to pain is an important aspect to be observed, certain kinds of information need to be elicited. The location and extent of the pain is, of course, significant. What kind of pain it is—dull, burning, sharp, stabbing, cramping, or throbbing? Is it steady or intermittent? When does the pain occur, and under what circumstances does it increase or decrease? To what extent does the pain interfere with the patient's ability to carry out his usual activities? For example, does it restrict his motor activities or his interactions with other people? Is it mild or intense? How does the patient describe his pain and how does he react to it? Is he frightened and anxious, indifferent, or proud of his ability "to take it"?

Some of this information can be gained from the patient's subjective complaints and some by observation of the patient's general appearance and behavior. An additional and valuable source of information is the patient's relatives and visitors who know him fairly well. Such persons usually have the advantage of knowing the patient when he was not in pain and therefore have a valuable comparative basis for observations.

The recording and reporting of the patient's pain should be based upon the patient's own description, using his own words, and the additional evidence gathered by the nurse that adds relevant facts to improve interpretations. For example, the patient may report, "I have a sharp pain in my abdomen about every five or ten minutes," and the nurse may add, "The pain is more severe when the patient turns to the left than when he turns to the right" or "The pain seems to be less before the patient eats and worse after he eats." A change in the nature of pain should always be promptly reported, and severe, intense pain should always be reported. In addition, the sudden cessation of pain should be reported immediately.

The nurse may be able to make a substantial contribution to the control or lessening of pain through the use of physical hygiene measures, positioning, support of the affected part, environmental manipulation, distraction, and alleviation of anxiety. A patient in pain and physically uncomfortable to boot will find the pain accentuated. Tight bottom sheets and top sheets that are loose enough for comfort, back rubs or skin care, good oral hygiene, and massage are samples of the kind of physical hygiene measures that promote physical comfort and make an indirect but real contribution to the control of pain. Positioning also can help. Placing the patient in the position most comfortable for him, unless definitely contraindicated by his health problem, is the usual measure. Any position, however, should usually not be maintained for too long a period, with the exception of immobilized parts. Change of position may be indicated even though the change itself may temporarily increase pain. Support can also add to the patient's comfort; a patient with recent major abdominal surgery is usually more comfortable on his side with his back supported by a pillow.

A noisy, disorganized, and unpleasant physical environment can increase the patient's perception and awareness of pain. Adequate ventilation, air temperature that avoids the extremes, the reduction of noise, the limitation of the number of personnel and the number of times they enter the patient's environment, the adjustment of light to the patient's needs, the control of unpleasant odors, and the placement of equipment and utilities in places convenient for the patient can reduce the environmental accentuation of his problems.

If at all possible, the patient's interest should be focused on something other than his pain. If he has only this, pain can become overwhelming. Although it is not intended to imply that a checker game is an antidote for severe and intense pain, there are many instances in which the provision of recreational or diversional activities, based upon the patient's past interests and abilities, make pain more bearable.

The alleviation of anxiety when a patient is in pain also constitutes a significant nursing measure. Handling anxiety requires listening, paraphrasing, reflecting, using open-end questions, and, above all, showing sufficient interest in the patient as a person to keep channels of communication open for the patient to use when he is ready. Pain itself can arouse a great deal of anxiety.

Carrying out medical orders to relieve pain is another nursing responsibility. Such orders are usually chemotherapeutic in nature and involve the administration of analgesics and tranquilizers. Opium and its derivatives, or similar compounds such as Demerol, are commonly used for pain. Acetylsalicylic acid is often used for pain of musculoskeletal origin. Barbiturates may be used to make patients more susceptible to analgesic action, while ataractics, or tranquilizers, are used to relieve anxiety. In the administration of medications to relieve pain, the nurse evaluates the patient's response to medication, evaluates the need for more or less medication, uses judgment in the utilization of p.r.n. orders, and is sufficiently alert to the dangers of addiction that she does not rely solely on the administration of medications to relieve pain.

In addition to the alleviation of pain, the nurse has many opportunities in the normal course of events to prevent the occurrence of pain. Making sure that drainage tubes are patent, for example, can prevent the collection of fluid in the affected area, resulting in increased pressure accompanied by pain. Observing beginning signs of urinary retention and taking action to promote excretion of urine can prevent the pain of a distended bladder. Careful checking of any immobilizing device, such as traction, splints, and casts, can prevent unnecessary pain. Securing the padding around the edges of a cast can prevent pain. The use of bedrails for a restless or disoriented patient may prevent the pain and anxiety associated with a fall and broken bones. Using only that equipment which is in good working order also contributes to the prevention of pain. Sensitivity to patients' feelings and acceptance conveyed to patients can also do much to prevent pain.

In performing the many functions and responsibilities involved in carrying out medical therapy, the nurse herself may cause pain. The administration of intramuscular or subcutaneous injections, the irrigation of a body cavity, or the necessary change of position that may cause pain are examples. When the nurse herself must inflict pain, she can utilize psychological skills to reduce the patient's trauma and to indicate her understanding while explaining, at the patient's level, the need for such therapeutic measures. As part of emotional support, she can also be gentle, swift, and manually dexterous.

Fever

The maintenance of body temperature is dependent upon a balance of heat produced and heat lost. Actually, the human body possesses a rather remarkable homeostatic mechanism that maintains temperature for the most part in the narrow temperature range of the comfort zone* of 82.4° F. (28° C.) and 87.8° F. (31° C.) for men and 80.6° F. (27° C.) and 91.4° F. (33° C.) for women.† The difference for women is due to the thicker subcutaneous fat, which provides greater insulation.

Heat is produced in the body by any metabolic activity, but particularly by muscular activity and by the chemical reactions that take place in the

---

*Comfort zone temperature in this sentence refers to temperature of the environment, not body temperature.

†Best, Charles Herbert, and Taylor, Norman Burke: Physiological basis of medical practice, ed. 7, Baltimore, 1961, Williams & Wilkins Co., p. 890.

liver. Body temperature can also rise from the absorption of heat from the environment or from the ingestion of hot foods or liquids. Heat is lost from the body by radiation, conduction, and convection from skin, by warming and humidifying inspired air, by the evaporation of sweat and insensible perspiration, and, to a lesser extent, through urine and feces. Basically, the loss of heat, primarily via the skin, is achieved by the redistribution of blood, by variations in blood volume, and by increased circulation rate. When the body temperature rises and an increasing amount of heat must be dissipated, the amount of blood at the skin surface is increased and the quantity in the viscera reduced. This increases heat loss. When the temperature rises the blood volume increases, and when the temperature drops the blood volume decreases. The former promotes heat loss, and the latter conserves heat in the body. The increased circulation rate brings greater quantities of blood to the skin surface and promotes heat dissipation.

The homeostatic mechanisms that control body heat regulation are both nervous and chemical. It has been rather clearly demonstrated that a center of heat regulation control is found in the hypothalamus. The thyroid and adrenal hormones also influence regulation of body temperature. Whenever body temperature rises, adaptive responses increase heat dissipation. Whenever body temperature drops, adaptive responses increase heat production. A fairly common example of the latter is shivering in response to cold, when the muscular activity involved in shivering produces heat. Incidentally, the heat-regulating mechanisms are not fully developed at birth, so that the body temperature of children is considerably more irregular and unstable than that of adults.

Fever, or pyrexia, is an increase in body temperature above "normal" (usually considered 100° F. or 37.8° C.). The body response is considered defensive in nature, designed to make the internal environment uncomfortable or unsuitable for invading organisms or toxins. Fever results from infectious processes as a result of invading organisms, from toxic secretions of tissues injured in surgical intervention, from injuries to the nervous system, from dehydration, and from drugs or chemical substances. Although fever is believed to be essentially defensive and protective, it can, if it becomes high enough, become a threat to life. Temperatures that begin to reach toward 107° F. (41.6° C.) may themselves cause death.

The infectious fever is produced through the operation of the regulatory mechanism that conserves heat. Blood vessels in the body constrict, reducing heat loss through radiation and conduction. The body surface thus feels cold, the well-known sensation of a chill. Following this, shivering accompanying the chill produces additional heat that is retained. As the fever reaches its height and continues, the body mechanisms continue to keep heat loss reduced, while heat production becomes secondary. Usually the skin is flushed but hot and dry. Sweating and chills may occur, however. If the temperature rises too high for the patient's safety, measures such as an alcohol sponge or antipyretic medication may be ordered. When the infection is overcome, the temperature returns to normal, and the body dissipates the excess heat. If this happens very quickly, the resolution is called a "crisis"; but if it happens slowly, the resolution is called a "lysis."

The signs and symptoms of fever are usually systemic, for the entire body is involved. The temperature, of course, is elevated, and pulse and respirations are increased. Skin changes occur, and the skin may be flushed, warm, and dry or pale, cold, and clammy. Excessive perspiration may or may not occur. If there is excessive fluid loss and if fluid is not replaced by adequate intake, dehydration will occur, resulting in dry mucous membranes, dryness of the skin and loss of skin turgor, and reduced and concentrated urinary output.

If the temperature remains elevated and if the entire body metabolism continues to be disturbed, delirium may occur. The patient then becomes confused and restless and usually suffers from hallucinations (imaginary sense perceptions, such as hearing voices). Delusions, or fixed false beliefs (that someone is conspiring against him), may occur and tend to produce fear. The patient frequently misinterprets what goes on about him. At times, convulsions may also occur. In addition to the overt sign of fever, the patient subjectively will indicate directly or indirectly considerable discomfort.

The major nursing responsibilities in regard to the care of a patient with an elevated temperature include the following:

1. Observing and evaluating patient status
2. Providing fluid and nutrition intake
3. Providing adequate rest
4. Using physical comfort measures to improve patient status
5. Using environmental manipulation to contribute to rest
6. Allaying patient anxiety
7. Carrying out medical orders

The observation of patients with an elevated temperature serves the primary purpose of evaluating patient status to determine "when" and "what type of" medical intervention is needed. Vital signs are important, including temperature. Temperature needs constant evaluation, because an elevation beyond 106° F. or a long-continued elevation may become a danger to life rather than a physiological defense that protects it. Pulse and respiration, which are increased in rate during fever, must be closely observed. If the pulse becomes thready, very weak, or irregular and if the body defenses give signs of weakening, it may be necessary to institute radical medical measures rather than to rely on the more conservative measures.

The patient's general appearance is significant, because signs of exhaustion, restlessness, irritability, tremors, or clouded consciousness may indicate that the patient is being overwhelmed. The condition of the patient's mucous membrane and skin, its color and turgor, and the extent of the loss of fluid through perspiration are also clues to the extent or change of direction of the elevated temperature and to the extent of the need for replacement of body fluids. Urinary output also may provide clues as to the degree of hydration, for the appearance of scanty, concentrated urine signals the deficiency of body fluid.

In almost any incidence of elevated temperature, increased fluid intake is necessary. Although the fever is the result of decreased heat loss, the increased respiratory rate increases the loss of fluids via expired air, and the increased perspiring adds to this. Fluid intake, therefore, must be increased to replace lost body fluid, and this can be done only by planning specifically and by carrying out the plan over a period of time. The occasional and sporadic attention to patient needs for fluids is seldom effective. Generally, the fluids selected are those that the patient tolerates well and that are not contraindicated by the patient's specific health problem. If the patient feels like eating bland foods, these are also given, if not specifically contraindicated. A state of dehydration is to be avoided at all costs, because this presents the patient with an additional health problem.

Equally as important as providing fluid intake is the provision of sufficient intake to maintain nutrition. Because the body metabolism is increased, the patient's energy consumption is well above normal. Caloric requirements are therefore above the usual, and the caloric intake should be in the form of easily digested and quickly utilized foods, such as liquids high in carbohydrate content. The state of the patient's nutrition requires close evaluation, for supplementary measures instituted in time provide an extra margin in keeping the patient's own defense mechanisms operating in his behalf.

In the light of the patient's energy expenditures through an increased metabolic rate that is part of the elevated temperature, adequate rest becomes an important nursing measure in husbanding the patient's reserve. Unnecessary activity on his part should be prevented. Activities that involve the patient should be planned not to disturb him any oftener than is necessary. Wherever and whenever possible, things should be done *for* the patient until the temperature subsides. Explanations should be brief and to the point. Activities should not be prolonged. The conservation of patient energy becomes a consistent nursing goal.

Keeping the patient physically comfortable promotes a more generalized sense of well-being and reduces some of the physical discomfort that accompanies an elevated temperature. Skin care and oral hygiene are particularly important. Positioning the patient comfortably with supportive devices, if needed, and changing position periodically are helpful.

The environment should be as quiet and restful as possible. Most hospital environments could be much quieter than they are. The reduction of external stimuli reduces the energy demands made upon the patient. Ventilation is particularly important. Although the patient needs adequate fresh air because of increased respiratory rate and oxygen need, he should be kept free of drafts to prevent chills and should be adequately covered to maintain warmth without unnecessarily increasing body heat retained.

Here again, sensitivity to patient feelings and the recognition of signs of anxiety and providing a channel for its expression contribute to the patient's conservation of the energy he needs to get well.

Medical directives relating specifically to an elevated temperature are primarily chemotherapeutic; antipyretics and antibiotics are the most commonly used. Acetylsalicylic acid is frequently utilized as an antipyretic. Antibiotics are specific in terms of the causative agent; penicillin, streptomycin, and Chloromycetin are examples. Other common medical directives include alcohol sponge and parenteral administration of fluids. The alcohol sponge reduces temperature by increasing heat dissipation. The alcohol evaporates more readily than water, consuming heat and increasing heat loss through radiation. Parenteral administration, most often intravenous, replaces body fluid and may include some nutritional replacement and/or electrolyte replacement. The physician normally starts the intravenous infusion, with the nurse being responsible for its maintenance and termination.

Hemorrhage and shock

Hemorrhage is the loss of blood from the circulatory system and may result from any cause that destroys the integrity of any part of the system. Trauma due to accidents or surgery, an ulcer that destroys a blood vessel wall, cancer that penetrates and breaks into blood vessels, burns that destroy blood vessels, or the tubercle bacillus that opens blood vessels in the lung are examples of the range of causes of hemorrhage. Wherever a nurse may be employed, the danger of hemorrhage is usually an ever-present threat.

Hemorrhage may occur externally and/or internally, and the latter is usually the most dangerous, because it may be more difficult to detect and because reaching the site of hemorrhage to control it is usually more complicated. Hemorrhage may also be arterial, venous, or capillary in origin. Arterial bleeding is usually the most dangerous, because it is more difficult to control. In external hemorrhage, arterial bleeding is readily identified by the spurting flow and by the bright red color. External venous bleeding is identified by the darker red color of the blood and by its more steady, even flow. Capillary bleeding tends to be oozing in type and is usually somewhat bluish in color.

Internal bleeding within the gastrointestinal tract may be identified through excreta. If the bleeding is close to the source of excretion or ejection, frank blood may appear. If the blood is not immediately ejected, the vomitus, sputum, or urine, for example, may appear brown in color. If the bleeding occurs some distance from the point of ejection or excretion, the color moves toward a darker brown or black. The so-called tarry stool, for example, is evidence of bleeding in the upper gastrointestinal tract.

Hemorrhage may be slight, moderate, or severe and massive. The detection of slight hemorrhage depends upon evidence that the bleeding has occurred and the evidence may be sought on the basis of patients' subjective complaints or through diagnostic tests. External severe or massive hemorrhage presents no problem in detection and demands immediate measures to stop the loss of blood. Internal severe or massive hemorrhage can be identified by characteristic symptoms presented by the patient. Typically, the symptoms of severe hemorrhage include apprehension and restlessness, increasing pulse and respiration with decreasing body temperature, thirst, and paleness combined with a cold, moist skin.

Shock is a state of circulatory collapse, of the peripheral circulatory system primarily, and may be caused by massive hemorrhage as well as many other factors. Anything that reduces sharply the circulating blood volume can produce shock. The loss of blood or plasma volume due to hemorrhage, trauma, or burns, for example, may produce shock.

Shock may be primary or secondary, with primary shock occurring at the time of injury and secondary shock usually developing several hours after injury. Characteristic symptoms include a dropping blood pressure, a weak and rapid pulse, and a pale, cold, and moist skin. The patient may be apathetic, or he may be apprehensive. He is especially likely to be apprehensive if shock results from hemorrhage. Respirations become rapid and shallow, the temperature drops, and, if shock is not reversed, cyanosis appears. The appearance of shock is a serious symptom, for if blood volume is not replaced rapidly, the shock becomes irreversible.

Different in cause from shock produced by trauma, burns, or crushing injuries is anaphylactic shock. Traumatic shock results from loss of blood volume and becomes irreversible because of damage caused to vital structures through the decreased blood flow. Anaphylactic shock follows the injection or administration of a foreign substance to a person who has been sensitized by a previous administration of the same substance. The first dose acts as an antigen and stimulates the production of antibodies. When the foreign substance is injected again, the antigen-antibody reaction liberates histamine in affected tissues, and the histamine is a factor in producing the anaphylactic response. When the action is severe, anaphylactic shock with circulatory collapse occurs.

Major nursing responsibilities in relation to hemorrhage and shock include the following:

1. Observation and assessment of patient status
2. The prevention of hemorrhage and shock
3. The immediate control of hemorrhage
4. Immediate measures to reverse shock
5. Allaying patient anxiety
6. Carrying out medical directives

The observation of patients is directed largely toward identifying the early signs of shock and hemorrhage, because early detection of either or both offers the patient the best opportunity to remain alive. Of particular importance are immediate postoperative patients (regardless of how minor the surgery), patients who have been injured in accidents of any kind, patients who have suffered burns, patients suffering severe pain, patients with carcinoma, patients who are seriously ill, or patients who are known as "bleeders" (hemophiliacs). The indication of external hemorrhage is, of course, the appearance of blood, and this is the reason for the frequent and conscientious observation of wound dressings. The signs of internal hemorrhage, and therefore the focus of observation, are (1) an increasingly rapid pulse that becomes weak, (2) increasing respiratory rate with air hunger, thirst, cold and pale skin, and (3) apprehension and restlessness. Shock may result as the blood volume decreases. The signs of shock are dropping blood pressure, a weak and rapid pulse, and cold and clammy skin.

In general, the prevention of shock and hemorrhage can be accomplished by the following:

1. Decreasing amount of stress, local or general, to which the patient must respond
2. Resting injured or diseased parts
3. Avoiding stress or strain in operated areas
4. The control of severe pain
5. Maintaining fluid intake and reducing fluid loss in order to maintain blood volume
6. Learning about and respecting patient sensitivity to foreign substances
7. Allaying patient anxiety

In the instance of evidence that would indicate internal hemorrhage, the physician should be notified immediately. This does not mean that the nurse drops everything and runs for the physician—she delegates the notification, requests the emergency drug and/or other setup kept in the clinical area, and takes care of the patient. The patient may be placed flat in bed or the nurse may elevate the foot of the bed in order to ensure a supply of blood to the brain. The patient should be kept as quiet as possible, and attention should be given to reassuring the patient to relieve anxiety and apprehension.

In the instance of external hemorrhage, any one of several measures may be appropriate, including the application of a tourniquet, pressure dressings, reinforcement of dressings, elevation of an extremity, or digital pressure. A tourniquet can be applied to an extremity above the point of hemorrhage; the tourniquet should be loosened periodically, and the usual period of toleration is between fifteen and twenty minutes. However, this is an individual matter, depending upon the circulatory adequacy of any given individual. If the skin in the area of circulatory deprivation becomes cyanotic and cold, the tourniquet should be released.

Pressure bandages may also be used, and these are applied directly to the source of hemorrhage. Such pressure bandages should, if at all possible, be applied over a sterile dressing. Again, careful observation of the area of circulatory deprivation is necessary, and the occurrence of cyanosis and skin coldness calls for the release of the bandage.

In addition to controlling blood supply to an extremity by compression of circulation, the part may be elevated, taking advantage of the force of gravity to reduce circulation to the area. In case of hemorrhage, dressings on flat surfaces, such as the abdomen, may be reinforced. The underlying purpose is to increase pressure, so the reinforcement to the original dressing should be firmly secured. Digital pressure may also be employed to control hemorrhage. If the bleeding is arterial, pressure should be applied to the major artery as near the wound as possible. In almost all instances, this is *above* the wound, and the pressure should be applied where the artery can be compressed against a bone. When the hemorrhage is venous in origin, pressure should be applied below the wound or directly on the wound.

In the instance of shock, the patient may be placed flat in bed before the arrival of the physician. Whether or not the patient will be placed in shock position, i.e., with the head lower than the trunk on an inclined plane, is a medical determination based on the cause of shock. In any case, a dropping blood pressure accompanied by a rapid, weak pulse and by a cold, clammy skin call for immediate medical attention. Provision should be made for intravenous procedures, because the early replacement of blood volume is prerequisite to the reversal of shock.

As might be guessed from the frequency with which apprehension is mentioned as a symptom in hemorrhage and shock, the ability to avoid increasing the patient's anxiety, to allay existing anxiety, and to function calmly have both physical and psychological contributions to make to the patient's well-being.

Medical directives will include primarily the administration of medications, intravenous infusions, or surgical intervention to control hemorrhage. What these may be specifically are determined by the cause of hemorrhage and/or shock. Commonly used are morphine or Demerol for their quieting effect on the patient. Vasopressors, such as Levophed and Aramine, are often used to combat the dropping blood pressure in shock. Also in shock, and sometimes in hemorrhage, the replacement of blood volume is attempted by the administration of whole blood, plasma, or isotonic solutions.

Anorexia, nausea, and vomiting

Nausea and vomiting are closely related, and nausea usually precedes vomiting, although either may occur alone. Increased tension upon the walls of the stomach or duodenum or distention of the lower part of the esophagus causes the sensation of nausea. Appetite, on the other hand, is not based on demonstrable visceral changes but is largely due to the anticipated pleasure of eating; it may be associated with hunger but frequently is not. Anorexia, the lack of appetite, may thus be due to visceral changes that militate against wanting to eat or to factors that relate to anticipation of eating, such as distasteful food or unpleasant surroundings. As a matter of fact, extreme hunger may reduce appetite, because it can produce nausea as a result of hunger contractions in the duodenum.

Anorexia, nausea, and vomiting are common responses to disease processes. Vomiting empties the upper gastrointestinal tract and results from irritation of either the organs themselves or the nerves that supply them, or from an unusual stimulation of the gastrointestinal tract. Vomiting can also be caused by unusual stimulation of the labyrinth of the ear when the sense of equilibrium is disturbed, as in seasickness and airsickness. Nausea and vomiting can also result from direct stimulation of the vomiting center in the medulla oblongata. There also exists a type of central vomiting, characterized by extremely forceful ejection known as projectile vomiting, that occurs with head injuries, increased intracranial pressure, and meningeal irritation.

In contrast to the vomiting center in the medulla, which is concerned with the ejection of the contents of the upper gastrointestinal tract, the hypothalamus contains centers that have to do with food intake. Although the feeding centers in the hypothalamus do not control food intake directly, they influence lower brain centers which control getting, consuming, and assimilating food. Also, the hypothalamus contains a "satiety" center that reacts by reducing the desire for food when a sufficient intake has been reached.

Thus, anorexia, nausea, and vomiting can be the result of local physical problems in the upper gastrointestinal tract, of general systemic difficulties that affect either the gastrointestinal tract or the central nervous system, or of difficulties in the central nervous system itself. In addition to physical sources that produce anorexia, nausea, and vomiting, cultural factors can also be influential. The intake of food is a significant aspect of social living, and eating is associated with strong feelings and many social taboos. The influence of cultural factors on eating habits and appetite has been discussed previously.

Although anorexia, nausea, and vomiting are frequently situational in nature in response to cultural, esthetic, and personal factors, they are also frequently presenting symptoms of physical disease. In this case, they are both symptoms and complications.

The maintenance of health is dependent upon adequate fluid and food intake. When the symptoms of disease complicate the maintenance of an adequate balanced diet and fluid intake, the therapy planned for the patient must be broadened to include this factor. Because intake and output are determining factors in maintaining fluid and electrolyte balance in the body, this balance may also present complications for therapy.

Vomiting, of course, is an obvious symptom—the ejection of the contents of the upper gastrointestinal tract (emesis). Nausea may be indicated by the patient's subjective complaints of a nauseous sensation or by gagging. Anorexia may be indicated by the patient's subjective complaints and by his refusal to eat. With the diminution of intake and the output via emesis, the resulting course of events leads to weight loss, dehydration, and fluid and electrolyte imbalance. The skin becomes dry, there is loss of skin turgor, and poor oral hygiene may lead to halitosis. The patient's subjective complaints usually go beyond specifics related to anorexia, nausea, and vomiting and include general symptoms of discomfort.

The major nursing responsibilities in providing nursing care for patients with anorexia and/or nausea and vomiting include the following:

1. Observation and assessment of patient status
2. Serving food to promote appetite

3. Respecting patients' cultural food patterns
4. Using physical comfort measures to improve appetite
5. Providing adequate rest
6. Manipulating environment to improve appetite
7. Nursing care related to symptoms of nausea and vomiting
8. Allaying anxiety
9. Carrying out medical directives

The observation and assessment of patient status when anorexia, nausea, and vomiting are present is concerned with four primary focuses:

1. The extent of the impact on the patient's total physical status
2. The identification of psychological factors that can be utilized to help the patient
3. The identification of cultural factors that can be utilized to help the patient
4. Patient response to therapeutic plans

In observing for the impact of the existence of anorexia and/or nausea and vomiting on the patient's total physical status, certain clues become significant. These include the patient's fluid and food intake, the relationship of intake and output, the loss of body weight, changes in skin color or turgor, character and amount of vomitus, the degree of activity the patient is able to exhibit, the extent of drying of the mucous membrane, and the amount and character of other excretions such as urine, stool, and perspiration. The dangers for the patient lie in nutritional deficiency, dehydration, and disturbance of fluid and electrolyte balance. The preceding clues give indications of these occurrences.

The second area of observation is directed toward finding psychological factors that may relieve nausea and vomiting or increase appetite. What are the patient's normal eating habits and preferences? How does he feel about food? Is it an important aspect of his life, i.e., does he live to eat or does he eat to live? When is he accustomed to eating, and when does he have his "heavy" meal? Does he react to problems, and has he before, by getting "sick"? Who usually feeds him? Any scrap of knowledge that can be gleaned regarding the patient's eating habits, preferences, or attitudes may be useful in providing nursing care. Relatives and friends may be as helpful as the patient, and sometimes even more helpful. In addition, the patient's specific reaction to eating in the hospital setting needs careful observation.

An additional focus of observation is the cultural taboos, rituals, and values about food and eating that are characteristic of the patient's background. Again, relatives and friends are as valuable a source of information as the patient. Such information provides the clues for many "do's" and "dont's" in planning nursing care. Although many northerners object to hominy grits with eggs for breakfast, a southern patient in a northern hospital may enjoy eating such a breakfast.

The fourth focus of observation is the patient's response to therapeutic plans to relieve the anorexia and/or nausea and vomiting. A patient on a milk and cream diet who cannot tolerate milk or cream, or who simply refuses it because he does not like it, needs some change in therapeutic plans, even if it is only someone to talk to him.

In serving food to patients who are not particularly hungry or overwhelmed with a desire for food, certain ground rules apply. Frequent small feedings are more effective than fewer, heavier ones. Food should be attractively served with meticulous attention to small details such as clean dishes, flatware in the right place, hot food hot and cold food cold, and food placed where the patient can reach it if he is to feed himself. Foods that the particular patient dislikes should be removed from his plate before he is served. A patient who is having difficulty with nausea and vomiting should not be forced to eat, nor should he be forced to look at a tray long after he has finished eating. The patient should be in a comfortable position to eat and in a comfortable position *after* eating. If he wants to complain about the food, he should be permitted to do so. The period before, during, and after eating should not be disturbed by painful or irritating procedures.

The patient's cultural attitudes and habits should be respected. For example, although an Orthodox Jew is not required to adhere to the dietary laws of his religion if he requires a different diet for health reasons, he will frequently adhere to his religious customs anyway. If he does, food that obviously violates his customs will not only not be eaten, but he may well be, and has every right to be, offended. Adaptations to cultural patterns can be made, and the patient's right to his own preferences can be respected. He should not be condemned, ridiculed, ignored, or forced.

Patients' physical comfort becomes especially significant when they have almost any symptom of physical illness, including nausea and vomiting. Physical discomfort increases the nausea and vomiting, and physical comfort can contribute somewhat to their alleviation. Therefore, attention to oral hygiene especially, but also to skin care, back rubs, massage, comfortable position, and comfortable bed linens are important.

Adequate rest is an important aspect of the control of nausea and vomiting. Actually, nausea and vomiting occurs in relatively healthy people as a result of inadequate sleep and rest. Therefore, rest for the patient becomes a nursing goal.

Patients with nausea and vomiting, like patients with pain or elevated temperature, tend to be extremely sensitive to the environment. In all instances, noise, overactivity, odors, confusion, and too many people tend to accentuate the symptoms. For patients with nausea and vomiting, odors, noise, and confusion are particularly disagreeable. Therefore, environmental control in the direction of a quieter and less disagreeable surrounding contributes to the alleviation of nausea and vomiting.

If a patient is nauseated but does not vomit, quiet, deep breathing and the reduction of environmental stimuli may help to control the nausea. Intake of fluid or foods to control nausea (which can result from excessive hunger) should be based on the patient's preference and tolerance. If the patient does vomit, the vomitus should be observed carefully and disposed of promptly. Of all things, it should not be left where the patient can see or smell it. The amount, consistency, color, and odor should be noted and charted. From the patient's point of view, oral hygiene becomes important.

Permitting the patient to express his feelings, accepting them, keeping channels of communication open, and allaying anxiety are especially significant. Anorexia, nausea, and vomiting are as frequently behavioral manifestations of feelings as they are symptoms of physical illness.

Medical directives usually relate to the administration of medications, diet adaptations, or adaptations in method of feeding, depending upon the causative factors. If anorexia, nausea, and vomiting are due to pain, analgesics may be ordered to relieve the pain. If anorexia, nausea, and vomiting are due to exhaustion, sedatives may be ordered; if they are due to tension and worry, tranquilizers may be ordered.

The diet may be adapted and range from nothing by mouth, to liquid, to semiliquid, to bland, to soft, etc. The method of feeding may also be adapted, and the patient may receive caloric intake and body fluid via intravenous infusion, or he may be fed via a Levin tube. The nurse may also collect specimens (such as fluid suctioned from the Levin tube for gastric analysis). Under many medical directives, the physician initiates the treatment, such as placing the Levin tube and inserting the intravenous needle, and the nurse carries through and completes the therapy.

Weakness and malaise

Common patient perceptions of disease processes are weakness and malaise, and these are frequent presenting complaints either when a patient seeks a physician or during the course of almost any frank illness. Malaise is defined by Webster as "an indefinite feeling of debility or lack of health often indicative of or accompanying the onset of an illness."*

Weakness and malaise of physical origin are usually systemic in nature and are responses to lack of adequate intake and/or output, lack of adequate rest and sleep, physical or emotional processes that require an unusually high proportion of body energy expenditure, or they indicate an overactive function of the central nervous system or the chemical endocrine-regulating hormones. Weakness and malaise can also occur as a result of prolonged emotional stress. Weakness and malaise, then, result when the energy balance of the body is not maintained and when there is less energy available than the individual requires for daily living activities. Inadequate food intake, for example, reduces metabolism and, thus, heat production and available energy. Inadequate rest and sleep increases energy consumption, because the activity that accompanies the waking hours increases energy needs. Fever raises the metabolic rate of the body, increases energy utilization, and therefore can, if prolonged, produce weakness and malaise. Thyroid hormone secretion below normal levels reduces the body metabolic rate and energy production, and thyroid hormone secretion above

---

*By permission. From Webster's Seventh New Collegiate Dictionary, copyright 1963 by G. & C. Merriam Co. Publishers of the Merriam-Webster Dictionaries.

normal levels increases energy production and utilization. Therefore, a most anything that disturbs the energy balance of the body can result i the symptoms of weakness and malaise.

The two symptoms are usually not difficult to identify—the patient general appearance and his subjective descriptions of how he feels are rela tively obvious. In addition to the weakness and feeling of disease or discom fort, the patient may be lethargic or restless and irritable. Tremors or dizz ness may occur, and loss of muscle tone is fairly common. The patient attention span may be and probably will be reduced. Effort syndrome i usually seen; for example, it takes a great deal of effort for the patient t undertake or initiate any activity.

Major nursing responsibilities for the patient with weakness and malais include the following:

1. Observation and assessment of patient status
2. Providing for rest
3. Use of physical comfort measures
4. Maintaining fluid and food intake
5. Allaying anxiety
6. Carrying out medical directives

Observation and assessment of patient status are focused primarily upo the extent to which the patient's symptoms limit his daily living activities This assessment then provides the basis for the nursing care plan for the pa tient and provides clues for needed medical intervention. Significant clue are the patient's general appearance, the degree of alertness or lethargy, th extent of interest in the environment, the condition of the skin and mucou membrane, the balance of intake and output, the extent to which the patien appears willing to make decisions, and the extent to which he can partic pate in his therapy.

The provision of rest for the patient is a significant aspect of nursin care. The disturbance in energy balance leaves the patient with a nee to conserve what he has for the effort to get well, and much of the respon sibility for energy production for the activities of daily living must be sup plied by the nurse. Care for the patient should be planned to provide hir with frequent rest periods. Decisions that he does not wish to make shoul be made for him (in his own interests, not those of getting things done and the decisions he does make should be respected. The environmen should be conducive to rest, and the patient should not be forced or pushe or pulled.

For the patient with weakness and malaise, physical comfort become an important nursing measure, because discomfort increases the patient energy consumption. Therefore, the usual attention to all the physical mea sures designed to promote comfort are indicated.

Fluid and food intake are often measures for attention, because patient who do not feel well or strong are usually not too interested in food. Th measures previously described in regard to food and its serving are equall appropriate for the patient suffering from weakness and malaise.

The patient who does not feel well or strong is certain to have feelings about his physical condition and feelings about himself. The open channel of communication and the measures to allay anxiety are important here, too.

Medical directives again are concerned primarily with the administration of medications. In this instance, sedatives and hypnotics, such as the barbiturates, are used to promote sleep and rest. Nutritional supplements such as vitamins and hematinics may be indicated. Selected tranquilizing agents are sometimes used clinically to produce a feeling of well-being in patients who are depressed. Depression is a fairly common concomitant of weakness and malaise. Therefore, the patient should be rewarded for every little success and not encouraged to reach for unrealistic goals but to feel better about the things he can do. Feelings of depression should be expressed by the patient if he so desires. Overcheerfulness on the part of the nurse can be most discouraging.

Edema and dehydration

Over half of the total body weight of a human being is composed of water. Approximately 65% of the total body weight of men is water; the percentage drops around 10 points for women. The body cells, to exist, must be bathed by tissue fluid. Body water is found within the cells themselves (intracellular water), in blood vessels (intravascular water), and in tissues between vascular spaces and cells (interstitial water). Intravascular and interstitial water are also called extracellular water. Intracellular fluid in adults is about two thirds of the total body water as compared to extracellular fluid, which is about one-third. In infants and young children, the distribution of intracellular and extracellular water is about even.

The maintenance of the fluid balance of the body is accomplished by the balance of water intake and output. When the intake exceeds the output, water is retained in the body (positive water balance); and when the output exceeds the intake, water content in the body is reduced and dehydration results (negative water balance).

Water intake is accomplished in two ways: by the ingestion of water, of liquids, and of solid foods that contain water, and by water formed in metabolism through the oxidation of foods. Water is absorbed, in decreasing order, in the small intestine, the large intestine, and the stomach. Water intake is regulated by thirst, which occurs when the volume of body water decreases.

Water is lost from the body through urine, feces, expired air from the lungs, and evaporation from the skin. The loss is greatest through the kidneys and next through the skin and expired air.

Thus, disturbance in water balance can result from reduced intake, increased output, or increased retention. When the balance is negative, dehydration occurs. When the balance is positive, water is retained, and edema (an excessive accumulation of fluids in the tissue spaces) occurs.

Dehydration may be caused by a wide variety of health problems. Simple lack of water intake may occur when a patient is unable to retain fluids or refuses to drink water because of emotional illness. The increased loss of fluid that results from persistent vomiting or diarrhea or excessive perspiration or urine excretion may also result in dehydration. When the basic cause is water depletion, the osmotic pressure in extracellular fluid rises, drawing water from the cells themselves.

Dehydration may also be caused by change in the quantity of electrolytes in body fluids. In fact, the electrolyte concentration of body fluid is controlled through the elimination or retention of water. For example, if the salt (NaCl) content of the tissues is reduced, water is lost, and if the salt content is increased, water is retained, thus maintaining the normal saline concentration of body fluids. In addition, dehydration can result from the injection of hypertonic solutions into the blood stream. (Hypertonic solutions are those containing a higher concentration of a substance, such as salt, than is normally found in body tissue.)

Dehydration is manifested by weight loss, disturbances in acid-base balance (usually increased acid), rise in the nonprotein nitrogen in the blood, rise in plasma protein concentration, rise in body temperature, increased pulse rate and reduced cardiac output, thirst, dryness, and wrinkling of the skin. Exhaustion and collapse may follow.

Edema, the accumulation of fluid in excess in tissue spaces, represents the opposite end of water imbalance. Edema is always due to an increase in the extracellular body fluid and may result from a variety of causes. In congestive heart failure, salt is retained and water accumulates in the body tissues. Measures to reduce edema are directed at this specific cause, i.e., reduced intake or medication that increases both salt and water excretion. Mechanical vein obstruction may reduce the return flow of blood from any part of the body and cause an accumulation of fluid in the affected part. Edema may also accompany renal disease, especially when the ability of the kidney to excrete salt may be reduced. As the salt is retained, fluid is retained to dilute it. Edema may also occur as a result of the inflammatory process. Other factors include anemias and malnutrition, especially in patients whose blood plasma protein is lowered, leading directly to an accumulation of fluid in the extracellular spaces. Edema may also occur in the presence of excessive heat.

Edema is manifested by swelling due to presence of increased fluid. It may be general or localized. The presence of fluid is often indicated by so-called pitting edema; i.e., when one presses on the body surface and then removes the pressure, a "pit" forms which slowly disappears as the fluid filters back into the area. The presence of lung edema can be identified by the sound of the fluid as the patient breathes.

Major nursing responsibilities for the patient who has edema include the following:

1. The observation and assessment of patient status
2. The use of physical comfort measures
3. Providing a balance of rest and exercise
4. Providing an intake-output balance that leans toward output

5. Allaying anxiety

6. Carrying out medical directives

The observation and assessment of patient status is directed toward identification of local or general edema, its extent, type, change in degree, intake-output balance, and the patient's response to therapy. Edema may occur in the extremities (dependent portions of the body) and may be localized or general. Of particular significance is the occurrence of edema in the lungs, which can result, for example, from "backing-up" in pulmonary circulation due to congestive heart failure. Lung edema is revealed by dyspnea, or shortness of breath, cough, moist sounds that accompany breathing, and expectoration of mucoid or frothy blood-tinged sputum.

Edema that appears on the body surface (for example, the feet or ankles) may range from a mild swelling, such as many people experience during hot weather, to such an extensive increase in tissue fluid that the swelling is marked and the skin is stretched until it is hard and shiny. Edema may disappear with elevation of the part or may be persistent despite change of position. Edema may be "hard" (i.e., it does not recede with pressure), "pitting" (i.e., pressure leaves a "pit" that fills in slowly as the fluid returns to the part), or elastic (i.e., pressure produces an indentation that fills as soon as the pressure is removed). Change in the extent toward increase indicates that therapy is not controlling the edema development; decrease in extent may indicate improvement. Changes in the extent of edema in relation to the patient's intake-output balance and medical therapy provide significant clues to the patient's response to therapy. In addition to measurable output, the respiratory rate and the extent of sweating provide additional clues to intake-output balance.

Here again, physical comfort measures have a significant implication for patient therapy. Edema is usually accompanied by a sense of discomfort and, in some situations, by a threat to the patient which produces anxiety. Patients tend to be sensitive to physical discomfort, and it increases the feeling of illness and disease. Skin care of the edematous part is especially important, because excessive prolonged swelling can lead to skin breaks, and these occur more readily when skin care is inadequate.

A balance of rest and exercise is indicated for the patient with surface edema. One basic guiding line is change of position at periodic intervals. The patient who has edematous ankles and feet, for example, should have them elevated, but they should periodically be let down at regular intervals. Edematous parts that are elevated should be comfortably supported. If edema occurs in dependent parts of the body, i.e., those parts that are lower than others, frequent change of position is indicated. If edema occurs in the lungs and pleura, positioning to make breathing as easy and effortless as possible should be employed. This is usually a supported, upright position. In general, in surface edema, it is wise to keep the patient in a position that promotes drainage of the part involved but not to keep any one position indefinitely.

The observation and control of intake and output are musts. If the patient is on restricted intake, the provision of foods and fluids should be planned at spaced intervals. Fluids or foods high in salt content are to be avoided, because the edema is a body defense that serves the purpose of diluting the salt content of body fluid. In evaluating output, as pointed out previously, the loss of fluid through expired air or sweat may be taken into account. Increased respiratory rate or sweating should be noted and reported. The recording of intake and output seems a relatively simple task and, yet, is one of the most difficult pieces of information to obtain accurately. Conscientious attention to the recording of intake and output is sorely needed.

As in any physical problem a patient experiences, the patient's feelings about himself and his health problems are an aspect of nursing care that has a direct influence upon the course of the patient's physical illness. Recognizing and accepting the patient's feelings and permitting him to express them or not express them as he wishes will help to allay anxiety.

Medical directives designed to reduce edema include the administration of medications, adaptations of diet, and specific local measures to reduce the edema, such as hypertonic saline solution soaks. Medications may include diuretics such as Diamox or Diuril, sedatives (such as the barbiturates) to promote rest and quiet, and drugs designed to regulate heart action (such as digitalis) if the edema is the result of cardiac disease. The usual diet restriction in the presence of edema is a low-salt diet. Other dietary adaptations may be ordered related to treatment of the cause of the edema. If the patient is receiving a diuretic drug, foods and fluids high in potassium should be included in the diet. Orange juice and bananas are prime examples. Hypertonic salt solutions (magnesium sulfate) may be used to reduce edema if the area of edema is localized. In such instances, through osmotic pressure, fluid in the edematous area moves into the solution with the strongest sodium concentration. Hypertonic solutions may be used as soaks or compresses.

The major nursing responsibilities in the care of patients who are in a state of negative water balance, or dehydration, include the following:

1. Observation and assessment of patient status
2. Utilization of physical comfort measures
3. Provision of fluid and nutrition intake
4. Provision of rest
5. Allaying anxiety
6. Carrying out medical directives

The observation and assessment of patient status for patients who are dehydrated relate primarily to vital signs, skin condition, general level of patient activity, and weight change. Dehydration is usually accompanied by rising temperature and increased pulse rate, by decrease in skin turgor, and by dryness of mucous membrane. The degree and extent of these symptoms become clues to the amount of dehydration. The patient's general level of activity is another significant clue. Weight loss occurs as a result of loss of body fluid, because body fluid constitutes a large proportion of body weight. Many patients in terminal stages of illness finally succumb to effects of dehydration, and some patients probably die unnecessarily from its effects. Therefore, accurate observation forms not only the basis for nursing measures, but may well indicate medical intervention.

Physical comfort measures are particularly important for the patient in negative water balance. Anyone who has suffered from even a mild degree of dehydration can attest to this fact. Oral hygiene and skin care are especially important. The patient's general sense of discomfort requires attention to ventilation, comfortable bed linens, back rubs, change in position, and other measures designed to promote patient comfort. Particular attention to support and protection for bony prominences, care in lifting and moving to avoid skin injury, and frequent change in position to reduce the chance of skin damage are needed.

Patient fluid intake, of course, is of the highest order of measures designed to improve patient status because all therapy is directed toward replacement of body fluids. In providing fluid intake, frequent and consistent administration of fluids is desirable. The selection of fluids is influenced by two factors: the possibility of disturbance of body acid-base balance, usually in the acid direction, and the need for easily digested and utilized nutrition content in order to conserve patient energy. A variety of fluids is much better than using any one fluid to excess, and a lot of water is always indicated. Intake and output are always checked. Urinary output should be carefully followed, because scanty, concentrated urine constitutes a danger signal.

The provision of adequate rest reduces the patient's energy consumption and permits him to use available energy for basal metabolic maintenance. Planned rest periods are valuable, and procedures or care should be spaced and carried through with a minimum of patient activity. Environmental factors that contribute to rest should be promoted.

Medical directives are usually concerned with the restoration of body fluid and with maintenance of nutrition and replacement of lost electrolytes. Such procedures are frequently intravenous, and the nurse is responsible for maintaining the therapy after it is instituted.

ORIENTATION AND LEVEL OF CONSCIOUSNESS

Man is a unitary being, endowed with awareness. Through a vast and complicated system of sensory receptors, nerve pathways, and chemical and nervous regulators and coordinators, he orients himself in time and space and reacts with more or less appropriate behavior. Anything that interferes with perception of the internal or external environment that makes appropriate response impossible can threaten the maintenance of homeostasis. The capacity to stay in touch with the environment and to interpret it relatively correctly is a characteristic of physical and mental health. The loss of the ability to orient oneself and to remain alert is a body response to many forms of disease processes.

Orientation includes knowing "who," "what," "when," and "where." In order to do this, the patient must be alert to his surroundings. Any loss or diminution in degree of consciousness makes orientation difficult or impossible. The level of consciousness may range from complete alertness to complete coma. Consciousness may be clouded as a result of a delirium resulting from fever or intoxication, and the patient perceives the environment inaccurately, seeming confused and restless, misinterpreting, but responding. The patient may be comatose, appearing to be in coma but responding to painful stimuli, as a result of shock, injury, diabetic acidosis, or serious infection.

In coma, the patient becomes unconscious and does not respond to any stimuli. Any injury, infection, or degenerative process that is overwhelming can produce disorientation and a reduced level of awareness. Any injury, infection, or degenerative process that affects the brain can do the same.

The major responsibilities in the nursing care of the patient whose orientation and level of consciousness are disturbed include the following:

1. Observation and assessment of patient status
2. Assumption of responsibility that the patient cannot assume for himself
3. Providing physical comfort
4. Providing understanding and acceptance of the patient
5. Carrying out medical directives

The observation and assessment of the patient's status has two primary focuses: the degree of adequacy and appropriateness of the patient's response to his environment and signs and symptoms of damage to the central nervous system. The patient's orientation is revealed by his knowledge or lack of knowledge of who he is, where he is, and when it is. This is within reason, of course. Persons who do not write dates or to whom the specific date is not important often do not know the exact date. The level of consciousness is determined by the patient's response to stimuli. If he responds readily and accurately, he is alert and conscious. If he responds, but misinterprets, i.e., thinks the bedpost is a flag pole or the nurse is a relative, consciousness is clouded. If he is comatose, he responds to strong or painful stimuli but seems otherwise unconscious. If he is in coma, he does not respond to stimuli.

Symptoms of cerebral damage are related to the area involved, but, in general, twitching, disturbances in motor activity, convulsions, disturbances in any of the sensory areas such as sight or hearing, or coma itself are samples of central nervous system damage. Depression of any of the vital centers that control such activities as respiration, heart action, or heat control will be revealed by the vital signs of temperature, pulse, and respiration and blood pressure.

Unless a patient is completely oriented and conscious, the nurse must assume complete responsibility for all patient activities and must especially provide for the safety measures that prevent the patient from injuring himself and others. Frequent observations, side rails, the reduction of external stimuli, including limiting the number of personnel, are all safety measures.

The completely unconscious patient demands a high order of nursing skills. Observation is geared toward assessment of the level of response, identification of the needs that will maintain normal functions, and evaluation of the measures required to prevent complications. The balance of intake-output, indications of central nervous system problems such as a rising blood pressure and slowing pulse (increasing intracranial pressure), the status of the vital signs, changes in motor activity (i.e., muscle flaccidity, twitching, convulsions), and the presence or absence of reflexes (i.e., swallowing, eye response to light and accommodation) are especially important.

The responsibility for the maintenance of normal function rests largely with the nurse, although medical directives may initiate specific measures. The maintenance of oxygen intake depends upon adequate ventilation and positioning the patient so that the airway is free and clear from pressure. Nutrition may be supplied orally if the patient's swallowing reflex remains. If it does, then fluid may be given orally with an Asepto syringe equipped with tubing to prevent the patient from accidentally biting the end of the syringe. Fluids should be given slowly, in small amounts, and the patient placed in a normal swallowing position. He should never be flat on his back.

Other means of providing nutrition include a Levin tube, hypodermoclysis, and intravenous infusion. When the Levin tube is used, again small amounts and more frequent feeding are employed to prevent overfilling the stomach as a measure to prevent vomiting and possible aspiration. Hypodermoclysis, or the injection of fluids into the subcutaneous tissue of the skin, is not frequently used because the intravenous method is more effective and less dangerous. However, when intravenous infusions are difficult or contraindicated or poor veins are being reserved for anticipated emergencies, the procedure may be used. Intravenous infusion is frequently used for both body fluid replacement and the maintenance of minimal nutrition. The total fluid intake planned for the patient will be influenced by the presence or absence of cerebral edema or increased intracranial pressure.

The maintenance of elimination is complicated by the occurrence of incontinence and the reduced muscle tone that predisposes to constipation and urinary retention. If the patient remains unconscious for any period of time, enemas on a routine schedule, i.e., every two or three days, will usually be instituted. The insertion of a Foley catheter is a common measure to avoid the difficulties the patient encounters from incontinence and to prevent bladder distention.

The normal need for a balance of rest and activity requires that the patient's exercise be provided by nursing personnel. Frequent and regular change of position, passive exercise, massage, and moving joints through the full range of motion at scheduled intervals are indicated. The routine physical comfort measures, such as the daily bath, are utilized to provide activity and stimulate circulation.

The possible complications that confront the unconscious patient are numerous: aspiration, decubitus ulcers, restriction of circulation, hypostatic pneumonia (pneumonia due to lying in the same position too long), atelectasis (lung collapse), deformities due to poor body alignment, and accidents are among the more common.

The prevention of aspiration of mucus, vomitus, or fluids into the lungs rests upon careful assessment of patient status and continuous measures to keep the mouth and pharynx clean and clear. The accumulation of mucus calls for suctioning, the prevention of vomiting calls for control of the amount and time of feeding (if by mouth or Levin tube), the avoidance of too much movement immediately before and after feeding, and the use of physical comfort measures to promote patient well-being.

The prevention of decubitus ulcers presents a major problem. Only minute, detailed, meticulously executed plans for skin care, the avoidance of pressure, frequent change of position, and immediate treatment of reddened areas will prevent decubitus ulcers. The skin should be kept clean, and the use of drying substances, such as alcohol, should be avoided in giving massage. Skin circulation may be stimuated by movement and by massage. Frequent change of position changes the surface area that supports the body weight, in addition to improving circulation. Key areas, such as the buttocks, heels, elbows, or shoulders, should be supported with devices that distribute pressure more evenly and should receive special attention, i.e., extra massage or application of emollients. If the patient is incontinent, immediate cleansing is indicated. Any schedule designed to prevent decubitus ulcers goes by the board unless it is regularly scheduled every hour or two and unless the schedule is rigorously carried out.

The restriction of circulation to a local area such as the hand, the arm, or the leg can be avoided by positioning patients correctly and providing support to keep one part of the body from cutting off circulation to another. An arm lying under the patient's body will soon show the blue, cold signs of reduced circulation. When the patient is on his side, the upper arm and leg must be supported to prevent their pressure upon the arm or leg on which the patient is lying. An additional safety measure is a careful check of any restriction to circulation from bed clothes or any restraining device, such as the bandage and/or adhesive that holds an intravenous infusion in place.

Hypostatic pneumonia can occur when the patient lies too long in the same position. It occurs as a result of pulmonary congestion when the blood stagnates in the lungs. The frequent change of position combats the danger, and one of the reasons for getting patients out of bed early and often is to prevent this particular complication. Atelectasis, or collapse of a portion or all of the lung, may result.

The maintenance of body alignment constitutes a major aspect of nursing care of the unconscious patient. It is of particular significance as a first step in rehabilitation, and neglect can lead to permanent damage. In all turning, moving, exercising, and positioning, body alignment must be maintained. For this reason, it is usually unwise to move an unconscious patient alone. Placing a folded sheet from above the shoulders to under the buttocks and using at least two persons to turn the patient makes the procedure easier. Drop foot can be prevented by using a footboard or sandbags to brace the foot in an anatomical position. The wrist can be supported to prevent wristdrop. A bandage roll can be inserted in the palm of the patient's hand if there is a tendency toward holding the fists clenched. The neck can be straight whether the patient is prone or on his side by the use of pillows. Extremities can be maintained in alignment by supports regardless of the position in which the patient is placed. The maintenance of body alignment should be frequently checked. Any deformity that follows a period of unconsciousness is an indication of poor nursing care.

The prevention of accidents involves identifying all possible sources of danger and guarding against them. The application of heat is usually contraindicated because of its potential for skin damage. Because the patient is not responsible, padded bedside rails reduce the danger of injury from restlessness and the danger of falling out of bed. Careful maintenance of body alignment reduces the danger of fractures. A padded mouth gag at the bedside may be useful in preventing tongue biting if the patient has a convulsion. The removal of dentures avoids possible difficulties of swallowing or choking on them. If restraining devices are used, securing them so that they are not too tight and cannot be accidentally pulled too tight by the patient can prevent cutting off circulation. The nurse must think and act completely for the unconscious patient.

Physical comfort measures are particularly important for the entire group of patients with disturbance in orientation and level of consciousness, ranging from the patient with clouded consciousness to the patient in coma. Since the patient is incapable of any self-care, the total responsibility for physical comfort rests with the nurse.

Understanding and acceptance of the patient are significant nursing measures for the patient with clouded consciousness. The recognition of the implications of the symptoms of the patient's inappropriate responses leads to gentle, firm, and understanding nursing responses to patient behavior.

Medical directives include administration of medications, intravenous fluid and food administration, and diagnostic tests. Medications may include tranquilizers, sedatives, and anticonvulsants. A spinal tap may be done for diagnostic purposes, as may an electroencephalogram or ventriculogram. Other medical therapy depends on the cause of disorientation or of disturbance in level of consciousness.

BIBLIOGRAPHY

1. Apperly, Frank L.: Patterns of disease, Philadelphia, 1951, J. B. Lippincott Co.
2. Best, Charles Herbert, and Taylor, Norman Burke: Physiological basis of medical practice, ed. 7, Baltimore, 1961, Williams & Wilkins Co., pp. 19-32, 39-41, 407-410, 733-739, 894-897, 1142-1144.
3. Crowle, Alfred J.: Delayed hypersensitivity, Scientific American **202**:129-138, April 1960.

4. Crowley, Dorothy M.: Pain and its alleviation, U.C.L.A. School of Nursing, Regents of the University of California, 1962.
5. Darlington, Charles G., and Davenport, Charlotte: Applied pathology, ed. 2, Philadelphia, 1958, J. B. Lippincott Co., pp. 18-72, 230-233.
6. Hunter, John: The mark of pain, American Journal of Nursing **61**:96-99, Oct. 1961.
7. Kaufman, Margaret A., and Brown, Dorothy E.: Pain wears many faces, American Journal of Nursing **61**:48-51, Jan. 1961.
8. Landells, John W.: Essential principles of pathology, Philadelphia, 1959, J. B. Lippincott Co., pp. 1-55, 89-93, 212-241.
9. Phelps, Elbert T.: Fever—its causes and effects, American Journal of Nursing **56**:319-321, March 1956.
10. Shafer, Kathleen Newton, Sawyer, Janet R., McCluskey, Audrey M., and Beck, Edna Lifgren: Medical-surgical nursing, ed. 2, St. Louis, 1961, The C. V. Mosby Co., pp. 69-76, 90-98, 107-127.

Chapter 17

Nursing care of patients with oxygen problems

Homeostasis is a relatively stable state of equilibrium. Man, as a unitary being, adapts to a changing external and internal environment to maintain such a state of equilibrium. The maintenance of an adequate supply of oxygen to all body cells is basic to existence. Cells cannot survive long without oxygen, particularly the cells in the gray matter of the brain. Therefore, anything that interferes with either local or general cell oxygenation constitutes an immediate threat to the life of a local part of the body or to life of the organism itself.

ESSENTIAL MECHANISMS

There are certain physiological and physical necessities basic to maintaining an oxygen supply to all body cells.
1. An adequate supply of oxygen available
2. A patent airway
3. An adequate absorption area
4. Adequate transportation of oxygen
5. Ability of body cells to utilize oxygen

The maintenance of an adequate oxygen supply, therefore, rests upon the integrity of the respiratory system, the cardiovascular system, and the central nervous system. The respiratory system provides the airway and the absorbing surface where the gaseous exchange involving oxygen and carbon dioxide between the air in the lungs and the blood in the circulatory system takes place. The cardiovascular system supplies both the means and the method of transportation of oxygen to all body cells. The oxygen combines with hemoglobin in the red blood cells, forming oxyhemoglobin, and is transported through the circulatory system to the body tissues. The central nervous system provides control and communication upon which respiration, cardiac function, and circulation depend.

WHAT CAN GO WRONG

Impairment of the respiratory, cardiovascular, or central nervous system, in addition to an inadequate oxygen supply in the environment, can present threats to the maintenance of oxygen.

It is an interesting fact that man can exist comfortably in his natural state within a relatively narrow atmospheric range in which the concentration of oxygen is suited to his physiological capacities. Too far above sea level the oxygen content of the atmosphere contains too little oxygen. For example, aviators cannot fly beyond the upper limits of 45,000 feet, even breathing 100% oxygen; beyond the range of 40,000 to 45,000 feet pressurized cabins in airplanes are required. Inadequacy of oxygen supply is one of the more common problems, although overoxygenation can occur. Hypoxia, or anoxia, means literally lack of oxygen supply to body tissues and is identical to oxygen lack or want. This can occur at high altitudes, or it can occur when the oxygen supply in the environment is reduced or cut off. Asphyxiation, a suspended state of animation due to decreased oxygen and increased carbon dioxide in the blood, can occur as a result of drowning or electric shock. The inhalation of inert gases that replace oxygen in the respiratory system, such as nitrogen or nitrous oxide, can also produce asphyxiation. Suffocation can also occur by intent, but probably occurs more often by accident. When asphyxiation or suffocation occurs, heroic emergency measures are usually indicated. In any instance, interference with an adequate oxygen supply in the immediate environment constitutes a major threat to life that leaves only a margin of minutes for action.

Overoxygenation, or hyperoxia, occurs when the oxygen concentration in the blood and in the tissues is raised and the carbon dioxide concentration is lowered. A fall in blood pressure results. Hyperoxia can be produced by voluntary hyperventilation or by administration of oxygen at concentrations that are too high.

Any number of pathological problems can interfere with the functioning or efficiency of the airway from the nose and mouth to the lung alveoli. From a mechanical point of view, obstruction can be partial or complete and can be caused by foreign objects inhaled or ingested from the external environment or by internal pathology that occludes the airway to some degree. For example, infections in any part of the airway may produce the characteristic responses of inflammation, including swelling. Abscesses may also occur. Cancer, a growth disturbance, can either partially or completely occlude any part of the airway. Any condition that results in increased secretion from the mucous membrane that lines the respiratory system may threaten the patency of the airway, including the common cold. Congenital defects can also impair the efficiency of the airway for oxygen intake.

The alveolar sacs of the lungs hold air with the oxygen concentration that supplies the blood stream with oxygen. The blood in the capillaries and the air in the alveoli are separated by two membranes, the alveolar and capillary walls, through which the diffusion of oxygen into the blood stream and carbon dioxide into the lungs takes place. Without this "absorbing" surface, the body's oxygen supply cannot be maintained. Inflammatory or infectious diseases of the lung, benign or malignant tumors of the lung, the introduction of fluid or air into the pleural cavity, or the accumulation of fluid in the alveoli as a result of circulatory difficulties will reduce the extent or the functioning of the absorbing surface and will consequently compromise the maintenance of an oxygen supply to all body cells.

Any number of pathological problems are included in the group that complicate the free exchange of oxygen and carbon dioxide between lungs and blood. Pneumonia is an infection of lung tissue, and the resulting inflammatory process reduces the extent of diffusion of the critical gases. Influenza and viral infections have the same result. Tuberculosis, which results in the destruction of lung tissues as body defenses wall off the area invaded by the bacillus, also interferes with oxygen absorption. Tumors, benign or malignant (and carcinoma of the lungs is becoming steadily higher in incidence), reduce lung space and efficiency. Congestive heart failure may cause inefficient pulmonary circulation, with a resultant accumulation of fluid within the alveolar spaces, and the patient can literally drown internally. Bronchiectasis, or the presence of dilated bronchi following inflammatory reactions, also interferes with the free diffusion of oxygen and carbon dioxide between alveolar air and capillaries. Air, fluid, or infection in the pleural cavity can decrease lung space. Any process that reduces lung space, covers the cellular lining of the alveoli, destroys lung tissue, or brings pressure to bear upon the alveolar lining poses a problem in adequate absorption of oxygen needed to maintain life.

For oxygen absorbed from the lungs to reach body tissues, the cardiovascular system provides both a means for carrying oxygen and the mechanical transportation that carries it to its ultimate destination. Thus, there are two aspects of cardiovascular system function that have implications for oxygen maintenance.

Anything that interferes with the union of oxygen and hemoglobin constitutes the first aspect. The amount of hemoglobin can be reduced by hemorrhage or blood volume loss, inadequate iron intake, anemia that results in a reduced number of red blood cells, or diseases of the blood-forming organs that result in reduced red blood cell formation. On the other hand, certain chemicals can interfere with the formation of oxyhemoglobin by forming a very stable union with hemoglobin so that the hemoglobin no longer can combine with oxygen. Carbon monoxide and cyanide are examples. Hemoglobin, contained in an adequate number of red blood cells, must be available if oxygen is to be transported to all body cells.

From the mechanical aspect of transportation of oxygen, effective heart pump action and an unimpaired state of the arteries, capillaries, and veins are essential to adequate function. Among the kinds of heart damage that present problems are (1) congestive heart failure, in which the inability to maintain blood flow results in widespread congestion; (2) hypertensive heart disease, in which increased blood pressure finally compromises efficient heart action; (3) coronary heart disease, such as acute myocardial infarction, caused by a sudden narrowing or obstruction of the coronary arteries; and (4) rheumatic heart disease, caused by the cardiac inflammation that accompanies rheumatic fever. Any actual damage to heart tissue makes the transportation of oxygen to body cells a major concern.

Peripheral vascular problems, i.e., disease of blood vessels outside the heart, can also embarrass oxygen transportation. Among the more common of such disorders are (1) thromboangiitis obliterans, or Buerger's disease, with inflammation, thrombus formation, and vessel destruction; (2) arteriosclerosis obliterans, in which artery changes result in a narrowed lumen; (3) Raynaud's disease, with its spasms of arteries in the extremities; (4) thrombophlebitis, with thrombus development, vein occlusion, and inflammation; and (5) varicose veins. Interference in the normal function of the vascular bed can cause local or general interference with oxygen supply.

The physiological action of both the respiratory system and the cardiovascular system is dependent upon the function of the central nervous system. In brain surgery, for example, it is not unusual for the surgeon to perform a tracheotomy, a surgical incision into the trachea into which a tube is inserted to maintain a patent airway. This procedure is done because edema, or swelling due to fluid retention, results from the trauma of surgery. The edema produces pressure within the cranium and affects the vital respiratory, as well as other, centers in this area. Thus, damage to the central nervous system, including the brain, spinal cord, or antonomic nervous system, can have implications for the maintenance of oxygen. Brain injury or trauma, brain hemorrhage, brain or spinal cord tumors, infections and inflammatory diseases (such as meningitis or poliomyelitis), or degenerative changes in the central nervous system can affect the function of the respiratory and cardiovascular systems and, in turn, affect the ability of the body to maintain an adequate oxygen supply to body cells.

As a last requirement, individual body cells must be able to utilize oxygen when it is delivered. Local trauma, local infections, chemicals that interfere with cell metabolism, and viral infections constitute examples of interference at the individual cell level. Another example would be a change in the acid-base balance in the fluid surrounding the cells—a change beyond the safety range in either the acid or the base direction.

The maintenance of an adequate supply of oxygen to all body cells thus requires adequate supply, intake, absorption, transportation, and utilization.

NURSING INTERVENTION

The treatment and care of patients whose supply of oxygen is threatened involves general measures directed toward preserving total hygiene and specific measures directed toward solving the individual oxygen problem. Nursing responsibility is divided into three categories:

1. Critical observation of vital symptoms
2. Dependent nursing function consisting of assisting with medical pro-

cedures, care of patients before, during, and after procedures, and carrying out specific therapeutic measures

3. The independent nursing functions, both general and specific

Dependent nursing functions are so called because they "depend" upon a directive received from someone else, usually a licensed medical practitioner. However, when carrying out a dependent function such as a treatment or medication prescribed by a physician, the nurse must independently use her own judgment. For example, the physician may order a medication, but the nurse is legally responsible for the preparation and administration of the medication and may be responsible for withholding a medication if the patient's condition so indicates. Even in the area of dependent functions, the nurse must independently make judgments based on a knowledge of cause and effect.

Observation

Whenever there is a health problem interfering with maintenance of oxygen supply to body cells, the existence of certain symptoms as compensatory mechanisms gives indication of the patient's level of security. Recognition of these signs and their implications with regard to patient safety is fundamental to nursing care. Overtly, observation is concerned with four basic physical facts:

1. Color, both local and general
2. Skin temperature
3. The mechanics of respiration
4. Cough

From the viewpoint of its significance as a key indicator of homeostatic deviation, color is of prime importance. This is equally true for local color changes that accompany obstruction, infectious processes, or inflammatory processes and for general, over-all color changes that accompany systemic problems. Systemic responses, i.e., those relating to the entire organism, will be discussed first.

Regardless of primary skin color, there are recognizable physiological indices of adequate oxygenation in the skin—buccal mucosa, orbital mucosa, and the digits and nail beds of both extremities. Color changes are related to normal and usual color tones, and deviations are measured in terms of inadequate supply or superfluous supply of oxygen systemically. Natural color results from the presence of the required oxygen concentration in the cells. This, in turn, is dependent upon (1) the requisite red blood cells and hemoglobin essential to supply all body cells, (2) an efficiently functioning circulatory system to transport blood, and (3) thoroughly patent respiratory system able to absorb the essential components and to excrete nonessentials.

Inadequate oxygenation is evidenced by pallor (a lack of natural color) and cyanosis, the addition of a bluish discoloration along with pallor. Pallor and cyanosis can span a range of quality and character from the insidious and discrete to the sudden and acute. Regardless of dramatic depth of the patient's appearance, recognition of significant changes is critical to patient safety. Color as an indication of "air hunger" can result from many physiological problems and is a systemic "S.O.S." dictating direct action for palliative, supportive, or restorative measures. The responsibility of the nurse lies in the identification of the existence of anoxia as evidenced by pallor and cyanosis, calculation of the significance of the degree of danger to the patient, and the implementation of independent and dependent nursing measures appropriate to the situation.

Impaired oxygenation of a local area is also characterized by pallor or by blanching and cyanosis. It occurs in a variety of health problems involving circulatory obstruction resulting from mechanical or pathological interference with blood flow. Accurate evaluation and reporting of the extent of circulatory impairment is essential to prevent degenerative changes in the tissue involved. Inadequate oxygenation of extremities, for example, can lead quickly to necrosis or to tissue death if measures are not taken to restore the oxygen supply.

Of particular concern to the nurse is frequent and accurate observation of color when supportive, palliative, or therapeutic measures employed have a potential for interference with circulation. Bandages and all types of immobilizing devices, such as casts, are examples of circulatory threats.

In contrast to pallor and cyanosis, hyperemia or redness indicates increased oxygenation of the tissues, locally or generally, where it is manifest. The increase of blood supply to the periphery may be at the expense of internal organs. It may occur in a local area as an indication of an inflammatory process. Systemic hyperemia may be the result of the body's homeostatic mechanism for maintaining body temperature. Increased peripheral circulation serves to dissipate heat and reduce body temperature. Here, again, the significant fact involved consists of noting the degree and the extent of hyperemia, assessing its significance, reporting, and undertaking independent nursing measures that will alleviate circulatory disturbance. If, for example, the hyperemia is due to fever, independent nursing care includes rest, administration of fluids, keeping the patient adequately warm, giving skin care, and maintenance of nutrition. The anticipated diaphoresis that accompanies the hyperemia just described would include a considerable loss of sodium as well as fluid. The nurse must therefore consider the need for sodium. Increased body metabolism that accompanies a rise in body temperature would call for increased carbohydrate and protein intake to supplement the greater internal utilization of these.

Thus color—red, white, and blue—is an area of critical observation for the nurse in assessing the adequacy of the patient's oxygen supply, either locally or systemically.

Skin temperature, either locally or generally, provides vital information regarding the status of oxygenation of body tissues. The feeling of cold or warmth (either described by the patient or perceived by the nurse's touch), when combined with color, is an important indication of anoxia or hyperemia. The combination of pallor and cyanosis of any degree in conjunction with a cold skin means a seriously reduced oxygen supply. The combination of warmth in conjunction with hyperemia means an increased oxygen supply. Both states require the use of discriminatory judgment in determining probable cause. In any event, both states call for direct reporting to the physician responsible for medical management.

Another area of critical observation in relation to the maintenance of oxygen is the rate, rhythm, and character of respiration. The rate, rhythm, and character of respirations can vary widely under normal conditions, such as the amount of physical exercise, emotional stress, altitude above sea level, and similar factors. Therefore, the evaluation of the patient's respiration must take into account all such factors. Of particular significance from the point of view of observation is dyspnea, or difficulty in breathing. This may take the form of any one of the kinds of respiration described previously, such as apnea, or it may take the form of orthopnea, Cheyne-Stokes respiration, or Kussmaul's respiration. (The latter two types are relatively serious symptoms.) The extent of any type of dyspnea can show a wide range of degree from slight difficulty in breathing to serious struggle to keep breathing.

In addition to observation of character, rate, and rhythm of respiration, the nurse needs to observe the extrinsic and intrinsic factors that appear to affect respiration. The combined observation of the respiratory mechanism and the factors that affect it form the basis for nursing action. Examples of extrinsic factors that may be significant are ventilation, position, emotional response, increased body metabolism, or pain.

Coughing is a defense mechanism that supports the function of the external respiratory tract and constitutes another critical area of observation for the nurse. Major points of observation in relation to cough include character, time of occurrence, frequency, duration, productivity, and associated pain.

Observation of the character of a cough includes answers to the following questions. Is the cough dry or "hacking"? Is it moist or loose? Is the cough paroxysmal or rhymic? Is it asthmatic or "wheezy"?

In regard to time of occurrence, observation relates to whether coughing is usual in the morning or evening, or occurs during the night. The frequency and duration of the occurrence is also pertinent. Is the coughing occasional, frequent, or almost continual? Is the cough chronic or acute? Does the patient have long periods of coughing with rests between them, or does he cough for short periods of time, but often.

The productivity of the cough is significant not only in terms of whether or not it is productive, but also in terms of the character of the sputum produced. Sputum, which is the most significant of cough products, comes from within the lungs themselves and is produced by deep coughing that is forcible enough to remove secretions from the lungs. This point is important in collection of sputum specimens. Specific areas of observation include consistency, amount, color, odor, and the presence or absence of blood. The presence of blood in any product resulting from a cough requires additional evaluation to determine the source of blood, whether it is coming from the upper or lower respiratory tract, and the severity of bleeding. Such factors as the color of blood, as an indication of whether it is old or frank, and its presence in or on the surface of the sputum are significant in making this determination.

Pain may or may not be associated with coughing. In addition to the patient's subjective description of the character and duration of pain, observation of the patient's position can provide clues about pain. The patient may "splint" the chest while coughing and will most often assume an upright or sitting position when he does so. As well as using position, he may support his chest with his hands. The patient who has pain will also try to suppress the cough to the extent that he is able to do so.

The critical observations that the nurse is required to make in relation to the maintenance of an adequate supply of oxygen to all body tissues are in the areas of color, skin temperature, respiration, and cough.

Dependent nursing functions

Dependent nursing functions in relation to the maintenance of oxygen include the following:

1. Preparation for, assistance with, or being responsible for seeing that procedures are carried out
2. Assistance with and care of the patient during or after medical procedures
3. Carrying out the physician's orders for medications and/or treatments

Diagnostic procedures

In general, in relation to diagnostic procedures concerned with determination of oxygen deficiency, the nurse is frequently not involved in the actual process of the testing procedure itself. She is, however, responsible for the preparation of the patient by means of explanation and supportive care in advance of and following the diagnostic test.

Included in the diagnostic category are chest x-ray films, sputum examination, determination of vital capacity of the lungs, bronchoscopy and bronchogram, blood tests, especially red blood cells, hemoglobin, and carbon dioxide combining power.

In regard to diagnostic procedures, direct nursing responsibility includes knowing the exact procedure ordered, arranging for or checking to ensure that a procedure is scheduled and carried out, having necessary preparation completed before the test, having the patient ready for the test, and observing the patient's reaction following the test. With regard to x-ray films, the nurse either arranges for or accompanies the patient to the x-ray department and is responsible for his total safety before, during, and after examination. When sputum examination is ordered, the nurse is responsible for collection of the specimen.

Although determination of vital capacity of the lungs is performed by the physician, the nurse needs to know the terminology used to describe lung capacity in order to understand results and to explain the test to the patient. Bronchoscopy, a medical diagnostic procedure, enables the physician to view the trachea and bronchi directly by insertion of an instrument called a bronchoscope. The nurse's responsibilities are considerable in the area of patient preparation since the procedure is impossible without the patient's cooperation. Explanation should emphasize that the mouth and throat will be anesthetized, that the room will be dark in order for the physician to see more clearly, that the patient's eyes will be covered to protect them from the introduction of foreign material, and that the patient will be able to breathe through the inserted tube. The patient should be encouraged to ask questions and express feelings freely about the procedure. Additional helpful measures would be to have the patient practice breathing through his nose with his mouth open and relaxing while lying flat on his back with his head hyperextended. All food and fluids are withheld for at least eight hours prior to the procedure to avoid problems that may arise due to vomiting. Sedation is normally ordered for the patient to lessen anxiety and discomfort. Meticulous oral hygiene before and after the procedure is indicated.

In bronchography, a medical diagnostic procedure similar to bronchoscopy, a radiopaque oil is introduced into the bronchus through a catheter inserted through a laryngeal cannula to permit visualization of the bronchial tree. Nursing care for the patient undergoing bronchography is essentially the same as that of a patient experiencing bronchoscopy, except for the additional measure of postural drainage after and frequently before the bronchogram is made. Postural drainage is indicated before a bronchogram in order to remove accumulated bronchial secretions that interfere with the radiopaque agent's reaching all surfaces of the area. It is indicated following the examination to ensure total removal of the opaque agent which otherwise becomes a foreign body constituting a threat to homeostasis by interfering with the function of the absorbing surface and predisposing to inflammatory and infectious processes.

Assisting with medical procedures

In addition to the specific diagnostic tests, medical treatments commonly used therapeutically or palliatively when patients have problems with maintenance of oxygen are (1) closed chest drainage, (2) thoracentesis, (3) therapeutic pneumothorax, (4) postural drainage, (5) tracheostomy, (6) dry phlebotomy, (7) radiation therapy, and (8) administration of oxygen.

Chest drainage is closed, because the tube used is attached to an air-sealed apparatus to prevent entrance of air into the pleural space. The purpose of closed drainage is to permit the release of fluid or air without collapsing the lung.

Thoracentesis is removal of fluid from the pleural space.

Pneumothorax is the introduction of air into the pleural space to collapse a lung partially or totally.

Postural drainage rests upon the law of gravity. The procedure is used to promote drainage from the bronchioles, usually in chronic lung problems.

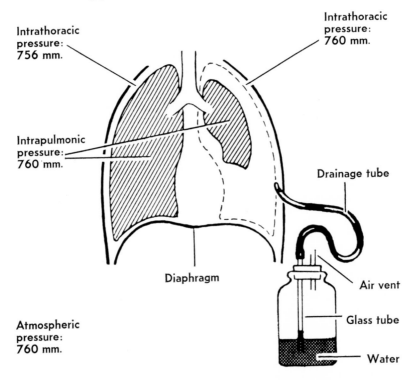

Fig. 31. The chest at rest, with lung pressure equaling atmospheric pressure. On inspiration and expiration, intrapulmonic pressure drops slightly. The need for closed drainage becomes obvious—neither air in the drainage system nor fluid should be permitted to enter the intrathoracic cavity. (Reprinted by permission from RN magazine, January, 1960. Copyright 1960, RN Publications, Inc., Oradell, N. J.)

The essence of the procedure is positioning the patient so that the chest is above the trachea and mouth to allow residual secretions to drain from a higher to a lower level.

In a variety of health problems a tracheostomy is often performed to maintain a patent airway for intake of oxygen. This procedure consists in making an incision directly into the trachea and inserting an especially designed trocar and cannula.

A dry phlebotomy or phlebostasis consists of the application of tourniquets to the extremities on a rotating basis, three extremities being occluded at one time. The procedure is used in acute pulmonary edema to reduce the work of the heart.

Radiation therapy consists of exposing body tissues to the emanations of radioactive agents to halt the growth of neoplasms.

The medical procedures mentioned here differ in nature in regard to the role of the nurse. Some procedures, such as postural drainage, are ordered by the physician, and the nurse is completely responsible for carrying them out at the time intervals prescribed. A second kind of procedure, such as the thoracentesis, is a "stat" type, i.e., ordered once, and the nurse is responsible for assisting the physician. With the third type of medical procedure, such as closed drainage of the chest, the nurse not only assists with the procedure, but also is responsible for the maintenance of the closed chest drainage after the treatment has been instituted.

In general, the nurse's responsibilities in relation to medical procedures include the care of the patient, the care of equipment and specimens, and assisting the physician. She prepares the patient through explanation and through specific preparation of the body area involved if this is necessary. She supports the patient during the procedure and observes carefully for any untoward signs that indicate the patient is not reacting well to therapy. She is then responsible for aftercare of the patient, leaving him as comfortable as possible. In addition, she is responsible for seeing that necessary equipment is available when needed, for disposal of any specimens collected, and for disposal of equipment.

Closed chest drainage. Specifically, in closed chest drainage, the nurse checks the drainage system frequently to be sure that (1) no air enters, (2) the tubes are patent, (3) the glass tube in the control bottle is below the water, (4) clamps are available to close the drainage tubes in case of emergency, and (5) the drainage system is never above chest level. Because the pleural space has a pressure below atmospheric pressure, the drainage system must be maintained as closed drainage to avoid air or fluid entering the pleural space and causing the lung to collapse.

Thoracentesis. When a patient is to have a thoracentesis* or therapeutic pneumothorax, specific nursing care includes careful explanation and permitting the patient to express his feelings in order that the procedure will be accepted as well as possible. Frequently the skin area will need to be shaved. The patient usually appreciates support during the procedure. In addition, the patient's pulse, respiration, color, and degree of apprehension should be observed throughout the treatment. The patient should be advised to try not to cough, if it is possible, to reduce potential incidence of lung trauma.

Postural drainage. Specific nursing care for a patient who is to receive postural drainage relates to position, support for the dependent part of the body, observation of patient reaction, timing, safety, and health teaching. The basic principle involved in position is to use gravity to promote drainage from the chest. This means that the patient should be literally "upside down." The choice of position will depend upon the patient's age, size, health problem, degree of illness, and personality make-up. The patient may lie across the bed with the head and chest lowered over the side or may lie jackknifed on a gatch bed. The foot of the bed may be elevated on blocks. Whatever the choice, support must be provided for the dependent portions of the body. The patient usually requires encouragement both to assume the position and to use the treatment effectively. He must be encouraged to breathe and cough deeply to facilitate the removal of secre-

---

*See Appendix, pages 326-328, Paracentesis.

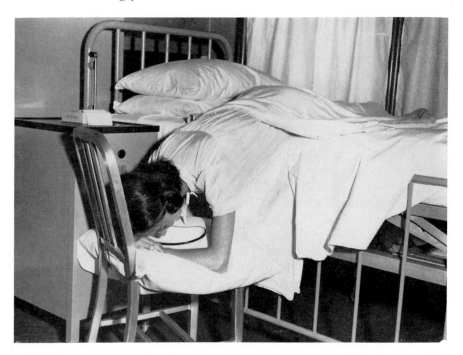

Fig. 32. Postural drainage depends on gravity to remove lung secretions. The patient lying over the side of the bed is in a frequently used position.

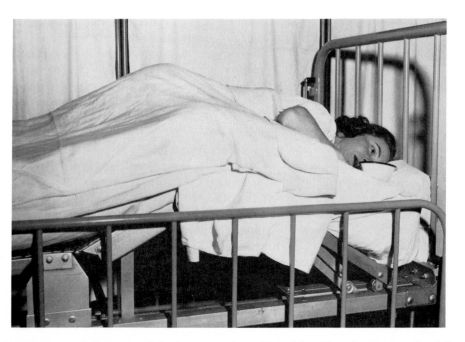

Fig. 33. Postural drainage of the lungs may be achieved by using the foot gatch of the bed. This is used most often for elderly or weak patients.

tions. Since most persons are not accustomed to being in an upside-down position, the procedure is usually not a very comfortable one.

Dizziness can be expected. Therefore, the nurse must stay with the patient to ensure his safety and to provide psychological support. The time the patient remains positioned may be increased gradually and may be as long as twenty to thirty minutes. This procedure should never be performed too close to mealtime and should be followed by thorough oral hygiene.

Because the patient frequently will be required to continue the procedure following its initiation in any health service, he should be taught how to position himself, how to protect himself, how to care for the discharge, how to attain maximum drainage, and the importance of timing and oral hygiene.

Tracheostomy. The key points in the nursing care of a patient with a tracheostomy are the reassurance of the patient, maintenance of a patent airway, and teaching the patient how to care for himself if the tracheostomy is permanent. Whether the tracheostomy is planned or is done in an emergency, the patient must be reassured that he will be able to breathe. Any threat to the oxygen supply has a deep psychological significance because man can exist only a few minutes without it. A tracheostomy, therefore, is a relatively frightening experience to most persons.

The patient needs all the reassurance that the nurse can give. In addition to what one tells the patient, a frequent check on his condition, prompt and effective suctioning, and a calm and quiet manner will contribute to the patient's feeling of security.

Of critical importance in the care of the tracheostomized patient is the use of suction to aspirate secretions and maintain the airway. A soft rubber

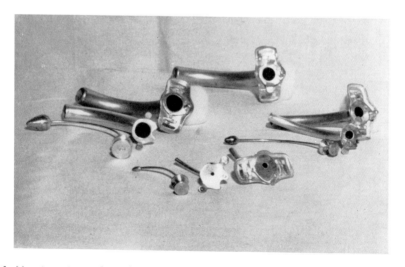

Fig. 34. Varying sizes of tracheostomy tubes. The top tube has the inner cannula in site.

catheter attached to a suction device is employed. When the catheter is inserted into the trachea more than four or five inches, or to a point where it is beyond the tracheostomy tube, care must be exercised to avoid applying the negative force of suction to the mucous membrane lining of the trachea for too long a period of time. If upper tracheal suction is not effectual, the physician must be notified, for deep tracheal suction is within the medical province. The inner tube should be removed and cleaned as often as necessary. If there is danger of the tube clogging, the patient should not be left alone. Moist gauze over the opening of the tube or steam inhalations may be ordered in the early stages to moisten the inspired air.

The wound should be managed as any postoperative wound, i.e., kept free from contamination and irritation.

The whole tracheostomy tube will need to be changed periodically, and the nurse should keep careful record of the times this is done in the interest of the patient's comfort and safety. The patient should be warned, if possible, that he will have some difficulty in speaking, and a means of communication should be provided—either pencil and paper or a system of signals. When a patient is conscious, the most comfortable and safest position is a sitting position with the head and neck supported to avoid tracheal irritation and to promote comfort and safety. The outer cannula is commonly secured around the neck with tapes. This should be checked frequently to ensure the retention of the tube in site.

If the tracheostomy is permanent, the patient will need to be taught how to care for the tubes and the tracheal opening. Referral to specialized health services following hospitalization is, of course, essential.

Whenever a tracheostomy is performed on a patient, two basic safety

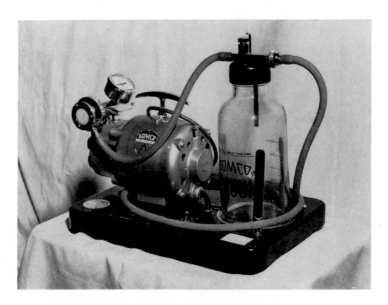

Fig. 35. An electrically powered suction machine.

factors must be provided. First, a hemostat should be within easy reach, because it can be used to maintain the tracheal opening in the event that the tube is inadvertently expelled. In addition, a sterile tracheostomy emergency tray should be readily accessible.

Dry phlebotomy. When dry phlebotomy is ordered, the nurse is usually responsible for carrying out the procedure. Tourniquets are applied to three extremities and rotated every 15 minutes. Each extremity is thus occluded for 45 minutes and free for 15 minutes. No extremity should be occluded for longer than 45 minutes because of the danger of permanent damage to tissues. The system of rotation, either clockwise or counterclockwise, must be established and must be adhered to rigidly. Skin temperature of the occluded extremities should be checked frequently, especially if the patient has any vascular problem.

Radiation therapy. If a patient is receiving radiation therapy, there are three special areas of concern to the nurse: (1) the patient's general reaction to the treatment, (2) skin care, and (3) psychological support.

The patient may react systemically with generalized symptoms such as nausea, vomiting, or mental depression. The extent of the patient's reaction should be promptly reported. Because most patients associate radiation with cancer and because cancer is a disease most patients fear, it is important for the nurse to know how much the physician has told the patient and how much he wants the patient to know.

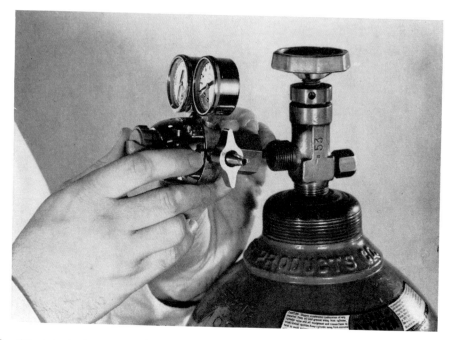

Fig. 36. A typical oxygen cylinder regulator. (Courtesy A. Linde Co., Division of Union Carbide Corporation, New York, N. Y.)

In regard to skin care, radiation dosage that is therapeutic almost always produces some skin damage. The parts involved should not be washed, and any marks on the patient's skin that are therapeutic guides should not be removed. The treatment of the skin reaction as well as routine skin care varies widely. Nothing should be used on the involved skin area unless medically prescribed.

From the psychological point of view, the nurse provides explanation of the routines of treatment, an opportunity for the patient to talk, and provides the patient with a sense of acceptance.

Administration of oxygen. The administration of oxygen on medical order is frequently the responsibility of the nurse. The selection of method of administration and the rate of desired concentration are usually included in the medical order. There are three basic methods of administration: the nasal catheter, the nasal or oronasal face mask, and the tent. Modifications of these have been designed for special situations. An example of this is the Croupette, an adaptation of the tent that is used to administer oxygen to

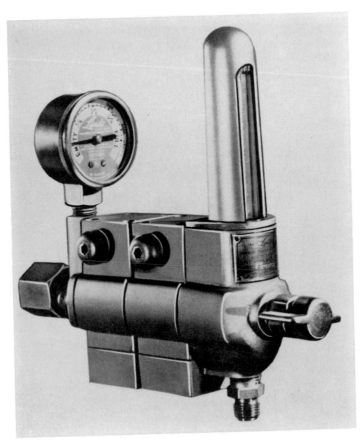

Fig. 37. A typical oxygen cylinder regulator. (Courtesy A. Linde Co., Division of Union Carbide Corporation, New York, N. Y.)

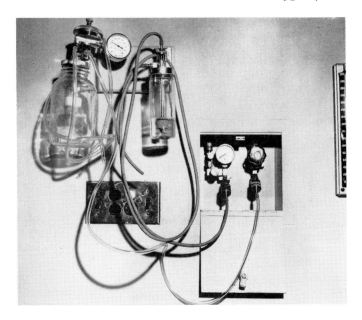

Fig. 38. Wall outlets for the administration of oxygen are becoming common.

infants. The actual selection of method is determined by the patient's need for oxygen concentration, the cause of the oxygen lack, and the patient's ability to cooperate with the treatment.

The oxygen is normally supplied in tanks or cylinders, in which the gas is contained under high pressure, or from wall outlets from a central supply source. The latter method is becoming increasingly popular in hospitals. In either case, a regulator that indicates the rate of liter flow will be present. This can be set at the desired level.

When oxygen is administered by nasal catheter, the catheter is inserted until it is just visible in the oropharynx, and then it is withdrawn about an inch. The catheter is attached to the patient's face with adhesive tape. The oxygen is humidified by being passed through water in a bottle attached to the regulator.

The face mask usually covers the mouth and nose and provides, in addition to oxygen intake, some means of control of the carbon dioxide exhaled. Oxygen may also be administered under positive pressure by this method. Positive pressure is used particularly when pulmonary edema is present, because the positive pressure increases the diffusion of oxygen into the capillaries.

Oxygen is administered by tent when a high concentration of oxygen is required in states of acute physiological distress. An oxygen tent consists of a refrigeration unit that cools and moistens the oxygen as it is propelled through it by means of a motor into the canopy that covers the patient. The tent usually operates on electrical power.

The nursing responsibilities in regard to oxygen therapy focus on safety,

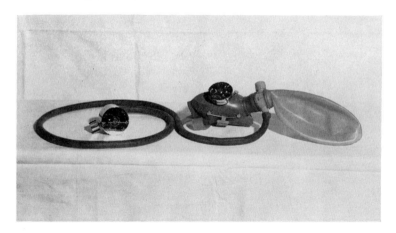

Fig. 39. Oxygen mask with positive pressure apparatus.

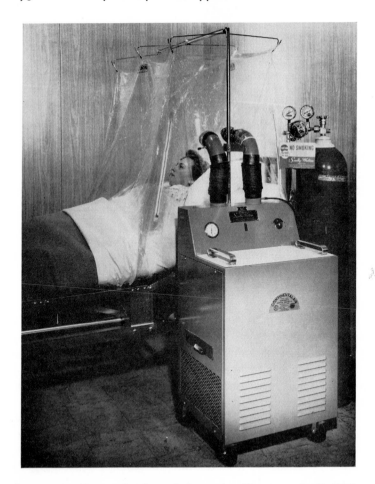

Fig. 40. Oxygen is often administered by tent. (Courtesy Scully-Walton Oxygen Therapy Service, New York, N. Y., and Chicago, Ill.)

the maintenance of oxygen, the maintenance of humidity, and the observation of the patient's reaction to oxygen therapy.

The major safety hazard in the use of oxygen is the danger of fire or explosion since oxygen supports combustion. Probably the greatest cause of danger is smoking, which cannot be permitted in rooms in which oxygen is in use. Another potential source of danger is static electricity. Electrical appliances of any type should be in good working order with insulating covering intact. In general, substances with an oil base may also be a source of danger.

The nurse is also responsible for the maintenance of the desired concentration of oxygen in any of the three methods of choice. The catheter and face mask should be adjusted to be as comfortable as possible for the patient. The mask should fit securely and the catheter should be inserted to the correct distance to prevent dissipation of inflow. The rate of oxygen flow should be frequently checked, and the intake supply should be maintained. Catheter and masks should be cleaned when necessary. The catheter is usually changed every forty-eight to seventy-two hours. The skin area around the nose and mouth requires particular care when a mask is employed. When oxygen is administered by tent, the canopy must be fitted securely under the mattress and across the patient's hips to retain the desired concentration. All nursing care should be planned to reduce the number of times and to decrease the amount of time the tent must be opened.

Because the administration of oxygen without moisture is iritating to mucous membranes of the respiratory tract, the nurse should assume responsibility for the effectiveness of whatever measure is used to humidify the oxygen. She should, for example, be sure that water is in the bottle attached to the regulator. She should be sure that the face mask fits tightly if it is one that depends upon moisture from the patient's exhaled air as a means of humidification.

One of the major responsibilities of the nurse in this area is observation of the patient's reaction to oxygen therapy. The patient's color, respiration, and pulse supply significant clues. In addition, the patient's apprehension, restlessness, excitability, and level of consciousness are important.

Independent nursing functions

In providing nursing care to patients with problems in the maintenance of oxygen, the nurse directs her efforts primarily toward supporting oxygen intake and reducing oxygen utilization.

There is a direct relationship between the patient's physical hygiene and comfort and the utilization of oxygen. When a patient is physically uncomfortable, he is restless and uneasy, and as a consequence the basic metabolic process is increased. When the metabolic rate is increased, the need for oxygen is also increased. Meticulous attention to physical hygiene measures, including skin care, oral hygiene, hair combing, nail care, etc., makes a direct contribution to reducing oxygen utilization. From this point of view, the promotion of elimination without stress or strain for the patient is also an important nursing measure. Constipation, for example, can lead to a considerable increase in metabolic activity as a result of physical and mental discomfort.

The management of activity and rest for the patient with problems of oxygen constitutes another significant nursing measure. While an immediate postoperative patient may need to be turned frequently to prevent the development of hypostatic pneumonia, the relationship of muscular activity to oxygen need is obvious. The problem for the nurse becomes one of balancing the patient's need for activity, which results in an increased utilization of oxygen, with the ability to absorb and transport oxygen. When the oxygen lack is serious, activity must be diminished. On the other hand, activity must be proportionate to the patient's ability to tolerate it. The reduction of activity for a patient calls for a great deal of thought on the part of the nurse particularly in regard to small details. Keeping things that the patient may need within reach, using help when moving the patient, assistance with feeding, assistance with physical hygiene, and planning care for the patient so that it takes as little time for the patient as possible are the kinds of small details that contribute much to patient comfort and rest.

Position of the patient is significant in relation to systemic oxygen want. From the point of view of systemic oxygen problems, the patient is most comfortable and breathing is facilitated when the position is upright, sitting, or in a semi-Fowler position. When the oxygen lack is a local one, as in Buerger's disease, the basic guiding rule is not to keep the affected part in any one position for too long a period. The nurse's responsibility is to see that the patient is placed in and maintained in the correct body position.

Another important nursing measure that contributes to a reduced utilization of oxygen is the prevention and the alleviation of anxiety. Anxiety, fear, anger, or apprehension can trigger the defense response that prepares the body for fight or flight. When oxygen supply is concerned, there is the additional factor that any threat to oxygen maintenance is a threat to life itself. Much can be done to prevent anxiety by clear explanation to the patient about what is going on around him and exactly and specifically what his limitations are. Any signs of worry or anxiety should immediately clue the nurse to the patient's need to explore whatever is bothering him. The management of anxiety is an important aspect of the nursing care of any patient with oxygen problems.

The supervision of the environment is an independent function of the nurse, and environmental control can be used to reduce oxygen utilization by the patient. Unpleasant sights, odors, and noises can increase body metabolism. Too many visitors or too many personnel functioning without regard to each other's activities can do the same thing. Therefore, the manipulation of the environment in the direction of peace and quiet in so far as possible makes a substantial contribution to the patient's well-being. In addition to reducing oxygen utilization, there must be an adequate supply of oxygen in the environment. Proper ventilation is therefore important.

Particular problems in health teaching for patients who have problems of

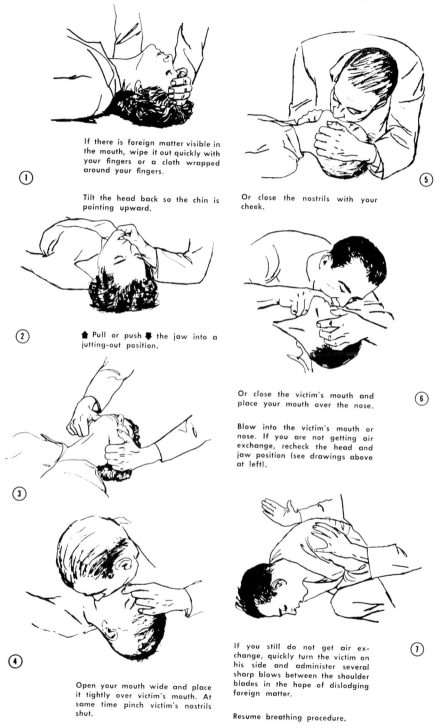

① If there is foreign matter visible in the mouth, wipe it out quickly with your fingers or a cloth wrapped around your fingers.

② Tilt the head back so the chin is pointing upward.

③ ⬆ Pull or push ⬇ the jaw into a jutting-out position.

④ Open your mouth wide and place it tightly over victim's mouth. At same time pinch victim's nostrils shut.

⑤ Or close the nostrils with your cheek.

⑥ Or close the victim's mouth and place your mouth over the nose.

Blow into the victim's mouth or nose. If you are not getting air exchange, recheck the head and jaw position (see drawings above at left).

⑦ If you still do not get air exchange, quickly turn the victim on his side and administer several sharp blows between the shoulder blades in the hope of dislodging foreign matter.

Resume breathing procedure.

Fig. 41. Artificial respiration—mouth-to-mouth (mouth-to-nose) method. (Courtesy American Red Cross.)

oxygenation will relate of course to specific health problems. Major areas of emphasis include teaching in regard to diet, medications, kinds and limitations of activity, diversional and occupational needs, and community resources. All such teaching should be done in considerable detail, being very specific. It is not enough for a patient to know, for example, that the local division of the American Cancer Society will provide help. The patient or a responsible family member should be taught exactly what services are available, where the organization is located, the name of its director, and when and how the organization can be contacted. If the patient is on a low-sodium diet, he should be taught not only what foods are low in sodium content, but also what foods are high in sodium content. He should further be taught how such foods can be prepared so that they are palatable.

Emergency nursing measures

In addition to the preceding measures, the nurse may also be called upon to perform certain essentially non-nursing measures in an emergency. Included are the administration of oxygen and various methods of resuscitation. When a patient appears to be in respiratory difficulty and there is a sudden increase in cyanosis, a nurse may begin the administration of oxygen, using the method of administration that can be instituted most rapidly.

Various methods of resuscitation are indicated if a patient suddenly ceases to breathe due to drowning, collapse, shock as a result of trauma or electrocution, asphyxiation, or chemical intoxication. Today, mouth-to-mouth resuscitation is considered by far the most effective method. The

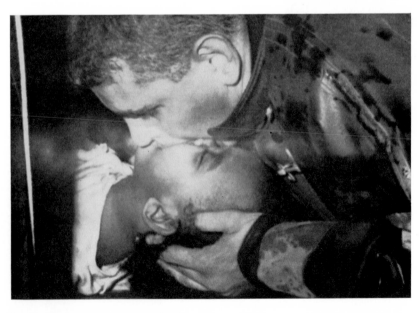

Fig. 42. Mouth-to-mouth resuscitation is often successful in emergencies. (Courtesy the New York Fire Department.)

effectiveness of this method depends upon the proper extension of the neck and the proper elevation of the jaw.

The patient is placed in a supine position with the head extended. The operator kneels at the side of the head. The lower jaw is grasped with the thumb and index finger and lifted upward vertically. The other thumb and index finger are used to close the nostrils. The operator inflates the patient's lungs with his own breath and then removes his mouth to permit the patient to exhale. This should be repeated 12 to 20 times per minute.

When mouth-to-mouth breathing is not possible, a method of artificial respiration called Holger-Nielson Manual method may be used. Briefly, the patient is placed in a prone position with the arms abducted at right angles to the trunk and bent at the elbows. The operator kneels at the patient's head with one knee on either side of the patient's head. Using both hands, the operator leans upon the patient's back, compressing the chest. As the operator straightens up, he slides his hand up along the patient's arms and raises them from the surface at the elbows. The double movement of compressing the chest and raising the arms is repeated about 12 times per minute.

BIBLIOGRAPHY

1. Creighton, Helen, and Coulter, William: The why of a pulmonary function test, American Journal of Nursing **60**:1771-1774, Dec. 1960.
2. M. Joanne De Vincenti, Sister, M. Bernadine Koenig, Sister, and M. Michele Carmody, Sister: Some reactions of cardiac patients to visitors, Nursing Outlook **8**:693-695, Dec. 1960.
3. Gilmore, Stuart I.: Rehabilitation after laryngectomy, American Journal of Nursing **61**:87-89, Jan. 1961.
4. Hoffman, Katherine B.: Chemistry for the applied sciences, Englewood Cliffs, N. J., 1963, Prentice-Hall, Inc., pp. 64-75.
5. Hughes, Edward C.: Life in inner space, American Journal of Nursing **63**:92-94, Jan. 1963.
6. Jensen, J. Trygne: Introduction to medical physics, Philadelphia, 1960, J. B. Lippincott Co., pp. 54-75.
7. Langby, Leroy L., and Cheraskin, E.: The physiology of man, ed. 2, New York, 1958, McGraw-Hill Book Co., Inc., pp. 363-409.
8. McClain, Esther M., and Gragg, Shirley H.: Scientific principles in nursing, ed. 4, St. Louis, 1962, The C. V. Mosby Co., pp. 225-243.
9. Nordmark, Madelyn T., and Rohweder, Anne W.: Scientific principles applied to nursing, Philadelphia, 1959, J. B. Lippincott Co., pp. 59-70.
10. Pons, Edward: Ambulatory use of oxygen, American Journal of Nursing **60**:1775, Dec. 1960.
11. Shafer, Kathleen Newton, Sawyer, Janet R., McCluskey, Audrey M., and Beck, Edna Lifgren: Medical-surgical nursing, ed. 2, St. Louis, 1961, The C. V. Mosby Co., pp. 219-265, 429-479.

Chapter 18

Nursing care of patients with nutritional problems

Nutrition (including the stages of mastication, deglutition, digestion, absorption, assimilation, and excretion) is a fundamental process resulting in tissue repair and building and in energy liberation that sustains life. Although one would die more slowly without food and water than without oxygen, the lack of food and water would make death no less certain. Thus, food contributes to the maintenance of internal homeostasis. While nutrition, elimination, and fluid and electrolyte balance are inextricably interwoven, they are separated here purely for convenience of organization. What is ingested forms the primary source of body water, electrolyte balance, and elimination.

ESSENTIAL REQUIREMENTS

If the nutrition of all body cells is to be maintained, certain criteria must be met.
1. Food intake must be adequate in amount and in the essential elements necessary to maintain optimum functioning of the human body.
2. The mechanical action and chemical substances necessary for digestion must be present and functioning effectively.
3. The absorption of digested food must take place.
4. The necessary food elements must be transported to all body cells.
5. The cells must be able to utilize the necessary elements of nutrition.
6. Storage must be provided for essential elements of nutrition to be available in times of need.

Thus, maintenance of nutrition to all body cells rests upon the integrity of the gastrointestinal tract, the liver and adjacent tissues, the pancreas, the cardiovascular system, and the central nervous system.

WHAT CAN GO WRONG

The adequate intake of food is influenced by a number of factors. Cultural standards and social custom, individual habits and preferences, food fads, socioeconomic standards, knowledge of nutritional needs, emotional problems, and the state of physical health constitute examples. Two very common nutritional problems in the United States are dieting and obesity. The majority of persons who diet do not do so under the direction of a physician, a practice which is a *sine qua non* for safe and sane dieting. Obesity has become a major health problem and is a serious one, because it predisposes its victims to early occurrence of other health problems, especially cardiovascular diseases.

Intake can present problems from both extremes—too little or too much. Too much, especially in the area of fat intake, is not an unusual occurrence. The relationship between high animal fat intake, overweight, high blood cholesterol, and coronary disease is under investigation, and although the evidence is not conclusive, it is suggestive enough that overweight persons with a high blood cholesterol are usually placed on a low cholesterol diet. Food fads are frequently dangerous, because they include excesses of one type of food at the expense of others, thus producing an unbalanced diet.

From a worldwide point of view, from the point of view of the underprivileged socioeconomic groups in our own society, and from the point of view of those with poor eating habits, the "too little" aspect of intake is most important. The results can be either general or specific. Systemic responses to underintake are weight loss, underactivity, lethargy, listlessness, loss of skin turgor, irritability, lack of ambition, and underachievement. Undernourished persons are readily susceptible to other health problems and tend to have a high sickness and absentee rate. Since body resistance is lowered, they succumb more readily to infections and take longer to recover from them.

Certain nutritional elements are so basic to the maintenance of homeostasis that their absence results in specific disease syndromes. A lack of iron can result in anemia, since iron is an essential constituent of red blood cells. An absence of vitamin C can produce scurvy, which is evidenced by loss of appetite, tender skin, sore mouth, bleeding gums and loosened teeth, pinpoint skin hemorrhages, and tenderness of knee joints. The lack of vitamin D in early years can result in rickets, in which bowed legs and malformation of teeth occur as a result of failure to absorb and utilize calcium. The absence of thiamine can produce beriberi. The absence of niacin can result in pellagra, with anorexia, dermatitis, diarrhea, weakness, and eventually dementia. The absence of carbohydrate in the presence of fat can result in acidosis. The absence of complete amino acids makes repair and rebuilding of body tissues impossible. Potassium deficiency results in generalized weakness and apprehension. There is no essential element in the balanced diet that can be long excluded from food intake without a reduced efficiency in physiological processes becoming apparent sooner or later.

The psychological and social influences on adequate nutritional patterns have been discussed previously. Their importance for the maintenance of a state of positive health cannot be overemphasized nor can the significance of maintaining adequate nutrition for emotional health be underestimated.

The mechanical aspects of digestion are dependent upon the ability to masticate, to swallow, and to provide digestive peristalsis in the stomach and the intestines. Anything that interferes at any one of these stages can affect nutrition. Thus, a tooth extraction, loss of dentures, a fractured jaw, or an inflammation of the mouth can limit or completely restrict the ability of the patient to chew and require dietary adaptation. Swallowing may be complicated by many factors such as a common cold, an inflammation of the mucous membrane lining the upper gastrointestinal tract, the presence of tumors or mechanical obstruction, a spasm of the cardiac sphincter muscle at the end of the esophagus, diverticula or pouching, injury or trauma, or damage to the vagus, hypoglossal, or glossopharyngeal nerves or the swallowing center in the floor of the fourth ventricle.

Normal digestive peristalsis which occurs in the stomach and the intestines is characterized by a constant rhythm. Strong emotional states may result in either hypermotility or hypomotility of the stomach muscles, either hurrying food through the stomach or holding it there for too long a period of time. Pyloric obstruction can also produce hyperperistalsis. The ability of the stomach to function mechanically can also be affected by the presence of cancerous growths, gastritis, or peptic ulcer.

The digestive peristaltic movements of the small and large intestines are dependent upon intact intestines and adequately functioning nervous control. Any obstruction of the intestine, whether due to cancer, kinking, intussusception, or strangulation, brings digestive processes to an end and constitutes, in addition, an immediate threat to life. Diverticulitis (pouching in the intestine), inflammation of the intestinal lining (including appendicitis), abscesses or fistulas, or hypomotility (constipation) can interfere with the normal peristaltic movements of the intestine and affect the mechanical efficiency of the total digestive process.

The clinical aspects of digestion involve adequate (neither too much nor too little) secretions from the salivary glands, the stomach mucosa, the liver and gallbladder, the pancreas, and the small intestines. The salivary glands supply the mucus and fluid to moisten food as well as salivary amylase, which begins carbohydrate digestion. Any pathological conditions affecting the mouth, throat, or salivary glands can therefore pose digestive problems. Examples include poor oral hygiene, periodontal disease (pyorrhea), stomatitis (inflammation of the mouth), Vincent's angina, fractured jaw, mumps, or traumatic injury. The stomach secretes hydrochloric acid (which creates the acid reaction within the stomach) and the enzymes that contribute to protein and fat digestion. (The action of salivary amylase continues in the stomach.) The enzymes secreted in the stomach are proteolytic and lipolytic: pepsinogen, which acts upon protein; rennin, which curdles milk and acts upon the milk protein casein; and lipase, which emulsifies fats other than those found in meat.

Any pathology involving the stomach has, of course, serious implications for the efficiency of the chemical digestive process. Gastritis (inflammation of the gastric mucosa) is a common problem. Another is peptic ulcer, one of the causative factors of which is believed to be the digestive action of the gastric mucosa secretions. In patients who develop ulcers in the duodenum, there is usually an increased secretion of hydrochloric acid, while this is not usually true for those who develop ulcers in the gastric area itself. In addition to gastritis and ulcers, another common stomach disorder is cancer. The stomach is also sensitive to emotional stress and emotional disorders and is an organ used often to express emotional discomfort. Statements such as "he makes me sick," "that nauseates me," and "I can't stomach that" are examples.

When partially digested food, known as chyme, moves into the small intestine, the secretions of the small intestine, liver, and pancreas join forces to complete the chemical process of digestion. The combined secretions, which are alkaline and therefore reverse the acid reaction of the stomach contents, act jointly to complete the digestion of proteins, carbohydrates, and fats. The liver secretes bile (stored in the gallbladder), and the bile emulsifies fats. The small intestine liberates secretin, which stimulates the release of pancreatic juices in addition to providing protease and peptidases which act on protein. The pancreatic juices contain proteolytic, amylolytic, and lipolytic enzymes: trypsin and chymotrypsin, which act on protein; lipase, which acts on fats; and amylase, which acts on carbohydrates. Again, any pathological process that involves the liver, gallbladder, pancreas, or small intestine has implications for the efficiency of the digestive process.

The small intestine is fairly often plagued with appendicitis, regional ileitis (inflammation of the ileum), intestinal obstruction, and cancer. The commonest of liver problems are trauma, viral hepatitis (inflammation caused by virus), carcinoma, abscess, and degenerative changes such as cirrhosis (fibrosis or sclerosis). The gallbladder is subject to cholecystitis (inflammation) and cholelithiasis (stone formation). The pancreas is prone to pancreatitis (inflammation) and the presence of carcinoma. Thus, the digestive process in the small intestine is subject to threat from a wide variety of causes.

In addition to secreting pancreatic juices, the pancreas is further involved in carbohydrate metabolism through the secretion of insulin from the islands of Langerhans. The insulin is secreted directly into the blood stream, and the failure of the pancreas to provide insulin results in diabetes mellitus, a disturbance in carbohydrate metabolism. Exactly how insulin works is uncertain, but it appears to limit sugar production and to facilitate its consumption.

Digestion in the large intestine is relatively limited. The colon receives the undigestible and undigested residue, reabsorbs water, and prepares the residue for evacuation. Problems here can arise from hypermotility (diarrhea, mucous colitis), hypomotility (constipation), obstruction, or cancer.

The entire gastrointestinal tract is under widespread chemical (hormonal) and nervous regulation. Plexuses of interconnected ganglia exist throughout the smooth muscle, there is abundant nerve supply from the autonomic nervous system, the pituitary-adrenal mechanism affects functioning, the varying vital centers in the brain affect certain aspects of nutrition and digestion, and both the more primitive and the neocortex are involved in regulation. Anything that affects almost any of the broad functions of the regulatory mechanisms of the body, as well as those parts of it that directly affect the gastrointestinal tract and other adjacent tissues involved in digestion, will have implications for the efficiency of the digestive process.

In addition to the previous generalization, the digestive organs and process are also extremely susceptible to the influence of emotional responses and emotional stress. This is not surprising, since the pituitary-adrenal-autonomic-hypothalamus-rhinencephalon mechanisms are involved in emotional expression, and this is "felt" largely in the viscera. Emotional responses and emotional distress thus affect the digestive process.

Absorption of digested products takes place primarily in the small intestine, with additional water being absorbed from the large intestine. The remarkably large absorbing surface in the small intestine, due to its length and relatively narrow lumen with the villi studding the entire mucosa, make it particularly well suited for this function. The direct route of absorption is through the epithelial cells of the villi to underlying capillaries, to the superior and inferior mesenteric veins, and thence to the portal vein. Fat, however, is absorbed by the lacteals and into the lymph system. Since the primary absorption area is the small intestine, any of the pathological processes occurring in the small intestine that were discussed in relation to digestion will also pose problems for absorption.

An intact cardiovascular system is essential for the adequate transportation of nutrition from the end products of digestion in the small intestine to all body cells. In the nursing problem of maintenance of nutrition, the major difficulties are in the mechanical aspects of transportation, general and local. Therefore, the pathological processes that are most likely to present complications are those discussed in the preceding chapter on oxygen. In terms of general nutritional problems, these include congestive heart failure, hypertensive heart disease, coronary heart disease (such as acute myocardial infarction), and rheumatic heart disease. Local problems in maintaining nutrition result from Buerger's disease, Raynaud's disease, thrombophlebitis, varicose veins, or mechanical interference with local circulation due to pressure or trauma.

In regard to circulatory integrity, one key aspect of circulation particularly significant in the area of the maintenance of nutrition is the portal circulation. Since the portal vein carries blood from the small and large intestines, spleen, and stomach to the liver before the nutrition-laden blood enters the general circulation, special problems are posed if the portal vein is blocked. This may occur in degenerative changes in liver, such as cirrhosis.

The ability of individual body cells to utilize nutrition when delivered depends upon the health of individual cells. Trauma, infection, necrosis, gangrene, or any factor impairing individual cell metabolism may result in inability to utilize nutritive substances brought to the cells.

Some of the nutrients taken into the body are stored for use when needed, and one of the important storage areas is the liver. Carbohydrates can be stored as glycogen in the liver, and glycogen can be reconverted to glucose and released as the body needs it. Also stored in the liver are iron, copper, and vitamins A, B complex, D, and K. Fat is stored in adipose tissue beneath the skin, in intermuscular connective tissue, and in the abdominal cavity. Any of the preceding possibilities of liver damage can increase the threat to nutrition since it may reduce the liver's vital storage capacity.

NURSING INTERVENTION

Nursing responsibilities with patients who have nutritional problems are broad in scope and range and, in addition, require the exercise of considerable judgment. Eating is a sensitive process for most people—its social and psychological significance is deep. The nurse who is aware of and respects the unity of the individual patient as a person will have the kind of foundation needed to provide quality nursing care for patients with nutritional problems.

Observation

Observation of patients with nutritional problems is focused upon assessing the patient's nutritional status in relation to difficulties that may complicate the maintenance of homeostasis.

The general appearance of the patient is of significance since malnutrition of any type is usually reflected in the total picture of the patient. Listlessness, lack of energy, change in color, indifference to personal appearance, dull eyes, skin change, loss of weight, slow response to stimuli, lack of interest in the environment, irritability, and poor eating habits may all be signs or symptoms of malnutrition. Obesity, preoccupation with food, constant "nibbling," irritability, and complaints of fullness may be indications of overeating.

Observation of the mouth and its ability to function in the mastication and moistening of food as the first step in digestion is another key area. Dental health problems are endemic in the United States and all too often dental hygiene (and its significance for total health) is ignored. The condition of teeth, gums, and the buccal mucosa, along with the moistness of the mouth generally, are key areas of observation. When the body water balance leans toward the negative, the secretions of the salivary glands are reduced and the mucous membrane of the mouth may be dry. The condition of the tongue is also important. The condition of the lips may interfere with eating, because cracked, sore lips may make the ingestion of food difficult or unpleasant. The mouth can also indicate the specific lack of vitamin C, since the symptoms of scurvy are revealed there by a sore mouth with edema and ulcerations of the gums and by loosened teeth. In general, the condition of mucous membrane—wherever it may be observed—may provide clues to the state of nutrition. Change in color toward pallor or reddish blue and a change in the state of moisture of the membrane are worthy of note.

The condition of the skin, hair, and nails are indicators of the state of nutrition, and they can also be indicators of specific dietary lacks. The skin in particular may indicate allergic response to food intake. Dry and brittle nails that break easily are usually a sign of poor nutrition that may be due to several causes, such as calcium or vitamin deficiency. Dry, lifeless hair and hair that grays prematurely may also be related to nutritional deficiency. A dry skin with a loss of turgor may also indicate poor nutrition or dehydration, and the appearance of rashes may indicate either an allergic response or a specific deficiency in intake.

The patient's level of energy is closely related to his state of nutrition. Basically, food intake provides the source of energy that makes activity possible. In short periods of food deprivation, the body can draw on its own reserve supplies, but this cannot continue for long. In addition, vitamins and minerals are essential regulators, catalysts, or moderators of specific types of body responses and their absence interferes with the body functions with which they are associated. Therefore, motor activity of any type becomes a focus of observation in relation to nutrition. Of critical importance is the amount of energy expended by patients. Nutritional lack is associated with a reduced level of energy consumption and is reflected in indifference, apathy, and lassitude. This may range from mild to severe. Because minerals are essential for maintaining the irritability of muscles, nerves, and the heart, their lack will be reflected in motor and cardiac activities. Bone formation depends upon the presence of adequate calcium, phosphorus, and vitamin D, and their absence in the very young will be reflected by the development of rickets.

Weight, of course, is usually very closely related to the nutritional state of the patient. Of most importance are extremes in weight—too much or too little—and sudden or marked weight change. The latter is particularly important, since patients who are overweight or underweight are likely to be weighed regularly, while the patient who has a weight change may go unnoticed for a period of time.

Another key area of observation is the patient's appetite and the factors that appear to affect it. If the patient's appetite is not good, more frequent, smaller feedings may be helpful. If the patient is always hungry, more closely spaced feedings may be helpful. The patient's subjective complaints may provide evidence concerning his appetite as well as evidence about how he approaches eating. If he picks at food, pushes it around, and eats little, it may be assumed that his appetite is poor. Examples of factors that affect appetite include patient preferences, time of feeding, attractiveness of serving, patient's physical state, patient's emotional reactions, and the state of the environment. To note that a patient's appetite is poor is simply a clue to seek the possible factors that are affecting the particular patient. To assume that because a patient is physically ill his appetite is bound to be poor is to assume more than the facts may support. Investigation is always indicated.

Specific symptoms in relation to eating that form a focus of observation are dysphagia, anorexia, nausea, and vomiting. Dysphagia (difficulty in swallowing) should be carefully noted in terms of kind of difficulty in swallowing, relationship to time of occurrence and the patient's feeling at the time, whether any particular position affects it, whether consistency of food or type of food increases or decreases the difficulty, and the patient's reaction to the dysphagia. Anorexia (refusal or inability to eat) should be evaluated in the light of the patient's subjective reason "why," physical status, capability to eat, emotional status, and all other factors that affect appetite. The occasion of nausea and/or vomiting should be carefully noted in terms of type, character, amount, and the setting in which it occurs. Readers are referred to the discussion on anorexia, nausea, and vomiting in Chapter 16.

Another point of observation is the patient's eating habits, including personal and cultural preferences. While these may indicate teaching needs in the light of the patient's health problems, they may also provide clues for ways to help the patient maintain nutrition. The patient's attitude toward food and eating are also significant, and these can be learned by encouraging patients to talk about eating and food, by learning about food and eating attitudes in the cultural background from which the patient comes, and by observation of the patient before, during, and after eating.

Noting the patient's total intake of food and fluid is a responsibility that rests primarily upon nursing personnel. Although the patient may be on a balanced or adjusted diet that is complete for the day when it is served to him, only those persons in and out of his room during and after meals are in a position to know how much of what food the patient actually consumes. Only those persons in and out of the patient's room between meals are in a position to know whether the patient is supplementing his diet from outside sources and what particular form the supplementation takes. This is especially important in patients with nutritional problems. Does the patient eat everything served him? Does he reject completely a diet he dislikes? Does he eat everything except liver, other organ meats, and muscle meats, egg yolks, grean leafy vegetables, and whole grain bread and cereals when his diet is intended to be high in iron? Does he eat the protein and fat and leave the carbohydrates? Is he surreptitiously supplementing a low-salt diet with salted peanuts? If he needs to build new tissues following surgery, does he eat everything but the proteins? Only careful observation and recording will detect those nutritional deficiencies that may not be obvious.

Certain colors play a significant role in the assessment of nutritional status and difficulties. These colors are white (pallor), blue (cyanosis), gray (cachexia), and yellow (jaundice). A state of malnutrition may be reflected in pallor or blanching of the skin. If the malnutrition involves a nutritional anemia with a lack of iron that affects the red blood cells, cyanosis due to the reduced oxygen content of the blood will be apparent. In cachexia, a general lack of nutrition and wasting which occurs primarily in chronic diseases, the concomitant pallor has a gray undertone. Disorders that involve an increased accumulation of bile in the blood stream are followed by the deposit of the pigment in the conjunctiva of eyes, the mucous membranes, and the skin, all of which become tinted yellow. Jaundice may be due to increased production of bile from the breakdown of hemoglobin, to damage to the liver cells from infections or toxins, or to obstruction of the bile passages. The extent, depth, and change in color are of importance.

Pain, of course, is always a symptom of significance that requires careful observation and evaluation in the light of individual and cultural differences in the response to the experience of pain. In nutritional difficulties, as in others, the nature of the pain, the time of its occurrence, duration, location, and the patient's reaction and subjective complaints should be carefully noted. The effect of activity and motion on the pain should also be determined. Of particular significance in nutritional problems is the relationship of pain to eating. Does it occur before, during, or after meals, and, if so, at what time intervals? Is the pain relieved or made worse by eating? Does the pain occur only after a long interval between eating, i.e., only before breakfast? Everything that can be learned about pain should be learned.

Because of its relationship to some of the more acute and dramatic threats to the maintenance of nutrition, the abdomen is also a key focus of observation. Distention, rigid and boardlike splinting, severe pain, and the accumulation of fluid are the symptoms of particular importance. Distention can occur from several causes, including those related to elimination, such as a full bladder. Distention can also occur as a result of an accumulation of gas in the intestines. A rigid, boardlike abdomen accompanied by intense pain may indicate intestinal obstruction or peritonitis, inflammation of the lining of the abdomen (peritoneum). Ascites, or an accumulation of fluid in the abdominal cavity, may accompany heart or liver disease.

The character of body excreta may provide clues as to the efficiency of the digestive apparatus. Vomitus may reveal bleeding in the gastrointestinal tract by the presence of frank (red) or old (brown) blood. Fecal matter or bile may also be contained in vomitus. Urine may be colored with evidence of blood or bile. The stool may contain frank (red) blood or old (brown or black) blood or may be clay-colored, indicating the absence of bile.

Another key area for observation is the water and acid-base balance. In the presence of inadequate intake, excessive output such as vomiting with the loss of hydrochloric acid, or the failure to excrete as in kidney damage, the balance in either water or acid-base balance can be disturbed. Both positive and negative water balance are evidenced by edema and dehydration (see Chapter 16). Acidosis is accompanied by increased respiration (to remove carbon dioxide), restlessness, rising temperature, and disorientation and coma. Unless reversed, death ensues. Alkalosis causes decreased respiration and temperature rise, resulting in death unless the balance is reversed.

If the patient has undergone surgery, if there is a possibility of perforation of the gastrointestinal tract, or if varices (such as esophageal varices resulting from a vein pressure exerted by a damaged liver) present a potential threat, careful observation for signs of hemorrhage and/or shock is in order. The classical signs of internal hemorrhage are apprehension and restlessness, increasing pulse and respiration, decreasing body temperature, thirst, pallor, and a cold, moist skin. The classical signs of shock are a falling blood pressure, a weak and rapid pulse, and a pale, cold, and moist skin.

The final area of particular importance in observation of patients with problems in nutrition is the patient's emotional reactions. There are several good reasons why emotional status and nutrition are related:

1. Food and eating have strong psychological and cultural implications
2. The innervation and chemical control of the viscera generally are closely associated with the endocrine and nervous system mechanisms through which emotions are expressed.
3. The gastrointestinal tract is often used to express emotions and feelings.
4. A number of physical problems believed to have at least partial psychological causation are found in the gastrointestinal tract (peptic ulcer and mucous colitis are examples).

Therefore, observation is directed toward finding out as much as possible about the patient: his likes and dislikes, his fears and worries, his satisfactions and dissatisfactions, his ambitions and dreams, his successes and failures, what his illness means to him, his self-concept and his concept of people significant to him, his dependence and independence, how he relates to others, and his acceptance or lack of acceptance of the situation in which he finds himself.

Dependent nursing functions

The dependent nursing functions (i.e., functions dependent upon a directive from others) involved in providing nursing care for patients with nutritional problems are found in five categories: diagnostic tests, medical treatments, feeding, diet adaptations, and the administration of medications.

Diagnostic tests

When assisting with diagnostic tests, the nurse's responsibilities include the following:

1. Preparation of the patient, including explanation of "what" and "why"
2. Obtaining or being responsible for obtaining the necessary equipment and supplies
3. Observing and supporting the patient during the test
4. Perhaps assisting the physician
5. Perhaps assistance by helping to collect or by collecting specimens
6. Aftercare of the patient
7. Perhaps disposal of the specimen or specimens

Among the more common of the diagnostic tests in this area are gastric analysis, gastrointestinal series, esophagoscopy, gastroscopy, gallbladder series, biliary and pancreatic drainage, and a group of liver function tests.

A gastric analysis consists of the removal of gastric contents for examination for diagnostic purposes primarily. Gastric contents may be examined for carcinoma cells, for large amounts of undigested food (pyloric stenosis or gastric hypomotility), increased hydrochloric acid (peptic ulcer), or lack of free hydrochloric acid (malignancy or pernicious anemia). The test is done on fasting contents, and food and fluid are withheld during the night before the test. The physician passes a gastric tube through the nostril or mouth into the stomach and aspirates all stomach contents with a syringe. This constitues the first specimen and may be the only one. If there is no free hydrochloric acid in the first specimen, histamine phosphate is usually given subcutaneously. The histamine stimulates gastric secretion. After the histamine injection, gastric specimens are collected at ten-minute to twenty-minute intervals until three or more, as desired, are obtained. The tube is then removed. Insulin may be used instead of histamine, since insulin produces a drop in blood sugar that stimulates the vagus nerve. If the patient has a peptic ulcer, the action of the vagus on stomach secretion will be accelerated and gastric output and free hydrochloric acid will increase.

A gastrointestinal series consists of a series of fluoroscopic and x-ray examinations after a patient has swallowed barium, which is a radiopaque substance. A gastrointestinal series is used to identify ulceration, tumor existence, or malformation of the upper tract, usually down through the duodenum. Again, food and fluid are withheld the night before the test. After the patient swallows the barium, the physician uses both fluoroscopic and x-ray examinations at periodic intervals to outline the upper gastrointestinal tract and to trace the progress of the barium through the tract. Food is, of course, withheld until the treatment is completed. After the treatment is completed, a cathartic is usually ordered to prevent stasis in or obstruction of the tract by the barium.

Esophagoscopy and gastroscopy consist of the insertion of a tube into the esophagus or stomach for the purpose of visualizing the mucosa in either site or for the removal of a small specimen for examination. In both procedures, food and fluid are withheld beginning the night before. Because the procedure is not exactly comfortable and because it arouses apprehension, the patient is given medication in advance at the appropriate time. In addition, atropine is usually given to decrease secretion from the mucous membrane. Because the danger of perforation is real, securing the patient's cooperation is essential, and the preparation of the patient through simple though not prolonged explanation and emotional support are especially significant. Before the tube is passed, the pharynx is sprayed with a local anesthetic to inactivate the gag reflex. The patient requires keen observation and strong emotional support during the esophagoscopy or gastroscopy procedure. The patient should also be instructed not to take food or fluids until the gag reflex has returned and, having been given medication prior to the treatment, may need supervision to ensure that this instruction is carried out.

A gallbladder series is performed to test the ability of the gallbladder to function normally. The test is based on the use of radiopaque dyes that outline the gallbladder on x-ray films. Oral dyes are commonly employed, but if the patient is unable to ingest the tablets or is too nauseated to retain them, the dye may be given intravenously. The patient receives a low-fat evening meal which is followed by the ordered number of tablets of Periodax or Telepaque (the radiopaque dye). On the morning of the test and until time for the next test meal, the patient may have only water, black coffee, or clear tea. The patient is x-rayed twice in the morning and at noon receives either a high-fat diet or some fatty substance. The fat should stimulate the flow of bile from the gallbladder to the intestinal tract. Further x-ray examinations follow. Normally, the gallbladder should empty after the stimulation of fat. If stones are present, they will also show on the x-ray film.

Tests for biliary and pancreatic drainage are done by passing a tube into the duodenum and collecting drainage at that point. The tests are done for the purpose of determining volume and analyzing the constituents of the secretion. Either Levin or Miller-Abbott tubes may be used. Again, intake (except for small sips of water) is withheld for twelve hours and breakfast delayed until the test is completed. Usually, several specimens are collected. After passing the tube into the stomach, the patient is placed on his right side with the hips slightly elevated so that gravity combines with the stomach peristalisis to move the end of the tube into the duodenum.

The glucose or galactose tolerance test is used for the purpose of determining liver function as it relates to carbohydrate metabolism. After withholding breakfast and having the patient void, the patient is given 50 mg. of galactose in 500 ml. of lemon-flavored water. Urine specimens are then collected every hour for five hours and the specimens examined individually and collectively for total sugar excreted. An excretion above 3 mg. is considered abnormal.

The hippuric acid test of the ability of liver to detoxify does not require fasting. After a breakfast of toast and coffee, the patient is given 6 Gm. of sodium benzoate dissolved in flavored water. The patient voids and the first specimen is discarded. Following this, four urine specimens are collected at hourly intervals. Since benzoic acid and aminoacetic acid are synthesized into hippuric acid by the liver and excreted through the urine, the failure to excrete or limited excretion of hippuric acid indicates liver damage.

A series of fasting blood tests are also made to test liver function. They include tests of alkaline phosphatase (elevated in biliary obstruction), plasma cholesterol (liver disease indicated by increased esters in relation to total cholesterol), cephalin-cholesterol flocculations (in which blood serum flocculation indicates jaundice due to liver disease), and icterus index (in which increased bile pigment in the blood indicates liver damage).

Nonfasting blood tests of liver function are serum albumin/globulin ratio (liver damage is indicated by an albumin drop and globulin rise) and the quantitative van den Bergh test (increased serum bilirubin indicates liver damage).

Medical treatments

The major medical therapies which the nurse will be required to assist with or to maintain include gastric lavage, decompression of the stomach or intestines, and the maintenance of drainage from the gallbladder, pancreas, and abdomen.

The gastric lavage is a washing out of the contents of the stomach. It is most commonly used as an emergency measure to remove stomach contents in instances of the ingestion of poison which has not damaged the mucosa lining of the upper gastrointestinal tract or to empty the stomach of accumulated undigested food. It may also be used to empty the stomach of its contents before an operation or to obtain cells for diagnostic study. Water is most often used for the irrigation, although antidotes may also be used in the instance of poisoning. The essence of the procedure is the insertion of a tube into the stomach, the insertion of small amounts of fluid at a time, and the withdrawal of stomach contents by means of gravity through placing the end of the tube below the

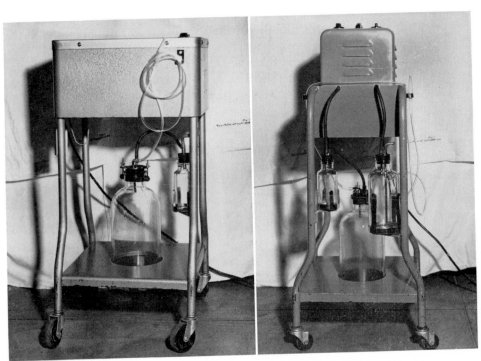

Fig. 43. Two examples of electrically operated machines used for decompression of the gastrointestinal tract.

level of the stomach. The nurse, of course, is responsible for the preparation of the patient, the preparation of the equipment and solution, the support of the patient, and his aftercare.

Gastric decompression means emptying the stomach contents, usually accomplished by the negative pressure of suction attached to a tube inserted into the stomach. The procedure prevents distention postoperatively, relieves nausea and vomiting, and prevents distention and distress in the presence of pyloric or intestinal obstruction. Gastric decompression may be used postoperatively for one, two, or three days or for a longer period of time when indicated. There are several types of electrically powered suction machines, all based on the principle of negative pressure that suctions the contents of the stomach into closed bottles that are part of the suction machine equipment.

Nursing responsibilities include patient comfort, maintaining the patency of tubes, accurate records of the amount of drainage, observation and reporting of patient reaction, and in replacing or having the suction machine repaired if it is not in proper working order. Patient comfort is especially important, since the patient is usually not too comfortable to begin with and the tube can be either uncomfortable or irritating. Oral hygiene is important—the portal of entry should be kept clean. Small sips of ice or warm gargles may be used to keep the mouth moist. Tubes should be carefully checked to be certain they are patent, and major sources of difficulty are blocking of the tube by drainage or pressure on the tube that occludes the lumen. The nurse may be required to irrigate the tube with small amounts of normal saline solution at periodic intervals. The actual amount of stomach drainage is important, because continuous drainage may lead to electrolyte imbalance. The patient's reaction should be noted and reported, and any problem with the procedure should be promptly reported, whether the difficulty is with the machine, the patency of the tubes, or the patient's difficulty in tolerating the procedure.

Intestinal decompression is similar to gastric decompression and is employed to drain fluids and gas from the intestines. It may be used before or after surgery, usually above intestinal obstruction or paralytic ileus. The Miller-Abbott and Cantor tubes are the most frequently used; both are longer than gastric tubes and have balloons at their tips that can be inflated to stimulate peristalsis and help gravity in the passage of the tube. Once in place, the tubes are taped to hold them in the desired position. In intestinal decompression, the tubes are usually left in place longer than gastric tubes. The nurse's responsibilities are the same as those in gastric decompression.

Following surgery, the nurse will be responsible for the care and maintenance of drainage from tubes left in the site of operation. Such drains are commonly placed following surgery on the gallbladder or pancreas, and sometimes following other abdominal operations. Following gallbladder surgery, dressings, drains, or T tubes may be used. Because bile must either drain to the exterior on dressings or through drains or tubes or drain to the interior through the intestine, key observation is directed toward signs of retention of bile in the general circulation. The sclera, mucous membrane, and skin are carefully checked for a yellow appearance. Dark yellowish color in urine may indicate the presence of bile, and a light-colored stool indicates an absence of bile pigment. Drainage should be carefully watched, recorded, and reported. Any sudden excess, increase, or diminution of drainage is cause for concern. In any abdominal surgery, drains may be used. The nurse observes and records the character and amount of drainage, reports promptly if drainage increases or decreases, and provides for the patient's comfort to the extent that is possible.

Feeding

Because many patients who have nutritional problems need adaptations in the method of feeding, the nurse generally carries more responsibility than usual for the actual process of feeding patients. Particular areas of responsibility include patients who cannot feed themselves, patients on diet adaptations that require feeding at other than regular feeding periods, patients who are fed via gastrostomy or enterostomy tubes, and patients receiving fluids and nutrition via intravenous infusion.

Patients who cannot feed themselves must be fed, and such feeding is not the simple procedure it might appear to be. Factors that affect successful feeding include the patient's ability to chew and swallow, the patient's appetite, the patient's food habits and preferences, the patient's feelings about being dependent, food that is palatably hot or cold, and the nurse's attitude toward feeding patients. Patients who have to be fed should be fed at a rate of speed and with an amount of food that is compatible with the patient's ability and level of energy. Hurrying or pushing can encourage the patient to plead lack of appetite to end the performance. Concern and interest in the patient can provide the basis for encouragement and support which are practically always necessary. Every physical measure should be employed as a supportive device with sensitivity to the significance of environmental effect upon appetite. The patient should be comfortable, unhurried, in a position that makes eating as easy as possible, and with adequate ventilation. Eating with a full bedpan on the chair beside the bed, with the bedside table piled high with paraphernalia for a procedure to follow soon, or with an unemptied emesis basin somewhere close is not the easiest thing in the world. Following feeding, the patient should have an opportunity to rest and should be left in a comfortable position.

Patients whose diet adaptations require feeding at supplementary or odd periods also tend to be at the mercy of nursing personnel. Examples are patients with gastric or peptic ulcers, patients suffering from malnutrition, and postoperative patients. For example, in the first stages of a peptic ulcer diet the patient may be receiving 2 ounces of a milk and cream mixture every hour. A patient with malnutrition may have high caloric supplemental feedings between meals and at bedtime. In such instances, the nurse is usually responsible for providing the proper nutrition at the correct time and encouraging the patient to take the prescribed diet. Timing becomes important in such instances. An eggnog spaced evenly between breakfast and lunch is more effective than an eggnog so close to lunch that the patient loses his appetite for the latter, and 4 ounces of milk and cream every two hours is not as effective as 2 ounces every hour.

Feeding via a tube inserted into the stomach (usually a Levin tube) is used when patients are resistive to eating or when the condition of the mouth or throat contraindicates the usual method of eating. In addition, where damage to the upper gastrointestinal tract above the stomach or down to and including the stomach (burns, poisons, or trauma) occurs, the stomach or intestine may be opened through the abdomen for the purpose of feeding. Feeding via all three methods have much in common, since all involve feeding via tubes. The nasal feeding is not permanent, while the gastrostomy or enterostomy feeding route is more likely to be, depending upon the reversibility or irreversibility of the damage suffered. In all three instances, the diet must be liquid or fine enough to pass through the tube. The patency of the tube must be assured. Feedings should be as ordered for the specific patient and are usually given frequently and in small amounts. Water following feeding will clear the tube of residue. Patients who have a permanent gastrostomy or enterostomy will also need to be taught how to feed themselves. The psychological impact of permanent gastrostomy or enterostomy is usually deep and profound, and the patient will require a great deal of emotional support.

In intravenous feeding, the nurse's responsibility is to prepare the patient, secure the necessary equipment, be sure the intravenous feeding given corresponds with that ordered, maintain the flow at the desired rate, add medications as ordered, check for infiltration and stop the flow if it occurs, and observe and support the patient during the procedure. In the provision of nutrition, the intravenous infusion is usually an emergency or stopgap measure. It is difficult to provide a complete and balanced diet by the intravenous infusion method.

Diet adaptations

Although the nurse is rarely, if ever, responsible for the actual preparation of special diets, she is often responsible for determining the extent to which the patient actually receives and utilizes the diet ordered and for knowing what is contraindicated so that she can help the patient stay within the limits of his diet. Diets are varied from normal in amount, in consistency, and in individual dietary elements such as carbohydrates, fats, proteins, and minerals. Among patients with nutritional disorders, almost every range of dietary variation may occur. Common are low-fat diet (gallbladder disease), restricted sodium diet (heart disease), low-cholesterol diet (gallbladder disease), restricted caloric diets (obesity), high-protein, high-carbohydrate, low-fat diets (hepatic disease), low-protein, low-fat, high-carbohydrate diets (hepatic disease), low-potassium diet (hepatic disease), dumping syndrome diet (postgastrectomy), peptic ulcer diet, soft diet, clear fluid diet, full fluid diet, and bland diet (postoperative).

Whenever a special diet is ordered for a patient, the nurse should check recent books on diet therapy or consult the dietary department to make sure she understands exactly what, what not, and when the patient should be fed, It is doubtful that any nurse has complete and accurate knowledge concerning all diets and the food sources of all nutritive elements. Even if there is a nurse who has memorized all this, she may well check her information anyway because increasing knowledge brings about changes. One of the great advances in knowledge that has resulted in the improved health status of our population has been in the field of nutrition. There is every indication that expansion of knowledge concerning nutrition will continue.

Administration of medications

The range of medications ordered for patients who have nutritional difficulties is wide. Vitamin supplements are common. Antacids, such as aluminum hydroxide gel or magnesium hydroxide, may be ordered. Anticholinergics that reduce stomach secretion and spasm, such as tincture of belladonna, may be employed. Atropine may be used for its antispasmodic action. Antibiotics of all types may be employed to treat or to prevent infection. Tranquilizers may be used to allay anxiety and apprehension. Cardiac drugs will be used if heart disease complicates the transportation of nutrition to all body cells, and the varying forms of digitalis are most commonly employed. Analgesics such as acetylsalicylic acid and sodium salicylate may be used. The sedative action of the barbiturates is utilized, and the narcotic group, including Demerol and morphine, are used to control pain. In the administration of medications, the nurse must use all physical measures to support the desired effect of the medication.

Independent nursing functions

The major focus of nursing goals in providing nursing care for patients with nutritional problems is upon measures that will strengthen the intake, digestion, and absorption of nutritive elements.

One of the major areas of nursing contribution can be the use of understanding of the complex factors that affect appetite or the desire to eat. Since cultural, psychological, personal, and environmental factors are involved, the promotion of positive support of the desire to eat is not always an easy matter. The attempt to enforce a preconceived idea of how, what, when, and where a patient should eat on the basis of "the doctor ordered it" or "it is good for the patient" is not usually effective. There may be a time when this can be said, but only when the groundwork has been laid by helping the patient become ready to accept this as consistent with his own judgment.

Respect for the patient's cultural patterns can be shown in many ways. He may not be able to have the sauerbraten and red cabbage he so dearly loves, but empathy for his wishes and encouragement to look forward to the day he may have it again may make it easier for him to endure its absence. Respect for and understanding of the meaning of food to the patient may also help. Possible adaptations in terms of personal preferences can contribute much to a patient's appetite. Acceptance of the patient's complaints about food and diet helps. Explanation of the "why" and "how" of dietary adaptations may be helpful, but only after matters that are of immediate concern to the patient have been taken care of or expressed.

Attractive serving of food, environmental manipulation to promote appetite, the nurse's understanding, the avoidance of procedures immediately before and after meals, and the preparation of the patient through such measures as oral hygiene and positioning can be sensitively used to promote the desire to eat. A knowledge of the patient as a person can also contribute to the nurse's ability to work with the patient.

The nurse may also provide the patient with help in adapting to variations in the dietary pattern. When intake is low, as in the postoperative patient or the patient with infection or pathology of the gastrointestinal tract, then energy consumption may need to be reduced. This can be accomplished in many ways: by the nurse assuming a more active part in physical hygiene, by having things where they are readily accessible for the patient, by planning so the patient has periods of rest, by keeping the patient physically comfortable, and by providing passive exercise to take the place of more active exercise. When frequent and smaller feedings are necessary, such feedings can be spaced at proper intervals and the relatively frequent patient contacts can be used to convey acceptance to the patient.

The relationship of physical comfort and the desire for and ability to tolerate food is an obvious one. Therefore, the comforting measures in nursing can contribute much to the patient's response to food. Comfort in position, in measures of hygiene (including oral hygiene), in sufficient change of position and movement to prevent hemostasis, in diversional activities that the patient can tolerate, and in comfortable relationships can all make a contribution.

As pointed out previously, the emotional and psychological aspects of nursing care of patients with nutritional problems is an extremely significant area. The nurse may encourage free expression of feelings, may remain nonjudgmental and nonpunitive, and may keep channels of communication open through which the patient can express his anxieties and his feelings. Alertness to facial expressions, body posture, recurring topics, complaints and projections, and reactions to other people (including visitors and personnel) may provide valuable guidelines in providing the patient with an opportunity to clarify his own feelings and thinking.

Patients with nutritional problems present real challenges in teaching nutrition. Many patients need to learn what constitutes a balanced diet, how to change eating habits, how to carry out a specific diet, or how to eat more or less. In teaching, the nurst must first be sure of the facts. Then, she must deal with what concerns the patient before trying to teach. She may also find out what the patient knows, teach in language and terminology he understands, and evaluate the patient's learning. No nurse can guarantee that a patient will use the knowledge he acquires, but it is certain he will not use it if he does not have it.

BIBLIOGRAPHY

1. Cunningham, Lyda Martin: The patient with ruptured esophageal varices, American Journal of Nursing **62**:69-71, Dec. 1962.
2. Fisk, Jean E.: Nursing care of the patient with surgery of the biliary tract, American Journal of Nursing **60**:53-55, Jan. 1960.
3. Garb, Solomon: Essentials of therapeutic nutrition, New York, 1958, Springer Publishing Co., Inc.
4. Heap, Beth: Sodium restricted diets, American Journal of Nursing **60**:206-209, Feb. 1960.
5. Burton, Benjamin T. (executive editor): Heinz handbook of nutrition, New York, 1959, McGraw-Hill Book Co., Inc.
6. Klug, Thomas J., Joyce, A., and Ellensohn, J.: Gastric resection, American Journal of Nursing **61**:73-77, Dec. 1961.
7. Krause, Marie V.: Food, nutrition and diet therapy, ed. 3, Philadelphia, 1961, W. B. Saunders Co.
8. Krug, Elsie E.: Pharmacology in nursing, ed. 8, St. Louis, 1960, The C. V. Mosby Co., pp. 13-136.
9. Mayer, Jean: Obesity: causes and treatment, American Journal of Nursing **59**:1132, Dec. 1959.
10. McClain, M. Esther, and Gragg, Shirley H.: Scientific principles in nursing, ed. 4, St. Louis, 1962, The C. V. Mosby Co., pp. 160-174.
11. Molander, David W., and Brosfield, Richard D.: Liver surgery, American Journal of Nursing **61**:72-74, July 1961.
12. Morris, Eva: How does a nurse teach nutrition to patients? American Journal of Nursing **60**:67-70, Jan. 1960.
13. Mowry, Lillian: Basic nutrition and diet therapy for nurses, ed. 2, St. Louis, 1962, The C. V. Mosby Co.
14. Nordmark, Madelyn T., and Rohweder, Anne W.: Scientific principles applied to nursing, Philadelphia, 1959, J. B. Lippincott Co., pp. 71-85.
15. Rynbergen, Henderika J.: In gastrointestinal disease—fewer diet restrictions, American Journal of Nursing **63**:86-89, Jan. 1963.
16. Shafer, Kathleen N., Sawyer, Janet R., McCluskey, Audrey M., and Beck, Edna Lifgren: Medical-surgical nursing, ed. 2, St. Louis, 1961, The C. V. Mosby Co., pp. 525-613.
17. Smith, Ann: Nasogastric tube feeding, American Journal of Nursing **57**:1451, Nov. 1957.
18. Virgadamo, Barbara T.: Care of the patient with liver surgery, American Journal of Nursing **61**:74-76, July 1961.

Chapter 19

Nursing care of patients with elimination problems

The maintenance of homeostasis is as dependent upon the excretion of waste products and toxic substances as it is upon adequate intake of fluid and nutrition. In fact, unless the intake-output balance is maintained within a relatively narrow range, life ceases. As complex as the human machinery is, its ability to maintain life with the fine adjustments necessary to maintain body temperature, osmotic pressure, and chemical composition within a very narrow range is remarkable. It is worthy of note that major functions such as nutrition and elimination are not dependent upon the functioning of one organ or one system alone. This fact, along with the amount of reserve tissue in vital organs, provides a flexibility that makes adaptation to malfunction in one area of the body possible. The "intellect" of the body as a unit often overshadows the level of intellectual activity of the man who inhabits it.

The responsibility for elimination is shared by the urinary system, the gastrointestinal tract, the respiratory system and the integumentary system. The skin, under ordinary circumstances, carries a minor excretory function, and the loss of water and sodium chloride are not usually great. Minute amounts of carbon dioxide, urea, and other salts are also eliminated. The excessive loss of water and sodium chloride in extremes of heat may require salt replacement. The major excretory products of the lung are water and carbon dioxide. Urine contains primarily water, urea, uric acids, creatinine, hippuric acids, ammonia salts, sodium chloride, and other salts and organic substances. Lost through the urine are nitrogenous substances, steroids, vitamins, electrolytes, and inorganic elements. Feces excreted from the gastrointestinal tract removes food residue, water, bacteria, gases, organic materials (cellulose, proteins, and fats), insoluble alkalines (calcium phosphate and iron phosphate), small quantities of enzymes, and bile pigment (partially responsible for color).

ESSENTIAL MECHANISMS

For adequate elimination to take place, the following conditions are necessary:

1. A balance in supply of essential elements
2. Absorption and utilization (metabolic activity)
3. Transportation of wastes to the excretory areas
4. Disposal of the wastes of metabolism

The ability to dispose of wastes is thus dependent upon the integrity of the lower gastrointestinal tract, the urinary system, the respiratory system, the integumentary system, the circulatory system (for transportation), and adequate regulatory mechanisms (both the endocrine system and the central nervous system).

WHAT CAN GO WRONG

The problems that may arise in the intake, digestion, and utilization of a balanced supply of nutritive substances have been discussed in the preceding chapter on nursing care of patients with nutritional problems. The problems that may arise in transportation, general and local, have been presented in both Chapters 17 and 18. The major consideration for this discussion, therefore, is the area of disposal of wastes.

The two systems that carry major responsibility for the excretion of wastes are the urinary system and the gastrointestinal system. The urinary system consists of the kidney (a complex and selective filtering system), the ureters (which transport the urine and its constituents to the storage compartment), and the bladder (from which urine is periodically discharged through the urethra). Damage to the kidney results in disorders of filtration, oversecretion or undersecretion of organic and inorganic substances (which result in accumulation of wastes or toxins in the body or depletion of normal body fluid constituents), or the presence of substances not normally found in urine, such as blood. Kidney functions include:

1. Excretion of harmful substances, including foreign proteins, urea, uric acid, and salts
2. Removal of excessive substances, such as glucose when it is present in excess
3. Maintaining osmotic pressure by removing water or salt as needed
4. Helping to maintain body acid-base balance

Kidney function can be negatively affected by infection, degenerative changes, tumors, the formation of calculi, poisons, emboli or thrombi, or decreased blood supply due to hypertensive vascular disease.

Among the more common pathological processes affecting the kidney are acute and chronic glomerulonephritis (Bright's disease, a diffuse inflammatory process involving the capillary loops in the glomeruli with a loss of function and degeneration of the tubules). The acute form usually follows a hemolytic streptococcal infection with an acute onset and is characterized by proteinuria and albuminuria, with edema and hypertension. The chronic form is similar but develops more slowly.

Nephrosclerosis results from renal hypertension and a decreased blood supply to the kidney, resulting in the loss of function of the glomeruli and tubules. Pyelonephritis is an inflammation of the kidney pelvis and parenchyma, and repeated attacks can result in degeneration of kidney tissue. Abscess formation in the soft kidney tissue is called a perinephritic abscess. Hydronephrosis (dilation of the kidney pelvis) can result from obstruction of the upper urinary tract. Renal calculi are readily formed, and although the majority are safely passed in the urine, the retention of calculi can lead to difficulties in any area of the urinary tract and may be one cause of hydronephrosis. Emboli or thrombi can interfere with circulation to or from the kidneys and result in loss of function. Certain metals or poisons, such as bichloride of mercury, may result in death because of their action upon the kidney. Tumors in the kidney are usually cancerous and destroy kidney tissue by infiltration. A nephrotic syndrome, not always clear as to causation, may occur; the serum protein level drops and generalized edema appears. Renal failure, such as uremia, occurs when the kidneys are seriously damaged and essential functions are lost.

The ureters are subject to partial or complete occlusion due to the presence of calculi or strictures. Strictures may be congenital malformations or may result from trauma or infection. Infection or inflammation of the urethra (urethritis) may also occur. Interference with the function of the ureter may well embarrass kidney function.

The bladder is a muscular organ that serves as a storage place for urine. Loss of muscle tone due to age, disease, trauma, or loss of control as a result of central nervous system damage presents a potential for infection in view of the location and normal contents of the bladder. Among the pathological processes relatively common to the bladder are cystitis (inflammation of the mucosa lining), diverticulosis (pouching of the wall that predisposes to retention and infection), calculi, tumors, and accidental injury, which may include rupture.

The urethra, of course, is subject to infection. In older men, the very common occurrence of prostatic hypertrophy may bring pressure to bear on the urethra and lead to urinary difficulty.

The gastrointestinal tract eliminates wastes and participates in the maintenance of fluid and electrolyte balance of the body. The large intestine is primarily concerned with elimination, but its function is dependent, of course, upon the function of the upper gastrointestinal tract and the small intestine. What can go wrong in these areas has been presented in the previous chapter, and all such pathological problems have their implications in the process of elimination.

The large intestine, and therefore its function, may be affected by infection or infestation, obstruction, change in motility, tumors, trauma, or pressure from and/or infection in the abdominal cavity. Ulcerative colitis is a relatively common disorder and may be due to bacillary or amebic infection and other chronic infections and is sometimes associated with personality disorders (mucous colitis). Obstruction may be due to foreign objects, pressures from adjacent organs, strictures, intussusception (telescoping of one part of the bowel into another), paralytic ileus, volvulus (looping of intestine on its mesenteric axis), or tumors. An acute and complete obstruction constitutes a surgical emergency. A chronic and partial obstruction is amenable to more conservative medical treatment. Tumors of the large intestine, especially malignant tumors, are common. A change in the normal peristaltic movements, either increased or decreased, may result from infection or any other pathological process, from dietary habits, from sedentary or overactive habit patterns, or from psychological factors. The abdomen, including the intestines, is a common site of traumatic injuries, both in automobile accidents and home accidents. Peritonitis or ascites can also affect the functioning of the large intestine.

The excretory function of the lung can be affected by anything that reduces the exchange of oxygen and carbon dioxide between the alveolar spaces and the lung capillaries and by anything that reduces or increases the rate of respiration. Common pathological processes that affect these functions have been described in Chapter 17.

The excretory function of the skin is limited, but it does take over some function when other areas of elimination are embarrassed. In renal failure, for example, urea and salt crystals may appear on the skin, the resulting "uremic frost" giving evidence of the skin's attempt to excrete substances normally excreted by the kidney. The maintenance of a major portion of the body surface intact therefore maintains this area of elimination. Some of the pathological processes that can interfere with the regulatory mechanisms (endocrine system and nervous system) that can also affect the control of elimination have been presented in previous chapters and will be discussed in more detail in Chapter 21.

NURSING INTERVENTION

Nursing intervention in the care of patients with problems in elimination is focused in the following three major areas: (1) maintaining optimum function, (2) helping to restore elimination through palliative (relief of symptoms) or restorative measures, and (3) teaching and rehabilitation.

Observation

The observation of the characteristics of excreta constitutes a significant nursing function. The amount, color, clarity, odor, and constituents of urine are an indication of major difficulties in elimination. Normally, the amount of urine is related to intake. It can, however, be retained, retained with overflow, or suppressed. In retention, the patient fails to excrete and suffers a sensation of fullness and discomfort, and the distended bladder can be felt. The patient may void small amounts frequently but fail to completely empty the bladder; this is known as retention with overflow. The patient experiences again a sense of fullness and discomfort, and sooner or later the bladder distention can be felt. Suppression is the failure to secrete urine. However, in suppression, the failure to void does not result in bladder distention and discomfort, but rather in systemic responses to the failure to excrete toxic substances and to electrolyte and fluid imbalance. Descriptive terms used in relation to voiding include anuria (suppression), oliguria (scanty urine), polyuria (unusually large amount), pyuria (pus in the urine), hematuria (blood in the urine), and dysuria (painful voiding). In addition to amounts, both for each voiding and for the twenty-four hour period, any degree of urgency or difficulty in voiding should be noted. Whether the urine is clear and transparent or is cloudy due to the presence of cells, casts, albumin, or other substances should also be observed. If cloudiness is due to an alkaline reaction, the urine will clear with heating or with the addition of acid. Freshly voided urine that smells of ammonia (which occurs after decomposition has taken place) or that has a sweetish smell (the result of the presence of acetone) should always be reported.

Elimination from the gastrointestinal tract may be either infrequent and difficult (constipation) or frequent and liquid (diarrhea). Flatus is the presence of gas in the intestine. Flatulence and tympanitis are terms used to describe the presence of flatus. Tenesmus is a term used to describe unsuccessful straining to produce a stool. Characteristics of the stool that are important to observe include number, consistency, shape, color, and odor. The stool should be formed—not hard, liquid, or loose. The color may indicate the absence of bile (clay colored) or the presence of fresh blood (red and on the outside of the stool) or old blood (black and mixed throughout). Any unusual odor or constituents (such as mucus, which causes a shiny appearance) should be observed and reported.

Whenever problems of elimination occur, are suspected, or are anticipated, the supplementary excretory functions of the skin and lungs should be observed and evaluated. The rate of respiration and the odor of expired air may be of significance. For example, in serious renal impairment or failure, the odor of expired air may be uriniferous, and air hunger may be present. In addition, the skin may have a white, powdery appearance due to the presence of urea and salt crystals. In cases of intestinal stasis, there may be a foul or fecal odor to the breath.

In addition to careful observation of the characteristics of excreta, the relationship of fluid and food intake to output becomes a significant point of attention. Dark, scanty, concentrated urine and constipation may result from inadequate fluid intake. In the presence of adequate fluid intake, the significance of these symptoms may change; for example, the concentrated urine may indicate renal problems, and the constipation may reflect a diet low in roughage or bulk.

A patient losing fluids continuously by vomiting and excessive perspiration would not be expected to excrete the same amount of urine as a patient on the same fluid intake who was neither vomiting nor perspiring excessively. It is the balance or relationship between the two that provides the significant clues in evaluating elimination. For this reason, the accurate recording of intake and output of fluids is extremely important. While keeping a careful record of all fluids the patient may receive by mouth, by tube feeding, or by intravenous infusion or any other method and a careful record of all output that is measurable such as urine, vomitus, or drainage, the summary for the shift or the day should include other relevant factors. If the patient is perspiring heavily, this should be noted on the intake-output record, as well as rapid respirations that would indicate increased carbon dioxide and water loss.

Related to intake and output, and above the significance of their amount, are the cardinal symptoms of water or fluid imbalance—edema and dehydration. These, particularly in relation to evaluating elimination, are important points of observation.

Dehydration may result from excessive elimination, and edema may result from failing or inadequate elimination. Edema is a classic symptom of renal difficulty. It may occur first as puffy eyelids or in dependent portions of the body (such as in the feet and legs of the ambulatory patient). It may occur as generalized edema involving the total body and, in instances of renal malfunction, is often pitting. Its location, extent, and character should be noted and recorded, because change in the edema in either a positive or negative direction will often provide clues to the success or failure of current therapy.

Dehydration, in addition to resulting from inadequate intake, can frequently be attributed to excessive elimination, either by the normal routes of excretion or by unusual ones, such as excessive vomiting. Diarrhea or polyuria can produce dehydration, for example. Edema is, of course, identified by the accumulation of fluid in the tissues with resultant swelling. Dehydration is identified by rise in body temperature, increased pulse rate and reduced cardiac output, thrist, dryness and wrinkling of the skin, and pallor. (See Chapter 16.)

The vital signs (temperature, pulse, respiration, and blood pressure) are of extreme importance. Nutrition, elimination, and fluid and electrolyte balance are complementary functions; what affects one affects the other, and these factors combined affect every aspect of physiology. Therefore, disturbances tend to be reflected in the vital signs. A rising blood pressure can be caused by renal impairment; on the other hand, hypertension can result in renal impairment. A rapid pulse can result from cardiac effort to maintain circulation to all areas, including the kidney, and failure of the kidney to excrete potassium can lead to an intoxication that may produce cardiac failure. Air hunger can be one of the symptoms of electrolyte imbalance that results from either overproduction or underproduction in elimination. If generalized edema exists as a result of failure to eliminate, a rising blood pressure and increasing pulse rate may signal the advent of cerebral edema. In any instance, the vital signs require close attention and prompt reporting of any evidence of change.

Many types and locations of pain characterize the range of disorders in elimination; therefore, pain is a primary focus of observation in providing nursing care for patients with problems with elimination. Appendicitis, for example, may show the typical rebound pain, i.e., the pain disappears when pressure is released. Pain from this source begins around the umbilicus, spreads throughout the abdomen, and localizes at McBurney's point midway between the umbilicus and the right iliac crest. An early symptom of intestinal obstruction is intermittent or cramping pain caused by increased peristaltic motion above the obstruction, followed by rigidity of the abdomen and continuous excruciating pain if the obstruction is complete. Diarrhea may be accompanied by sharp, cramping abdominal pain.

A kidney stone or calculus that is too large to pass but is forced into the ureter may cause renal colic, a severe pain in the abdomen or flank that may radiate to the genitalia and thigh. A distended bladder may cause dull to sharp pain associated with a feeling of fullness. A slowly developing hydronephrosis, dilatation of the kidney pelvis, may produce a dull flank pain.

In all instances, a complete description of the pain, its nature, location, extent, duration, its association with patient and environmental activities, and the patient's reaction to the pain should be obtained. (See Chapter 16.)

As might be noted from the preceding discussion, the abdomen is one area of focus for observation. This includes not only pain, but the state of muscle tone. The abdomen may be flaccid, distended, or tense and rigid. Whether accompanied by pain or not, such symptoms are worth noting and recording.

Anorexia, nausea, and vomiting, to some degree, are usual concomitants of all types of problems in elimination. The occurrence of anorexia, nausea, and vomiting and related patient and environmental activities should be observed, and the patient's subjective complaints should be combined with the overt observations. The amount, odor, color, and other characteristics of the vomitus should be observed and reported. Changes in characteristics should be promptly reported; for example, the appearance of frank blood in vomitus when it has not been seen before would call for immediate reporting.

Motor function and level of consciousness are also important areas of observation for patients with problems in elimination. Disturbances in electrolyte balance or cerebral edema may impinge upon cerebral efficiency. Twitching, muscle irritability, or convulsions may appear, and points of observation are location, type of motion, extent, and duration of motor activity. Headache, blurred vision, dizziness, or irritability may also occur and indicate cerebral irritation. Slowed mental processes, followed by drowsiness and leading into coma, may indicate progression toward death in renal failure.

Observation for signs of internal hemorrhage or shock is indicated for patients with problems in elimination following surgery, in acute intestinal obstruction, in excruciating pain, or under severe emotional stress. (See Chapter 16.)

Another very important aspect of observation is the emotional status and the personality pattern of the patient. Like nutrition, elimination is inextricably interwoven with cultural and personal value systems. In fact, the mouth, used in obtaining nutrition, and the two major organs of excretion are so significant that Freud used them as key factors in the foundation of his theory of psychosexual development.

There are two aspects to the social and psychological significance of the processes of elimination—the patient's and the nurse's. In regard to the patient, the nurse needs to look for and respond sensitively to the patient's feelings about elimination. She needs to protect privacy in addition to providing measures to make elimination as comfortable as possible. She also needs to be aware of the fact that interference with elimination is considered by most persons as a serious threat and tends to produce anxiety and fear. As a basis for planning nursing care for such patients, the nurse needs to learn about the patient's value system, his reactions to his health problem, his feelings about and attitudes toward elimination, the situations and people who alleviate his symptoms, and the situations and people who aggravate his symptoms. Elimination, like eating, can be used to express emotional conflicts, as well as causing emotional conflicts when it presents a health problem for a patient. Therefore, the greater the knowledge about the patient as a person, the better source the nurse has for planning nursing care. Here, the value of information that relatives or friends may provide is obvious.

Dependent nursing functions

Dependent nursing functions that the nurse may perform, provide for, or assist with include diagnostic tests, medical therapy, dietary modification, and the administration of medications.

Diagnostic tests

One of the more common diagnostic tests is urinalysis, and the nurse is responsible for the collection of the specimen. Nursing responsibilities include:
1. Knowing the reason for the urinalysis
2. Securing the patient's participation (it is frustrating to both the patient and nurse when the nurse comes dashing in and requests a specimen just after the patient has voided)
3. Providing the means for collecting (bedpan or urinal)
4. Placing the specimen in the proper receptacle (test tube or bottle)
5. Labeling the specimen with the patient's name, kind of specimen, date, and purpose of test
6. Routing the specimen to the proper laboratory at the right time

Any or all of these functions may be delegated under certain circumstances, but the responsibility rests with the nurse.

The urine may be examined for specific gravity, color, sugar acetone, plasma proteins (albumin, globulin, fibrogen), hemoglobin, blood, bacteria, pus, or cells. Sugar and acetone are usually related to diabetes, although acetone may be associated with starvation. Proteins suggest kidney disorders, as does a lowered or increased specific gravity. Sometimes a voided urine specimen may contain unusual substances, and a catheterized specimen may be requested to be certain the constituents are present in the urine rather than introduced extraneously. The procedure is usually carried out in women by female nurses and in men by a physician or a male nurse. When a urine culture is desired, the specimen is always obtained by catheterization, using sterile technique, including a sterile tube for collection.

In addition to the analysis of the urine that provides clues to the effectiveness of the kidney, there are a number of other renal function tests. Blood tests will often reveal an increased retention of urea in blood when the kidney is damaged. The BUN (blood urea nitrogen) and NPN (nonprotein nitrogen) tests are frequently used and are valueless unless done on a specimen obtained after fasting. Renal ability to concentrate and dilute urine may be tested in several ways and is significant because the normal kidney adjusts these functions to body conditions. Severe kidney damage impairs this ability, and the specific gravity of urine tends to stay at the same level.

Commonly used are the Fishberg dilution test, Addis test and Mosenthal test. In the Fishberg dilution test, the patient empties the bladder and drinks 1200 ml. of fluid within one-half hour and urine specimens are collected every half hour for three hours. The patient remains inactive until the test is completed.

In all concentration tests, urine specimens are collected at periodic intervals with or without fluid or intake variation. In one test, intake is withheld during the night and three spaced early-morning specimens are collected. In another, a twenty-four hour specimen is collected, followed by several individual specimens. The nurse should check the desired hours of collection.

A urea clearance test involves the analysis of both urine and blood for urea. The fasting patient voids and one hour later is asked to void again, at which time a blood specimen is also taken. An hour later an additional urine specimen is taken. The patient drinks water after the discard of the first specimen. Since the kidney is the usual route of excretion of urea, an increased blood urea and decreased urine urea signal renal impairment.

The phenolsulfonphthalein (PSP) test may be used to determine renal function, since the dye is normally excreted by the kidney. The patient voids, and after the specimen is discarded, exactly 1 ml. of the dye is injected intravenously. Since specimens are collected at fifteen minutes, thirty minutes, one hour, and two hours after the injection, fluids may need to be forced. About 80% of the dye should be excreted in two hours.

An intravenous pyelogram may also be taken for the purpose of assessing renal function. Foods and fluids are omitted during the night, and because the bowels must be empty to visualize the urinary tract, laxatives, cathartics, or an enema may be employed to clear the lower gastrointestinal tract. A radiopaque dye containing iodine (Diodrast, for example) is injected slowly after an x-ray film of the abdomen is taken. Roentgenograms of the urinary system are taken seven and fifteen minutes later and may be repeated in two hours or at later intervals. Since allergic responses to the iodine in the dyes used constitute a danger, sensitivity to iodine should be determined in advance. The patient should be observed for respiratory distress, urticaria, excessive perspiration, or clamminess. Any unusual sensation calls for immediate medical supervision.

A cystoscopic examination may also be used for diagnostic purposes. A cystoscope is introduced into the bladder in order to visualize its interior. In preparation for the examination, the patient should have an explanation of the procedure and an opportunity to discuss it and his feelings about it, for relaxation will reduce pain and discomfort. Fluids are forced, and the patient is usually sedated. The patient is placed in lithotomy position* and the cystoscope inserted. At this point the patient will usually need emotional support, and his reactions must be carefully observed. The bladder is filled with distilled water to aid visualization. In some instances, ureteral catheters may be passed through the ureters or into the kidney pelvis. Urine specimens at varying levels may be collected or dyes may be injected and their excretion noted. If radiopaque dyes are used, an x-ray examination of the ureters (retrograde pyelogram) may be done when the cystoscope is removed. Aftercare of the patient is important and includes promoting comfort and explaining to the patient what he may expect, such as some hematuria or the secretion of dyes.

Stool examination is to elimination via the gastrointestinal tract what urinalysis is to elimination via the urinary tract. Stool specimens may be collected by the patient himself or by the nurse or by other nursing service personnel. The responsibility, however, rests with the nurse. Most agencies provide a specimen box adapted to the purpose, and spatulas or tongue depressors may be used to place the specimen in the box. In addition to ordered specimens, any abnormal stool in regard to color, consistency, odor, or any other aspect of appearance should be saved for examination. The nurse's responsibilities are the same as those for the collection of urine specimens.

"Oscopies" involving visual examination of the lower end of the gastrointestinal tract include anoscopy (anus), protoscopy (rectum), and sigmoidoscopy (sigmoid). Usually, intake is reduced the evening before the procedure, and enemas are given to clear the area before examination. The psychological preparation of the patient is important, since his cooperation is essential for the examination. (This, in reality, is true of all effective examinations. They are worth more with the patient's free participation.) The appropriate instrument is inserted after the patient assumes a knee-chest position or a side-lying position. The nurse's emotional support, if given with sensitivity to the patient as a person, may help promote relaxation, and the nurse may also assist the patient in maintaining the correct position to facilitate maximum ease and comfort during the examination. Careful ob-

---

*For anatomical positions used for treatment and examination, see Appendix.

servation of the patient during the procedure is indicated, and any untoward signs revealed by color, respiration, pulse, or general appearance should be promptly reported.

Biopsy, or the removal of living tissue for diagnostic examination, may be done during any of the "oscopies" or may be taken from other areas of the systems involved in elimination. A biopsy is normally used to determine the nature (benign or malignant) of suspected or obvious tumors.

Medical therapies

The assistance with medical therapies for patients with problems in elimination are focused primarily in the areas of catheterization, irrigation, and maintenance of drainage.

Catheterization is the removal of urine through a catheter introduced into the bladder, using aseptic technique. The purpose is to obtain a specimen, relieve pressure if the patient cannot void, or to prepare for surgery. The nurse's responsibility includes preparation of the patient, cleansing the part, inserting the catheter, and ensuring patient safety, disposing of the specimen, and providing aftercare of the patient to ensure patient comfort. Disposable catheterization sets are now available, and, if they are not, sterile catheterization sets containing all necessary equipment are usually available from a central supply room.

Irrigations* are varied in location but widely used for patients with problems in elimination. Irrigations of the bladder and the colon are relatively common. In addition, irrigations of the intestines may be done through surgical openings that bring varying parts of the intestine to the outer aspect of the abdomen—colostomy, cecostomy, or ileostomy. A colostomy is an artificial opening into the colon, a cecostomy into the cecum, and an ileostomy into the ileum. The "ostomy" may be temporary or permanent. In all irrigations, certain generalizations apply. The nurse's responsibilities include:

1. Preparing the patient adequately through explanation and providing a channel for the patient to express himself if he wishes
2. Collecting and preparing equipment and supplies
3. Protecting the patient during the irrigation
4. Completing the procedure
5. Aftercare of the patient to ensure his comfort
6. Disposing of irrigation products
7. Cleansing and disposal of equipment
8. Charting of the time, effect, character of drainage, and patient reaction to the irrigation

The basic equipment for any irrigation includes (1) a container with the appropriate solution in sufficient quantity, (2) a means of irrigating (can with tube, tube with funnel, Asepto syringe, etc.), (3) lubricant for insertion if needed, (4) a receptacle for the return flow, (5) protection for the pa-

---

*For a summary of irrigations, see Appendix.

tient (rubber sheet or square with cover), and (6) materials for any necessary clean-up. If the procedure is sterile, additional necessary equipment is necessary: clean-up (alcohol sponge, sterile soap, and cotton balls), forceps for handling equipment, and/or rubber gloves. An appropriate cover for the set-up while being transported to and from the patient is included.

In general, the following factors are taken into consideration in giving irrigations.

1. The solution is the one ordered or the one appropriate.
2. The source of the irrigation is above the area to be irrigated, but not so high as to cause too much pressure from the flow of the solution.
3. The amount of solution introduced is not beyond the anatomical capacity of the area to be irrigated or beyond the patient's ability to tolerate it.
4. The temperature of the solution is appropriate to the anatomical area to be irrigated and the purpose of the irrigation. (An ice-cold enema may be used to help reduce temperature but would complicate achieving the purpose of a cleansing enema.)
5. The tube used for irrigation is appropriate in size for the orifice involved, i.e., a catheter is used for bladder irrigation and a rectal tube for an enema.
6. The receptacle for the return flow is appropriate to the site and amount of solution used for the irrigation.

A patient who has had a cecostomy usually has a tube left in situ. Irrigations may be employed to keep the tube patent and draining. If so, usually a limited amount of fluid (specified by the physician's order) is used, and the fluid is returned by gravity (lowering the Asepto syringe after removing the bulb). Pressure or suction is avoided to prevent further trauma.

A colostomy may be double (two openings, proximal and distal, on the abdomen) as well as single. The latter normally is lower in the intestinal tract (sigmoid), feces are more formed, and the patient can learn to control the colostomy evacuation through enemas and establishing habit patterns. Irrigation is done with a catheter, and the patient may need to be taught to do his own irrigations if the colostomy is permanent. If the colostomy is double, irrigations to promote fecal removal are through the proximal end, although irrigations of the distal end may be done to remove fecal matter previously accumulated. If there is no obstruction, or at least not complete obstruction, the irrigating solution introduced into the distal opening may be expelled through the rectum.

The maintenance of drainage is a common nursing responsibility in the care of patients with problems in elimination, especially when the urinary system is involved. Drainage from the bladder, the ureters, or the kidney pelvis may be established by inserting a retention catheter (Foley or Gilbert) directly into the bladder or by inserting catheters into the ureters or kidney pelvis via a cystoscope. In some instances, surgical openings may be made to insert the drainage tube. In the maintenance of drainage via the various tubes from the various sites most commonly drained. certain generalizations apply.

1. The tube must be retained in the site of intended drainage. The type of catheter may accomplish this, such as the Foley, with its balloon that can be inflated to hold it in the bladder. Otherwise, the drainage tube must be secured in place from the outside, with transparent tape or adhesive tape or by pinning to a dressing, or similar means.

2. The patency of the tube must be maintained. Following are the major sources of difficulty:
   (a) Clogging from mucus, blood clots, or sediment from an internal source
   (b) Pressure from the outside that occludes the lumen, such as kinking or the weight of the patient's body

3. The patency of drainage tubes should be frequently checked.

4. Suction or pressure should not be used to attempt to reestablish the patency of tubes.

5. The receptacle into which drainage flows must be below the level of the site being drained, since drainage depends upon the force of gravity.

6. Drainage bottles or other drainage receptacles should be changed and cleansed often enough to control odors.

7. The area of exit of the drainage tube should be kept clean.

8. All equipment used in the drainage apparatus should be maintained in the highest state of cleanliness possible to avoid infection.

9. The amount of drainage anticipated should be estimated, so that too much or too little can be noted and reported promptly.

10. The amount, color, consistency, odor, and span of time covered by the drainage should be noted and recorded.

11. Any change in the nature of the drainage should be promptly reported.

12. Drainage tubes, such as the Foley catheter, should be changed as often as necessary. The scheduled changes should be ascertained and checked, and the accumulation of crystals, a sandy feeling, or unclean appearance of the tube should be reported, since change is indicated.

If the catheter is to be irrigated and is in place for the purpose of drainage only, the amount of irrigation solution should be regulated by the fact that the primary purpose is to maintain patency. Therefore, small amounts are instilled and returns continued at intervals until clear.

Tidal drainage (or irrigation) consists of filling the bladder slowly with and irrigating solution and periodically emptying it. It is used primarily with patients with incontinence due to neurological disorders and, in addition to irrigating and draining, is employed to help reestablish a normal habit pattern of voiding.

Dietary adaptation

The range of dietary adaptations used for patients with problems in elimination includes practically the entire scope of diet therapy. The nurse therefore needs to check specific diet orders, verify the consistency and nutritional elements included, verify those *not* included, and evaluate the extent to which the patient partakes of that ordered and the patient's reaction to diet therapy. The latter should include the patient's personal and feeling responses as well as physical status.

Administration of medications

Commonly ordered medications include (1) sedatives, such as chloral hydrate and the barbiturates, (2) analgesics for the relief of pain, such as morphine and Demerol, (3) diuretics, such as meralluride (Mercuhydrin) or chlorothiazide (Diuril), (4) antispasmodics, such as atropine, (5) laxatives and cathartics, and (6) antibiotics.

Independent nursing functions

Because of the cultural, social, and psychological significance of the processes of elimination, the provision of emotional support is a major nursing responsibility. The matter-of-fact approach, keeping channels of communication open so that the patient can explore and express his feelings and thus, perhaps, come to grips with them, and indirect and nondirective approaches are of particular value.

Respect for privacy when possible, the invasion of privacy with an understanding of its implications for the patient when it is necessary, and a sincere interest in the patient as a person to create a basis for a satisfactory relationship to support him through his difficulties are indicated. The use of listening, open-end questions, paraphrasing, and reflecting and focusing on feeling areas are significant nursing measures. (See Chapter 7.) Anticipating patient needs in regard to elimination can also contribute to the patient's security. If the patient is having trouble voiding or defecating, providing fluids in advance, bedpan or urinal at regular intervals or especially appropriate times (bedpan after eating to take advantage of increased peristalsis), providing time and privacy, correct positioning, and, above all, not keeping the patient waiting may contribute to patient comfort. If the patient is eliminating at excessively frequent intervals, provision should be made for having the bedpan or urinal readily available, and they should be removed as soon as used. The reassurance of attention as needed, based on anticipation rather than patient request, makes a solid contribution to the patient's feeling of acceptance.

There are many independent measures that the nurse can provide to support the processes of elimination. For example, to assist the patient trying to void, turning on a faucet or pouring warm water over the external genitalia may help. Position is important; if the patient can be supported in the normal anatomical position for elimination, this should be done. The provision of fluids and encouragement to drink them regularly, if permitted, may also help. If the patient is weak or restless and confused, a regular schedule for providing fluids may be set up and followed. A balance of rest and activity is important for elimination, since most diseases cause some restriction of normal activity and may result in elimination problems because of reduced activity.

For the patient who is unable to control elimination, the nurse bears a heavy responsibility—the maintenance of cleanliness and the integrity of the skin. Only conscientious, frequent, and meticulous cleansing gives the patient a chance to avoid complications such as skin breakdown. Protection of the skin with emollients and prompt care of reddened areas are imperative. In addition to the physical aspects of care, the conscious patient who is incontinent needs considerable understanding and support.

Provisions of safety measures are frequently necessary. If the patient has a headache, or become drowsy or dizzy, or if there is any other indication of decreasing cerebral competence, padded bedside rails may be indicated. If the patient is weak, but adamant about navigating to the bathroom, an escort should be provided. After treatments or diagnostic tests that may be somewhat strenuous or unpleasant, the patient should be protected from attempting to resume activities at his previous level until he has time to recover from the effects of the procedure. If the patient is to continue drainage but moves from bed rest to ambulatory status, he will need both physical and psychological assistance in learning to adjust to "up" drainage. An accurate assessment of the patient's physical capacities and his willingness to function within his limits forms the guideline for ensuring patient safety.

The nurse can utilize her knowledge of the interrelatedness of the excretory functions of the four areas of elimination to support supplementary elimination when one organ or system is not functioning adequately. For example, if renal excretion is limited, positioning to maintain adequate and free respiration and good skin care to promote elimination by that route will be helpful.

Although orders for recording intake and output may be written, the nurse need not and should not restrict attention to simply recording as and when ordered. The prevention of difficulties in elimination can often be attributed to a recognition of an imbalance between intake and output. Alertness to and reporting factors in intake and output that cannot be measured, such as perspiration, are indicated. The nutritional and fluid balance of the body are basic to the maintenance of homeostasis and deserve detailed attention. One of the major difficulties is ensuring adequate fluid intake, for this cannot be done at one time or on a sporadic basis.

Physical comfort bears a direct relationship to the maintenance or control of elimination. Physical hygiene measures such as cleanliness, comfortable position, change of position, oral hygiene, and attention to the small details of comfort (such as hair, nails, tight bottom sheets) can avoid unnecessary increased or decreased elimination due to tension or discomfort. Such measures can also promote normal elimination and contribute to the avoidance of retention or constipation. The control of excessive elimination such as polyuria and diarrhea can also be influenced by physical comfort, since discomfort tends to increase both.

The balance of rest and exercise is an independent nursing measure that contributes to the maintenance of elimination. The completely inactive patient is predisposed to stasis of all types, particularly in the intestinal tract. Therefore, evaluation of patient capacity and provision for rest and activity at the level of patient needs is required. The nurse may need to provide change of position and passive exercise.

A major area of nursing intervention in providing nursing care for patients with problems in elimination is the area of teaching. The teaching needs of every patient should be identified and plans made to begin teaching as soon as the patient is ready for it. One of the quickest ways to get patients ready for teaching is to deal with the matters that are of greatest concern to them, no matter how irrelevant they may appear to someone else. There is little point in trying to teach a patient the relationship between diet and elimination if the patient is deeply concerned about what the nextdoor neighbors will tell his other neighbors about the nature of his illness.

Common teaching needs include the relationship of a balanced diet, fluid intake, and the establishment of regular habit patterns to elimination and the care of adaptations of life patterns that result from the patient's health problem, such as the care of a permanent colostomy. It can be fairly safely assumed that every patient with elimination problems has some teaching needs. It is the nurse's responsibility, with the patient's or his relatives' help, to identify the specific need or needs and to plan with the patient to help meet them.

BIBLIOGRAPHY

1. A cancer source book for nurses, New York, 1950, American Cancer Society.
2. Ansell, Julian S., and Taufic, Marjorie R.: Nephrectomy and nephrostomy: nursing the patient after nephrectomy, American Journal of Nursing **58**:1394-1398, Oct. 1958.
3. Anthony, Catherine P.: What makes fluids flow, American Journal of Nursing **56**:1256-1258, Oct. 1956.
4. Best, Charles H., and Taylor, Norman B.: Physiological basis of medical practice, ed. 7, Baltimore, 1961, Williams and Wilkins Co., pp. 570-582, 711-722.
5. Creevy, D. Donald, and Tollefson, Dorothy: Iliac diversion of the urine: nursing care of the patient with iliac diversion of the urine, American Journal of Nursing **59**:530-536, April 1959.
6. Fuerst, Elinor V., and Wolff, La Verne: Fundamentals of nursing, ed. 2, Philadelphia, 1959, J. B. Lippincott Co., pp. 335-398.
7. Hand, John R.: Infections of the urinary tract, American Journal of Nursing **57**:1008-1010, Aug. 1957.
8. Harmer, Bertha, and Henderson, Virginia: Textbook of the principles and practice of nursing, ed. 5, New York, 1955, The Macmillan Co., pp. 429-507, 840-895.
9. Ingles, Thelma, and Campbell, Emily: The patient with a colostomy, American Journal of Nursing **58**:1544-1546, Nov. 1958.

10. Jackson, Arlene F.: Cancer of the bladder, American Journal of Nursing **58**:249-250, Feb. 1958.
11. Jensen, J. Trygve: Introduction to medical physics, Philadelphia, 1960, J. B. Lippincott Co., pp. 76-96.
12. Linder, Janet: Inexpensive colostomy irrigation equipment, American Journal of Nursing **58**:844, June 1958.
13. Nordmark, Madelyn T., and Rohweder, Anne W.: Scientific principles applied to nursing, Philadelphia, 1959, J. B. Lippincott Co., pp. 124-129.
14. Shafer, Kathleen N., Sawyer, Janet R., McCluskey, Audrey M., and Beck, Edna L.: Medical-surgical nursing, ed. 2, St. Louis, 1961, The C. V. Mosby Co., pp. 313-375, 525-586.
15. Steigman, Frederick: Are laxatives necessary? American Journal of Nursing **62**:90-93, Oct. 1962.
16. Walsh, Michael, Ebner, Marion, and Casey, Joseph W.: Neo-bladder, American Journal of Nursing **63**:107-110, April 1963.
17. Weiss, Edward, and English, O. Spurgeon: Psychosomatic medicine, ed. 3, Philadelphia, 1957, W. B. Saunders Co., pp. 254-306.

Chapter 20

Nursing care of patients with fluid and electrolyte imbalance

Every body cell lives in a fluid environment with a hydrogen ion concentration that normally ranges from pH 7.35 to pH 7.45. If the pH concentration drops below 6.8 or goes above 8, death ensues. The maintenance of fluid, electrolyte, and acid-base balance is dependent upon a complex homeostatic mechanism that regulates within a narrow range the environment of individual body cells. Metabolic activity and survival depend on this.

Water is essential to life. Much of the body consists of water, and it represents approximately one half of the total body weight of adults and approximately three fourths of the total body weight of newborn infants. Water that is intracellular, i.e., within the cells, constitutes about two thirds of the total water found in the adult; about one third is extracellular, i.e., in the vascular system or between cells (interstitial). In infants and young children this distribution is approximately 50/50. Sources of water are fluid intake, water contained in solid foods, and water derived from the metabolic process. Water is lost primarily through the kidneys, lungs, and skin. Minor losses occur through saliva and the intestinal tract.

Electrolytes are compounds that dissociate into ions in solution, and the ions carry a positive or negative charge. The significant positive ions (cations) in normal body fluid are sodium, potassium, calcium, and magnesium. The significant negative ions (anions) include chloride, bicarbonate, phosphate, sulfate, and ions of organic acids and proteins. The electrolytes have several functions: (1) assist in the regulation of some metabolic activities, (2) are active in maintaining acid-base balance, and (3) participate in the control of body water volume.

The acid-base balance of body fluids is measured by the concentration of hydrogen ions. Body fluid is normally slightly alkaline. An increase in hydrogen ions makes body fluid more acid than normal, and a decrease in hydrogen ions makes body fluid more alkaline than normal. The human body cannot tolerate too marked deviations in either direction. The essence of maintaining acid-base balance, therefore, is controlling or changing the hydrogen ion concentration. This is accomplished by "buffers" which combine with surplus hydrogen ions or release them. The most important of the buffer systems is the carbonic acid-sodium bicarbonate system which is found in the extracellular fluid. Carbonic acid, H_2CO_3, ionizes to free a small quantity of hydrogen ion (H^+) and the bicarbonate ion (HCO_3^-). The bicarbonate hydrolyzes to H_2CO_3 (carbonic acid) and the hydroxyl ion (OH). In normal extracellular fluid, carbonic acid and base bicarbonate are present in a ratio of 1:20. Disturbance in this ratio means disturbance in the acid-base balance.

The maintenance of the delicately balanced fluid and electrolyte environment of body cells is a homeostatic must. Any immediate threat to the balance is a threat to life.

PROPORTION OF BODY WEIGHT REPRESENTED BY WATER

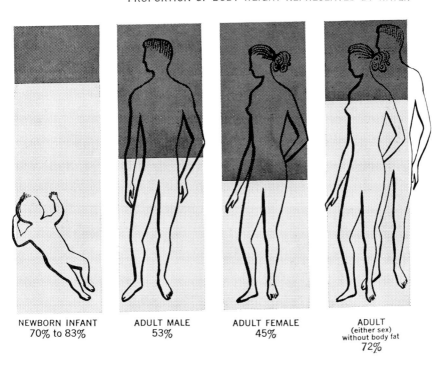

NEWBORN INFANT	ADULT MALE	ADULT FEMALE	ADULT
70% to 83%	53%	45%	(either sex) without body fat 72%

Fig. 44. Much of the body consists of water. It represents 53% of the body weight of the average adult male and 45% of the body weight of the average female. Since fat is essentially water free, the proportion of water to body weight is greater in the lean individual. Excluding the fatty tissues, about 72% of the body weight of adults is made up of water.

Infants have more water in comparison to body weight than adults. In the newborn infant, water comprises 70% to 83% of the total weight. The most rapid decline in the proportion of body water to body weight occurs during the first six months of life. (Courtesy Abbott Laboratories, North Chicago, Ill.)

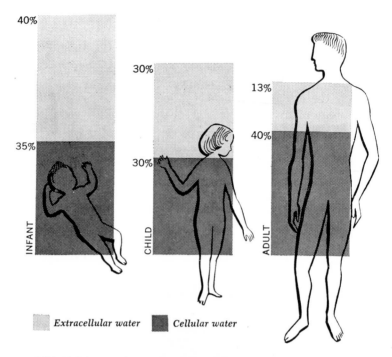

40%

30%

13%

35%

30%

40%

INFANT

CHILD

ADULT

▒ *Extracellular water*   ■ *Cellular water*

BODY WATER EXPRESSED AS A PERCENTAGE OF BODY WEIGHT

Fig. 45. The store of water in the body is replenished in two ways. (1) *By ingestion—* the most obvious mechanism is the consumption of liquids, but in addition solids such as meat and vegetables contain 60% to 97% water. (2) *By metabolism—*the breakdown of foodstuffs yields water of oxidation. This process releases about 12 ml. of water from the metabolism of each 100 calories of fat, carbohydrate, or protein. (Courtesy Abbot Laboratories, North Chicago, Ill.)

ESSENTIAL MECHANISMS

The maintenance of fluid and electrolyte balance depends upon a number of interrelated factors. There must be an adequate intake of fluid and foodstuffs that contain the necessary ingredients to support metabolic activity. There must be adequate transportation of oxygen, water, food, and wastes. The buffering system must be functioning. Elimination not only must be adequate in amount but must be selectively tuned to special needs for elimination of excesses and retention of depleted elements. Regulatory mechanisms must be functioning to bring about adjustment to compensate for any threatened or impending imbalance. As can be readily seen, the maintenance of fluid, electrolyte, and acid-base balance is related to the total function of the human body.

WHAT CAN GO WRONG

Almost any of the health problems previously discussed can affect fluid and particularly electrolyte balance. Of particular importance are nutrition and elimination, since the basic elements that form ions (such as proteins,

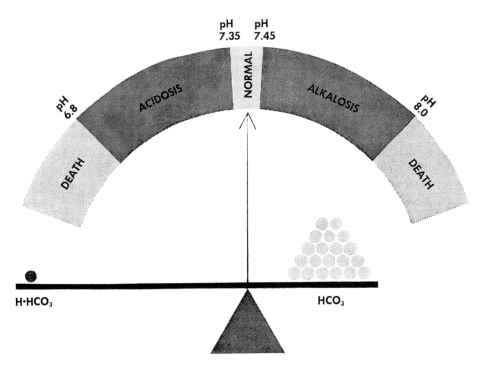

Fig. 46. Normally, these bicarbonates are present in the extracellular fluid in a ratio of 1 part of carbonic acid to 20 parts of base bicarbonate. When this ratio is disturbed, the acid-base equilibrium is also upset, and there is a deviation from the normal pH of the body fluid. The maintenance of health and life requires that the hydrogen ion concentration of body fluid varies only within a narrow range. (Courtesy Abbott Laboratories, North Chicago, Ill.)

calcium, potassium, and sodium chloride) must first be ingested. Deficiencies or excesses can affect both fluid and electrolyte balance. Of equal importance, if not greater, is the role of elimination; the kidneys, lungs, and skin make contributions to the maintenance of balance by adjusting excretion to body conditions. For example, if carbon dioxide (which forms carbonic acid in solution) accumulates in the blood stream, respirations increase to speed up the elimination of carbon dioxide. The kidney, in particular, is a major factor in stabilizing electrolyte balance. Any basic pathological process that affects nutrition or elimination also affects fluid and electrolyte balance.

The major health problems that directly affect electrolyte and acid-base balance, in addition to intake and utilization, are those problems in which considerable fluid loss occurs or in which adrenal or pituitary regulation of kidney function is impaired. Fluid loss can result from a number of causes. Hemorrhage is one obvious one, and major surgery is another. The increased knowledge of electrolytes is one of the factors that has made more extensive surgery possible.

Burns of the body surface cause extensive loss of fluid, electrolytes, and proteins to the interstitial space around the affected area. With the increased osmotic pressure in this area, water continues to be drawn from general body resources and sodium enters the edematous area. Since bicarbonate goes with the sodium, acidosis may develop. A major therapeutic problem in the management of burns is replacement of fluids and electrolytes.

Excessive vomiting leads to excessive water and chloride loss. In addition to water loss, diarrhea may result in the loss of potassium and bicarbonate. Excessive perspiration leads to the loss of sodium chloride, and it is the resulting electrolyte imbalance that is fundamentally responsible for heat cramps (severe cramping of the skeletal muscles). Excessive urine output can threaten the concentration of electrolytes, although this is not likely to occur with normal kidney function. Kidney damage can seriously impair electrolyte and acid-base balance, and renal failure is accompanied by severe acidosis which is often irreversible. Alkalosis can be produced by overmedication and sometimes by diet, such as the early diet for peptic ulcer, which is heavy in alkali residue.

NURSING INTERVENTION

In all nursing, regardless of the basic health problem, the prevention or detection of early signs of fluid, electrolyte, and/or acid-base balance is a matter of concern. Water imbalance is always serious, and electrolyte and acid-base imbalance constitute medical emergencies.

Observation

Observational skills are critical in this area. One focus, of course, is upon the cardinal signs of water imbalance—dehydration and edema. These have been discussed previously, but significant indications of edema are swelling and puffiness, weight gain, and, if the edema is progressive, dyspnea, headache, confusion, or coma. Dehydration is revealed by dryness of the skin and mucous membrane, thirst, temperature rise, decreased and concentrated urine, loss of weight, and, if the dehydration is progressive, exhaustion and collapse.

Acid-base balance may vary in either direction, and significant clues are usually evident when this does occur.

Signs of acidosis include (1) heavy forced breathing, designed to reduce carbon dioxide concentration, (2) diuresis, due to increased sodium excretion, (3) sweet odor to the breath, caused by acetone, and (4) lethargy, muscular weakness, or changed cardiac action, caused by potassium deficiency. Normal cellular function alters and may be reflected in reduced cerebral competence with drowsiness, irritability, clouded consciousness, or coma.

Signs of alkalosis include (1) slow and shallow respirations, due to reduced carbon dioxide concentration, (2) diuresis, due to increased sodium excretion, and (3) muscle twitching or tetany, due to calcium deficiency. Interference with usual cellular function may lead to coma.

Evidence of electrolyte imbalance may be reflected by any of the occurrences described in the preceding paragraphs. The absence or excess of specific electrolytes may also be detected by symptoms related to their specific function. Increased sodium chloride retention may be indicated by edema since water is retained to keep body fluid isotonic. The loss of sodium beyond safe limits leads to headache, muscle weakness, nausea and vomiting, abdominal cramps, and diarrhea. Potassium deficiency may cause muscular weakness, lethargy, intestinal distention, and changes in heart activity. Potassium intoxication is evidenced by nausea, muscle weakness, diarrhea, and cardiac arrest. Potassium is usually not safe for administration in electrolyte therapy unless renal function is adequate, since postassium is excreted by the kidney and renal disease can thus result in potassium intoxication. Calcium excess rarely presents problems, but calcium deficiency results in a tingling sensation in the fingers, toes, or nose, followed by muscular twitching, and then by jerking muscular contractions.

The observations discussed here must be included along with observations to be made on every patient to whom nursing care is given.

Dependent nursing functions

Specific dependent nursing functions in negative fluid and electrolyte balance are related primarily to the intravenous administration of fluid and electrolytes to replace losses and provide maintenance requirements.

In positive water balance, reduction of fluids and sodium intake are usual measures.

Independent nursing functions

Guide lines to providing nursing care for patients with fluid and/or electrolyte imbalance are as follows:

1. Encouragement and support for the patient to maintain adequate nutrition and elimination may prevent either fluid and/or electrolyte imbalance.
2. Intake and output must always be recorded.
3. Developing signs of fluid or electrolyte imbalance should be promptly reported.
4. Fluids are forced in the presence of dehydration, infections, or elevated temperature unless they are specifically contraindicated.
5. The presence of edema calls for restricted fluids unless otherwise ordered.
6. When fluids are restricted, they should be spaced to promote patient comfort.
7. Oral hygiene needs careful attention in the presence of water imbalance.
8. Unless contraindicated, sodium chloride intake should be encouraged in the presence of profuse perspiration or the loss of tissue fluid.
9. The administration of potassium should be questioned when urinary output is reduced.
10. Rest and activity should be balanced in the light of the patient's

physical condition, and both should be provided to conserve patient energy resources.

11. Good physical and environmental hygiene should be provided to prevent infection.

12. Good skin care and change of position should be provided to prevent skin damage in the presence of water imbalance.

13. If symptoms indicate any cerebral interference or damage, the patient's safety rests with the nurse. Bedside rails and/or continuous observation may be needed.

14. Emotional support is significant since fluid and electrolyte imbalance are serious threats to life.

BIBLIOGRAPHY

1. Abbott Laboratories: Fluid and electrolytes, North Chicago, 1960.
2. Brooks, Stewart M.: Basic facts of body water and ions, New York, 1960, Springer Pub. Co., Inc.
3. Collentine, G. E.: How to calculate fluids for burned patients, American Journal of Nursing 62:77-79, March 1962.
4. Editorial: Potassium intoxication in renal failure, Journal of the American Medical Association 175:703-704, Feb. 1961.
5. Hoffman, Katherine B.: Chemistry for the applied sciences, Englewood Cliffs, N. J., 1963, Prentice-Hall, Inc., pp. 98-110, 128-141.
6. McKittrick, J. B., and Shotkin, J. M.: Ulcerative colitis, American Journal of Nursing 62:60-64, Aug. 1962.
7. Nordmark, Madelyn T., and Rohweder, Anne W.: Scientific principles applied to nursing, Philadelphia, 1959, J. B. Lippincott Co., pp. 86-107.
8. Shafer, Kathleen N., Sawyer, Janet R., McCluskey, Audrey M., and Beck, Edna L.: Medical-surgical nursing, ed. 2, St. Louis, 1961, The C. V. Mosby Co., pp. 55-68, 664-674.
9. Snively, William D., and Brown, Barbara J.: In the balance, American Journal of Nursing 58:55-57, Jan. 1958.
10. Statland, Harry: Fluid and electrolytes in practice, ed. 2, Philadelphia, 1957, J. B. Lippincott Co., pp. 1-112.
11. Tuttle, W. W., and Schottelius, Byron A.: Textbook of physiology, ed. 14, St. Louis, 1961, The C. V. Mosby Co., pp. 321-330.

Chapter 21

Nursing care of patients with disturbances of regulatory and sensory mechanisms

Man's ability to maintain homeostasis in the face of a constantly changing environment necessitates the most perfect coordination of bodily function. Such coordination is dependent, in part, on an organized method of communication. Transmitting messages from the external environment or internally from one organ to another is accomplished by two methods: (1) the nervous system provides a mechanism by which rapid communication is established, and this communication is basically electrical in nature and (2) chemical substances, called hormones, are liberated into the blood stream and carried to distant structures on which they exert specific influences. In general, the nervous or electrical system is more rapid and controls finer adjustments, whereas the hormonal or chemical system is slower but its action is maintained longer.

ESSENTIAL MECHANISM

To maintain communication via the nervous system, there must be a means of receiving, coordinating, and transmitting impulses. This means that nerve fibers, the brain, and the spinal cord must be intact. Generally speaking, afferent nerves, which carry impulses to the central nervous system, are sensory in nature; efferent nerves, which carry impulses away from the central nervous system to the periphery, are motor in nature. Some nerves, however, may be both motor and sensory in function. Stimulus to the nervous system may arise from the external or internal environment and may be electrical, thermal, chemical, or mechanical in nature. Response to stimulus may manifest itself by perception and/or movement and/or secretion.

Control over this system of communication may be voluntary or involuntary (reflex) or, in some instances, both. For example, respiration is an involuntary function. Yet it is possible to alter rate and rhythm of respiration by voluntary control. This voluntary control, however, has limitations. When deliberate cessation of respiration sufficiently elevates the level of carbon dioxide in the blood, the central nervous system is stimulated so that respiration begins involuntarily.

The primary adaptive mechanism of the body involves two closely integrated systems: the endocrine (ductless) glands and the autonomic nervous system. Integration of these two systems is under the control of the hypothalamus.

The maintenance of communication via this adaptive mechanism is dependent on the integrity of the hypothalamus, autonomic nerve fibers, and the pituitary gland and other endocrine glands with their battery of hormones. Control over this system is involuntary and self-regulating and uses both electrical and chemical means of communication.

The reception, coordination, and transmission of impulses is essential for the acquisition of knowledge, for reasoning, pleasure, movement, and protection, and for the integration of bodily functions. Without this organized system of communication, life as we know it would be impossible.

WHAT CAN GO WRONG—CENTRAL NERVOUS SYSTEM

As with electricity, any interference with electrical impulses impairs or completely blocks the system of communication. The result is partial or total loss of sensory and/or motor function or, more rarely, exaggerated function. Generally speaking, interference is mechanical in nature and may occur between the point of stimulus and the central nervous system (afferent pathways), within the central nervous system itself, or between the central nervous system and the periphery (efferent pathways). Since there are specific receptors, nerve fibers, and higher brain centers for each type of stimulus, only specific functions may be lost or impaired. For example, awareness of changes in temperature may be lost in a localized area while the ability to respond to pressure changes in the same area may be intact. Interference may result from any one or a combination of the basic types of pathology (Chapter 16). The most common types of interference result from vascular disturbances, traumatic injury, inflammation and infection, tumor growth, and degenerative processes.

Vascular disturbances

Impairment of circulation to any tissue poses a threat to the life of the tissue. This is particularly true of brain tissue (Chapter 16) and may result from atherosclerosis, aneurysm (weakening and outpouching of a vessel wall), embolus, thrombosis, or cerebral vascular accident (hemorrhage).

The latter is the most common cause of impaired function of the nervous system and, as with the others, is often associated with vascular disease elsewhere in the body (heart, kidneys, peripheral vessels). Cerebral hemorrhage results from the rupture of a weakened vessel (aneurysm) or the rupture of a sclerosed vessel in persons with high blood pressure. Rupture of a vessel (stroke) results in extravasation of blood into the tissue on one side of the brain, leading to partial or complete paralysis of the opposite side of the body (hemiplegia). Briefly, there is interference with blood supply immediately beyond the site of the rupture; external pressure is exerted on surrounding tissue, including sensory and motor nerve fibers and nerve centers. This external pressure is due to the extravasation of blood, the development of edema, and increased intracranial pressure. The nonelastic bony framework (skull) in which the brain is encased leaves little or no room for expansion in the presence of this increased pressure. All of this results in a break in the transmission of impulses to and from that particular part of the brain.

The size of the vessel, the extent of hemorrhage, and the size and specific area of the brain involved determine the extent of impaired function. The impairment may vary from only a temporary clouding of consciousness and temporary sensory and motor weakness to severe shock, total loss of consciousness, complete paralysis, loss of vital function (heart and respiratory), and death.

Traumatic injury

Impaired function of the nervous system resulting from traumatic injury may be caused by laceration, compression, or concussion. The most common areas involved as a result of accidents are the head and spinal cord.

Head injury may vary from a simple scalp laceration, with control of hemorrhage and prevention of infection the only problem, to an open fracture with extensive brain damage that imperils life itself. However, there may be serious injury to the brain even although there is no visible evidence of laceration or fracture. As a result of a severe blow to the skull, the soft tissues within the cranial cavity may strike the bony covering with great force and may cause serious injury. This is known as concussion and is suspected where there is even momentary loss of consciousness at the time of an accident.

Fracture of the skull may cause little damage to the brain or may cause very serious damage to vital nerve pathways, such as occurs in a basal skull fracture.

Laceration of the spinal cord may result from fracture of the vertebrae, with tearing of the cord, or from a stab wound, which may partially or completely sever the cord. Injury is most often sustained as a result of compression from surrounding structures. The most common of these are rupture of an intervertebral disc with protrusion into the spinal canal, tumor growth, and fractures with the accompanying edema. Partial or complete severing or partial or total compression of the spinal cord results in partial or total paralysis below the level of the injury. For example, injury at the cervical level may result in paralysis of all four extremities and the trunk (quadriplegia), and injury at the thoracic or lumbar level may result in paralysis of the lower trunk and lower extremities (paraplegia). Injury of nerve fibers outside the brain and spinal cord may also occur as a result of laceration or compression. The result will be interference with motor or sensory function of a localized area such as part or all of one extremity.

Impaired function occurs, not uncommonly, as a result of benign or malignant tumor growth. Damage may be caused by the actual invasion of afferent or efferent nerve fibers, the brain, and/or spinal cord, which may result in actual destruction of nerve tissue itself. Damage may result, however, not from invasion of nerve tissue but from compression of nerve tissue by the growth of a tumor. The presence of a growing tumor within the nonelastic cranial cavity and spinal canal soon results in increased pressure, impaired circulation, edema, and/or necrosis of tissue. Here, again, the location and extent of the area involved determine the particular functions that may be lost or impaired.

Interruption of nerve pathways from degenerative involvement is generally slow in progression and usually of unknown cause. The involvement may be confined to a specific area, as in Parkinson's disease (paralysis agitans), in which there is destruction of the basal ganglia of the brain. The areas of degeneration may, however, be widely distributed, as in multiple sclerosis, in which there are patchy areas of degeneration in the white matter of the brain and outer myelin sheath of the spinal cord. As one might expect, the loss or impairment of specific functions is more limited in scope in the former and more widely varied in the latter.

Infections involving the nervous system are becoming less common as health problems since the advent of antibiotics and vaccines. A variety of organisms and viruses, however, may attack the nervous system by introduction at the site of an injury and by direct spread from surrounding tissue, but more commonly via the blood and lymph systems. Infections may involve only the meninges of the brain and spinal cord (meningitis), primarily the brain and its coverings (encephalitis), or be walled off and result in an abscess. Perhaps most common of the infections is poliomyelitis, in which the involvement is limited to the anterior horn cells of the spinal cord where the motor pathways are located.

In the discussion of the mechanism of inflammation and infection in Chapter 16, it was noted that there is impairment or loss of function of the part. Within the nervous system the impaired function becomes more generalized and may be temporary or permanent or partial or total, depending again on the extent and the particular areas involved.

Generally speaking, interference with transmission of impulses via the nervous system comes about because of impaired circulation to the area (lack of oxygen and nutrition), compression of nerve tissue, edema, depressed fracture, tumor, etc.), or direct injury or destruction (laceration, concussion, bacterial or viral infection, degenerative disease, etc.). These may involve only the nervous system or be associated with pathology elsewhere in the body.

Because the nervous system has either direct or indirect control over both vital and nonvital bodily function, interference with impulses leads to some loss of function. The impairment may be temporary or permanent, partial or total, motor and/or sensory. The degree of impairment may be so minimal as to have little or no effect on homeostasis or so severe as to constitute a threat to life itself.

WHAT CAN GO WRONG—ENDOCRINE SYSTEM

In the maintenance of homeostasis, activities and functions of the body's adaptive mechanisms (autonomic nervous system and endocrine glands with hypothalamus control) are so interrelated that what affects one structure has its reprecussions, in varying degrees, on every other structure in this self-regulating system. Such a complex interrelationship would seem to make this system exceptionally susceptible to breakdown. Yet, except for the thyroid gland, the islands of Langerhans in the pancreas, and, less often, the pituitary and adrenal glands, there is surprisingly little impairment. The interrelationships and self-regulating characteristics provide an extensive system of checks and balances that compensate for many impairments.

Impaired function of the autonomic nervous system and hypothalamus may result from any of the previously discussed types of interference with the transmission of impulses via the nervous system. Impaired function of the endocrine glands may be due to any of the basic types of pathology (Chapter 16) and is manifested by increased secretion of hormones (hyperactivity) or decreased secretion (hypoactivity).

Normal function of the thyroid gland is dependent upon a regulated stimulus from the anterior pituitary gland and, in turn, the hypothalamus and sufficient materials (namely, iodine) to form enough thyroxin to maintain body metabolism. Failure of either results in enlargement of the thyroid gland (goiter) and may be associated with overproduction of thyroxin (hyperthyroidism), deficient production (hypothyroidism), or neither. In the presence of hyperthyroidism (exopthalmic goiter or Graves' disease), all phases of body metabolism are speeded up. Hypothyroidism, in which there is a low metabolic rate, is evidenced in children as cretinism and in adults as myxedema.

Impaired function of the islands of Langerhans in the pancreas is most commonly evidenced by deficient secretion of insulin (diabetes mellitus). The resultant impaired carbohydrate metabolism leads to hyperglycemia. Since glucose is not stored or wholly utilized, it is lost in the urine (glycosuria). In the body's attempt to compensate, it calls on other sources (fats and ketones) with the result that these appear in excess in the blood and may also escape in the urine (ketonuria).

Impaired function of the pituitary gland is evidenced by hyperactivity or hypoactivity. The pituitary gland secretes a wide variety of hormones affecting growth, metabolism, reproduction, etc., either directly or indirectly through its influence on other endocrine glands. Deficiencies may be manifested by stunted growth in children (dwarfism) or pituitary cachexia (Simmonds' disease) in adults, by excessive urine loss (diabetes insipidus), and/or by hypoactivity of any of the other endocrine glands.

Hyperfunction of the pituitary gland may be evidenced by excessive growth (gigantism in children and acromegaly in adults) and by the results of overstimulation of other endocrine glands.

Function of the adrenal glands may be impaired through involvement of the adrenal glands directly or indirectly through the hypothalamus and pituitary. Secretion of hormones by the adrenal medulla is, however, under direct nervous control, is activated by demand for the body to meet an emergency ("flight or fight"), and is believed to reinforce the sympathetic nervous system. While this phase of man's adaptive mechanism is certainly advantageous, it is not essential to life. Excess or deficient secretion is, therefore, not significant as a health problem.

Hormones secreted by the adrenal cortex, known as steroids, exert an influence over a wide variety of bodily functions. Hyperactivity is evidenced primarily by alteration in sex characteristics (Cushing's syndrome) and hypoactivity by impaired carbohydrate metabolism and mineral and water metabolism (Addison's disease).

• • •

In summary, it can be said that interference with communication (chemical or electrical) via the adaptive mechanisms results in excessive or deficient activity of the organs or tissues involved which can and does alter function of other organs and tissues. The impairment may be so minimal as to be barely perceptible or so severe as to pose a threat to life itself.

NURSING INTERVENTION—SENSORY AND MOTOR DISTURBANCES

Nursing intervention in the care of patients with problems of sensory and motor function is focused around the maintenance of optimal function, restoration of function through palliative and restorative measures, and teaching and rehabilitation.

Observation

The observation of the level of consciousness is a significant nursing function. The degree of consciousness and development of changes are indications of the seriousness, progression, or resolution of damage. Altered consciousness may range from mere lethargy, with or without clouding of consciousness, to deep coma. The development of change in relation to the onset of pathology is of major importance. For example, the development of altered consciousness, after regaining consciousness, following a head injury may be indicative of an extradural hemorrhage. The development of altered consciousness several weeks or months later may indicate a subdural hematoma. Critical observations relating to levels of consciousness are discussed in detail in Chapter 16.

The vital signs (temperature, pulse, respiration, and blood pressure) are of critical importance. Since there are central nervous system centers that affect control of these vital functions, any pathological process interfering with the nervous system can seriously alter them. A rising blood pressure and slowing of pulse and respirations may be indicative of the development of increasing intracranial pressure. Change in the character of respiration in the presence of poliomyelitis may indicate sudden progress toward respiratory paralysis. Respiratory difficulty in the comatose patient may be indicative of blocking of the airway. A sudden rise in temperature indicates disturbance of the heat regulatory center in the hypothalamus that may occur as a result of trauma to vital centers. Hypothermia may occur when vital centers are depressed but control is not yet lost. In any case, the vital signs require close observation and prompt reporting of evidence of change since they serve as clues to diagnosis, progression, or resolution of impairment and may require emergency measures to sustain life.

Alterations of motor function are of major significance since some loss of function and control is common in most nervous system disorders. Absence of motor function (paralysis) may involve a major portion of the body (hemiplegia, paraplegia, or quadriplegia) or may be limited to particular groups or individual muscles. The location and type of paralysis are key factors in observation. Terms to describe the types are related to the status of muscle. Flaccid (limp and relaxed) and spastic (rigid and tense) describe the most common types of paralysis. Partial or total paralysis of a major portion of the body is readily recognized. Involvement of more limited areas or even isolated muscles may be less obvious but of equal significance. These may be evidenced by a wide variety of symptoms, such as difficulty in using fingers and hands for fine movements, changes in gait, difficulty in swallowing (dysphagia), inability to speak (motor aphasia), drooping of the eyelid (ptosis), etc.

Change in the character of movement is of equal significance. Tremor (involuntary, rhythmical oscillation) is usually manifested in the presence of degenerative changes as in Parkinson's disease. It may be evidenced only when voluntary movement is attempted (intentioned tremor) or when at rest (nonintentioned tremor). Sudden, involuntary movement or convulsive muscular contraction is referred to as a spasm. When such movement becomes generalized, it is termed a convulsion. The development of convulsive seizures may be indicative of increasing intracranial pressure and may accompany extreme temperature elevations and toxic states but most commonly occurs as a result of epilepsy. Key observations relative to convulsive seizures include type of convulsive movement, extent of involvement, and duration of seizure. Terms to describe the type of convulsion are tonic (all muscles contract at once) and clonic (alternating contraction and relaxation of opposing muscle groups), which results in jerking bodily movement. When a convulsion starts in one area and spreads to other areas or to the whole body, it is identified as a Jacksonian seizure. Involvement may be more pronounced in one area than in another and this fact should be noted. Other significant related changes may occur during a seizure that should be observed. These include rotation of the eyes to one side or the other, dilatation or contraction of the pupils, alteration in pulse and respirations, changes in skin color, diaphoresis, presence of incontinence, and grinding or clenching of teeth. Other related information must be gleaned following the seizure. These include state of consciousness, orientation, headache, etc.

Other alterations in motor function may be apparent not by loss or control of motor activities but by weakness (paresis) of particular muscles, groups of muscles, or a major portion of the body (hemiparesis, quadriparesis, etc.).

Changes in motor function require close observation, prompt reporting, and recording with accurate descriptions. The location, type, and extent of impaired function and the character, onset, and duration of unusual movement are significant since they serve as clues to diagnosis, location of lesion, and progression or resolution of impairment and may require emergency intervention.

Observation of sensory function is of equal importance and may be related to alterations in motor function or be evidenced as an isolated impairment. Changes in sensory function are most often subjective in nature. They may sometimes be apparent through the patient's lack of awareness or response to particular stimuli but require verification from the patient.

Complete absence of sensation is an area of anesthesia. This may be limited to an isolated area, indicating a blocking of a particular nerve, or may be more generalized, as in the presence of paralysis. The fact that there is loss of response to temperature and pressure changes is of particular significance for patient safety. Sensation may be intensified (hyperesthesia), may be painful (paralgesia), or may be abnormal (paresthesia), such as burning or itching. These changes may be indicative of cerebral irritation (as in toxic states), of degenerative changes, or invasion of nerve tissue by tumor growth. Many variations in vision may occur. Slight dimming of vision or double vision (diplopia) may result from papilledema or choked disc (swelling of the optic nerve head) and may be indicative of increasing intracranial pressure. Sensations of smell and taste may be altered. Unpleasant or unusual odors may be indicative of frontal lobe tumor. Sensory aphasia (inability to comprehend the spoken or written word) may occur singly or in combination with motor aphasia. Aphasia is indicative of damage to the speech center. Very astute observation is required since it may be evidenced by an inability to comprehend and/or an inability to speak and may be misinterpreted as loss of hearing.

Changes in sensory function require accurate observation, reporting, and recording since they serve as aids in diagnosis, progression, or resolution of impairment.

The type and location of pain are major points of observation in caring for patients with disorders of the nervous system. Headache is perhaps the most commonly experienced pain in human existence. In the presence of nervous system disorders, it is of major significance. A dull persistent headache may be indicative of increasing intracranial pressure. A sudden explosive headache may indicate the rupture of a cerebral aneurysm. Headache coupled with vertigo may be indicative of impending cerebral vascular accident. Hyperesthesia may occur locally or generally and may be mild in character or so extreme as to make contact with clothing, linen, and even movement of air currents an excruciating experience. When this does occur, it is usually the result of irritation of sensory nerves or, more often, actual invasion by malignancy. A complete and accurate description of pain should be obtained, reported, and recorded. (See Chapter 16.)

Anorexia, nausea, and vomiting are particularly significant observations. Since the vomiting center is in the medulla, it may be stimulated by many disorders of the central nervous system. Sudden and projectile vomiting are usually indicative of increased intracranial pressure or traumatic injury sustained in or near the vomiting center. An accurate description of all characteristics should be reported. (See Chapter 16.)

Observations for signs of shock and hemorrhage (see Chapter 16) are indicated in the care of patients with nervous system disorders. They are particularly significant following neurosurgery, cerebral vascular accident, or traumatic injury. Hemorrhage from the nose and ears is a critical observation following head injury and is suggestive of a basal skull fracture.

Careful observations relative to elimination (see Chapter 19) are also significant. Incontinence is commonly evidenced as an indication of loss of motor and sensory control. Urinary retention and constipation may, however, occur in the presence of spinal cord injury.

Another very important aspect of observation is the emotional status of the patient. The loss of one's ability to function or to predict one's movements constitutes, to some degree, a loss of one's independence and, as such, is a threat to emotional security. See Chapter 7 for the significance, recognition, and nursing implications relative to emotional responses evidenced by patients in the presence of illness.

Dependent nursing functions

Dependent nursing functions are centered around nursing responsibilities relative to diagnostic procedures, medical therapy, diet adaptations, and administration of medications.

Diagnostic procedures

Generally speaking, diagnostic procedures concerned with the functioning of the nervous system include neurological examination, x-ray studies, measurement of electrical waves, and spinal fluid examinations.

Neurological examination is concerned with testing for areas of abnormal response to a variety of stimuli, as well as testing specific nerves and groups of nerves. The nurse usually does not actively participate in this examination but needs to be familiar with a special vocabulary in order that results of the examination have meaning for her. Some of the terms which must be learned include Babinski, Romberg, Kernig, and Brudzinski. These tests have no meaning unless response is positive. Babinski refers to toe extension; Romberg, to loss of equilibrium; Brudzinski, to involuntary flexion of the lower extremities; and Kernig, to painful extension of the lower leg. The patellar reflex (knee jerk) and Achilles tendon reflex (foot flexion) are significant only when response is negative.

X-ray studies of the spinal cord and brain include pneumoencephalography (the injection of air into the spinal canal to replace spinal fluid that is withdrawn), ventriculography (the injection of air directly into the ventricles through trephine openings [burr holes]), arteriography, (the injection of radiopaque substance into the carotid artery), and myelography (the injection of a radiopaque substance into the subarachnoid space usually in the lumbar area). Depending on the area of injection, air or radiopaque substance permits visualization of the contour of the ventricles, blood vessels, or the spinal canal.

An electroencephalogram is an electrical recording of brain activity and is similar in method to an electrocardiogram.

Nursing responsibilities concerned with these diagnostic procedures include preparation of the patient by means of explanation and supportive care and specific physical care both before and after the procedures.

Lumbar puncture* (spinal puncture or tap) is entry into the spinal canal for the purpose of measuring pressure and removal of spinal fluid for examination. Nursing responsibility usually involves active participation with this diagnostic procedure. In addition to preparation of the patient through explanation and supportive care, the nurse is concerned with safety factors and participation during the procedure. She is responsible for securing the equipment, assisting the physician, and assisting the patient. Major safety measures include the maintenance of aseptic technique, the proper position for the patient (acute flexion of the head and knees) to avoid sudden movement and to permit easier insertion of the needle by the physician, and acute observation of the patient's reaction both during and after the procedure. During the procedure, the nurse may hold the manometer for recording spinal fluid pressure and may compress the jugular veins (singly and together) for additional pressure readings (Queckenstedt test). The nurse is responsible for accurate labeling and disposition of specimens obtained. A similar procedure is the cisternal puncture, in which the needle is inserted directly into the cisterna magna.

The nurse should be aware that with the exception of the neurological examination and electroencephalogram, it is not uncommon for the patient to experience headache following any of these diagnostic procedures.

Assisting with medical therapy

In addition to the specific diagnostic tests, medical treatments commonly used for patients with problems in motor or sensory function are administration of oxygen, tracheostomy, radiation, immobilization through the use of traction or application of a cast, and surgery. Specific nursing responsibilities relative to these therapies have been discussed previously. (See Chapters 12 and 17.)

---

*See Appendix for paracentesis (surgical puncture of a body cavity).

In general, specific nursing responsibilities relative to medical therapy include care of the patient, care of the equipment, and assisting the physician.

Diet adaptations

Specific dietary adaptations relative to patients with motor and sensory dysfunction are concerned primarily with consistency and method of feeding since mechanical problems are common. Patients often have major difficulty chewing and swallowing. For specific measures and related nursing responsibilities, see Chapter 18.

Administration of medications

Specific nursing responsibilities relative to the administration of medications are given in Chapter 15. The most common types of drugs used for altered function of the nervous system include anticonvulsants, muscle relaxants, anticoagulants, analgesics, antibiotics, and tranquilizers.

Independent nursing functions

In providing nursing care for patients with problems of motor and sensory function, the nurse directs her efforts primarily toward safety through the prevention of deformity, the prevention accidents, and attention to pressure areas, emotional support for the patient and family, and rehabilitation.

Nursing measures in regard to safety are based upon the following guidelines:

1. If there is interference with the patient's level of consciousness, safety devices such as side rails should be used.
2. Positioning of the patient in proper body alignment to prevent deformities may be achieved by the use of footboards, pillows, sandbags, and other supportive devices.
3. The prevention of skin breakdown (pressure areas) and pulmonary complications is accomplished by the use of sponge rubber mattresses, alternating pressure mattresses, and frequent changes in position.
4. Moving and turning patients at frequent and regularly scheduled intervals and the use of turning sheets are necessary to prevent skin irritation. These procedures require several persons.
5. Incontinence necessitates meticulous skin care to prevent skin breakdown. Incontinence should be reported, since a Foley catheter may be inserted as additional protection against skin breakdown.
6. Lifting patients requires several persons, lifting sheets, or especially designed hydraulic lifts when available.
7. Passive exercise and active exercise, when feasible, should be instituted.
8. If there is cerebral irritation, environmental stimuli such as noise and light should be reduced.
9. In convulsive seizures the patient must be protected from injury by

lowering him gently to the floor (if he is in a precarious position), moving equipment out of reach, and inserting a mouth gag (rubber wedge or padded tongue blade) between the back teeth to prevent biting of the tongue.

10. In the presence of edema, dehydration, or other impaired fluid balance, an accurate record of intake and output is indicated.

11. Since discomfort serves to intensify existing problems, general hygiene and comfort measures are imperative. Some aspects (oral hygiene and hair and nail care) may need to be done entirely by the nurse since many patients are unable to manage by themselves.

12. Prompt reporting of varied signs of change in the patient's condition is imperative.

13. In the presence of aphasia, a simple method of communication with the patient must be established.

14. Maintenance of all functions at optimal level will contribute to eventual rehabilitation.

15. Because disorders of motor or sensory function have deep psychological import for the concept of self, emotional support is a critical aspect in the provision of nursing care to patients and their families.

NURSING INTERVENTION—ENDOCRINE DISTURBANCES

Nursing intervention in the care of patients with problems of adaptive function is focused around maintenance of optimal function, restoration of function through palliative and restorative measures, and teaching rehabilitation measures.

Observation

Observation of vital signs (temperature, pulse, respiration, and blood pressure) is of major importance. A rising blood pressure and slowing pulse and respirations may be indicative of increasing intracranial pressure in the presence of a tumor of the pituitary gland or hypothalamus. Change in the character of respirations may indicate pressure on the trachea as a result of enlargement of the thyroid gland. A rise in blood pressure to dangerous heights may indicate the development of an adrenal tumor. Specific changes in vital signs, coupled with changes in color, serve as critical differentiating measures between diabetic coma and insulin shock (see Appendix).

Changes in growth and physical appearance are of major significance. Enlargement in the neck region is suggestive of thyroid pathology. Thinning hair, dry skin, changes in skin pigmentation, and generalized atrophy usually are indications of endocrine deficiency. Enlarged, coarse features, widening of the hands and feet, changes in secondary sex characteristics (growth of hair, deepening of voice) and "moon" face may indicate overactivity of one or more of the endocrine glands. These same signs of overactivity may evidence themselves in the presence of prolonged steroid therapy.

Observations relative to activity are significant. Restlessness, nervousness, tremor, and loss of emotional control may be evidence of increased metabolic rate, whereas lassitude, drowsiness, and slowing of speech may be indicative of decreased metabolic rate.

Since the endocrine glands exert a definite control over water balance, observations of excessive or decreased output are of major importance.

Generally speaking, changes in vital signs, in growth and appearance, in activity, and in emotional control require accurate observation, reporting, and recording since they serve as clues to diagnosis, progression, or resolution of impairment and may require emergency measures to sustain life.

Dependent nursing functions

Dependent nursing functions are centered around nursing responsibilities relative to diagnostic tests, medical therapy, diet adaptations, and administration of medications.

Diagnostic procedures

Generally speaking, diagnostic procedures concerned with endocrine function involve determinations of over-all metabolism and the metabolism of specific substances through chemical analysis of blood and urine.

Tests to determine the state of metabolic activity are basal metabolic rate (BMR), protein-bound iodine test (PBI), and radioactive iodine uptake test (RAD). The basal metabolic rate is determined by the amount of oxygen utilized when at rest. The protein-bound iodine test measures the amount of iodine that can be precipitated by plasma proteins. The radioactive iodine uptake determines the ability of the thyroid gland to accumulate iodine following ingestion of a tracer dose of radioactive iodine.

Nursing responsibilities concerned with these diagnostic tests include preparation of the patient through explanation and supportive care and specific physical preparation, when indicated, both before and after the procedures.

Specific blood chemistries to determine the degree of metabolism of particular substances include blood sugar, glucose tolerance, carbon dioxide combining power, and blood electrolytes.

Urinalyses are done to determine excessive loss or retention of specific substances related to metabolism. These tests include determination of sugar, acetone, and electrolytes.

Nursing responsibilities for these diagnostic tests include preparation of the patient by means of explanation and supportive measures and by specific physical care when indicated both before and after the procedures. The collection, accurate labeling, and disposition of specimens are also a major nursing responsibility.

Assisting with medical therapy

In addition to diagnostic procedures, medical therapy primarily involves prescribing hormones to supply deficiencies, agents to control excesses, and, where indicated, partial or total surgical removal of malfunctioning organs. Specific nursing responsibilities related to therapy are discussed later in this chapter.

Diet adaptations

Specific diet adaptations relative to patients with impaired metabolism are concerned primarily with supplementing deficiencies, eliminating or decreasing in amount those substances that cannot be utilized or are currently in excess. For specific nursing measures and related nursing responsibilities, see Chapter 18.

Administration of medications

The most common types of drugs used for altered function of the endocrine system include hormones, steroids, antibiotics, tranquilizers, vasodilators (antihypertensive agents), and analgesics.

Independent nursing functions

In providing nursing care for patients with problems of adaptive or endocrine function, the nurse directs her efforts primarily toward patient and family education and emotional support for both.

Nursing measures related to these areas are based on the following guidelines:

1. The pattern of rest and activity must be adapted to patients' limitations. Since rest and activity are influenced by and have an influence on metabolism, an increase or decrease in metabolic rate has definite implications for rest and activity.
2. Education of the patient to his limitations and to the kind of adaptation with which he must live is of major importance. Knowledge and understanding of and the ability to follow the special diet in the presence of diabetes mellitus is of critical importance, for example.
3. Education of the patient to specific symptoms (diabetic acidosis, insulin shock) which require immediate attention is essential.
4. Since many patients are maintained on chemotherapy for prolonged periods and, in some instances, for life, knowledge of the drug and its method of administration are critical. Insulin, for example, is essential to the life of a patient with diabetes mellitus. As a result, the patient must be able to administer his own insulin and be able to test his urine for sugar and acetone since this affects the amount of insulin required.
5. Education of the patient to specific measures necessary for prevention of complications is of major significance. Meticulous hygiene measures (skin, feet, hands) are critical in the presence of diabetes mellitus to prevent infection and skin breakdown.
6. Since adaptations to living are necessary in varying degrees with endocrine dysfunction, emotional support of the patient and family is a critical aspect in the provision of care.
7. Emotional support of the patient and family is of equal importance

because of changes in appearance which also have deep psychological import.

BIBLIOGRAPHY

1. Apperly, Frank: Patterns of disease, Philadelphia, 1951, J. B. Lippincott Co., pp. 367-421.
2. Best, Charles H., and Taylor, Norman B.: The physiological basis of medical practice, Baltimore, 1961, Williams & Wilkins Co., pp. 950-956, 1115-1136.
3. de Gutierrez-Mahoney, C. G., and Carini, Esta: Neurological and neurosurgical nursing, ed. 3, St. Louis, 1960, The C. V. Mosby Co.
4. Frohman, I. P.: The steroids, American Journal of Nursing **59**:518-521, April 1959.
5. Garb, Solomon, and Crim, Betty J.: Pharmacology and patient care, New York, 1962, Springer Publishing Co., Inc., pp. 83-108, 123-142.
6. Gleason, A. M.: Cerebral edema—care of the patient, American Journal of Nursing **61**: 92-94, March 1961.
7. Greenblatt, R. B., and Metts, J. C.: Addison's disease, American Journal of Nursing **60**: 1249-1252, Sept. 1960.
8. Lubic, R. W.: Nursing care after adrenalectomy or hypophysectomy, American Journal of Nursing **62**:84-86, April 1962.
9. MacKenzie, M., and Baldwin, M.: Cerebral seizures, American Journal of Nursing **57**: 312-316, March 1957.
10. Reich, B. H., and Ault, L. P.: Nursing care of the patient with Addison's disease, American Journal of Nursing **60**:1252-1255, Sept. 1960.
11. Shafer, K. N., Sawyer, J. R., McCluskey A. M., and Beck, E. F.: Medical-surgical nursing, ed. 2, St. Louis, 1961, The C. V. Mosby Co., pp. 614-642, 727-801.

Rehabilitation problems

Chapter 22

Implications of long-term illness for patients and nursing personnel

Up to this point, the student of fundamentals of nursing has been most concerned with learning about the immediate nursing care problems of the patients for whom she will be caring. This chapter will provide an overview of the long-range nursing problems of patients who have long-term, chronic, disabling illnesses. Long-term illness affects not only the individual person who is sick, but also his family and his community, since it represents prolonged dysfunction of a total individual.

With the increased knowledge provided by advances in the social, biological, and medical sciences, care of people who are disabled and/or chronically ill has changed radically from passive custodial supervision to a dynamic process which seeks to help each person achieve the most he is capable of being—physically, socially, and emotionally. Thus, the major objective of the nurse who is working with a patient who has a long-term (and often life-long) illness is to help the patient move from complete dependence to as much independence as he can realistically assume within the limitations and life modifications which his illness imposes upon his body. For example, the patient who is admitted to the hospital in diabetic coma is completely dependent. He has a disease which, at this time, can never be cured. Nevertheless, if he can learn to live within the prescribed limitations of diet, medication, and hygiene, he can become an independent, productive member of our society.

For the patient, this is a growing, developmental process, similar to that which we all experience in the progression from infancy to adulthood. It will involve new learnings about his body and its needs, new emotional reactions to himself and others, and the development of new physical skills. The nurse's role is to nurture this growth, much as a good mother fosters the development of her children. Patients with acute, brief illnesses probably experience this same phenomenon (i.e., the shift from dependence to independence) but over a shorter time span. In addition, the patient who becomes ill, receives treatment, and is cured undoubtedly has internal and external resources which are not available to the person with a long-term illness.

Long-term disabling illness is probably the major health problem in the United States today. Looked at from a very pragmatic viewpoint, it is also a major economic problem for our country in terms of expenditure for institutional care, drugs, appliances, and personnel.

In the early part of this century, the number one cause of death in the United States was infectious disease. Today, cardiovascular diseases head the list, not only as the primary cause of death in the United States but also as one of the major morbidity problems. In addition, cancer of all forms is now an important morbidity and mortality problem for all age groups. For most of the age groups under 65, accidents rank high among the morbidity-mortality statistics, with victims often incurring life-long disabilities as a result.

Population changes within the United States also serve to accentuate the problems of chronic illness. In the 1960 census, 16.6 million of our 180 million population were 65 or more years of age. This represents 9½% of the total population. In 1940, only 6½% of the population of the United States were 65 or older. It is estimated that by 1970, over 10% percent of the people living in the United States will be over 65.

As a group, persons over 65 years of age are often more susceptible to the development of degenerative, disabling, long-term illnesses. It is a mistake, however, to equate aging and chronic illness. At least 25% of patients with long-term illness are under 25 years of age. A 1955 survey of chronically ill patients revealed that only 21% were over 65; however, a greater percentage (41%) of the severely disabled were in this age group. As the number and proportion of people over 65 years of age increases in our total population, it is to be expected that a greater percentage of patients with chronic illness will be elderly. Unfortunately, the elderly person is likely to have more than one long-term illness which increases the complexity of his nursing problems and care.

As the people in our nation move from farms to cities in an urban population shift, they move into smaller dwelling places, and the structure and organization of families change. This poses very real difficulties when a grandparent or an aged aunt develops a long-term illness. The spatial limitations of a compact city apartment or suburban house may make it impossible for a nuclear family (i.e., mother, father, and growing children) to take in a sick, aged relative. Or, if they do, the patterns of their daily lives may undergo radical changes which can place many emotional stresses upon individual members of the family. It is difficult to imagine the home of growing children in which doors are never slammed, radios or hi-fi's never blare, and voices are never raised!

An additional problem for patients with long-term illness is the ever-increasing cost of medical care in the United States. The Consumer Price Index estimated the total cost of medical care in 1940 at 72.7; in 1960 it had risen to 158. Price index for hospital room rates had risen from 50.4 in 1940 to 228.7 in 1960.

There are very few people in the United States who can afford a long illness! If the person who becomes ill is the family wage earner, this financial burden is compounded by the loss of his salary. For the elderly person who may be living on a small pension and social security allotments, the economic strain of a protracted illness which may require hospitalization, drugs, appliances, etc. is often intolerable. In September 1961, over 16 million people in the United States were receiving monthly benefits from Federal Old Age, Survivors and Disability Insurance. Fifty-four percent were collecting old age insurance, with an average monthly benefit of $75.71. The financial problems of elderly persons are further magnified when one considers the fact that health insurance rates often increase markedly at the age of 65 and that eligibility for and benefits from health insurance usually decrease sharply.

What is a long-term illness? Why use the words "long-term" in place of "chronic" or "handicapped"? A long-term illness is any disruption of a person's life which necessitates modifications of that life—physically, psychosocially, or economically. The words "chronic," "handicapped," "crippled" have unfortunate connotations in our society and often impart feelings of hopelessness and despair. They are words which offer pity and sympathy but little constructive help or hope. On the other hand, a person with a long-term illness can often learn to use all of his remaining abilities and to become increasingly responsible for himself, and often for his family.

From a medical standpoint, the person with a chronic illness is easily identified. In 1949 the American Medical Association, the American Public Health Association, the American Public Welfare Association, and the American Hospital Association established the Joint Commission on Chronic Illness. The Commission has broadly defined chronic illness as "any illness of three or more months' duration" and established the following list of diagnoses classified as chronic diseases:

1. Cancer, all sites
2. Nonmalignant tumors and tumors, nature unspecified
3. Acute rheumatic fever
4. Chronic rheumatism, arthritis, and gout
5. Diabetes mellitus
6. Disease of the thyroid gland, including all types of goiter and parathyroid disease
7. Anemia, all forms
8. Other general diseases
9. Cerebral hemorrhage (apoplexy), embolism, and thrombosis
10. Paralysis
11. Chorea
12. Neuralgia and neuritis
13. Diseases of the eye and blindness
14. Diseases of the ear and deafness

15. Diseases of the heart and coronary arteries
16. Arteriosclerosis and high blood pressure
17. Tuberculosis (all forms)
18. Hemorrhoids
19. Varicose veins or ulcer, and varicocele
20. Sinusitis
21. Asthma
22. Hay fever
23. Ulcer of the stomach or duodenum
24. Hernia
25. Diseases of the gallbladder and liver
26. Nephritis and other diseases of the kidney, including kidney, unspecified
27. Diseases of the bladder, urethra, and urinary passages
28. Nonvenereal disease of the male genital organs
29. Cysts of the ovaries, uterus, and tubes
30. Eczema
31. Diseases of the bones and joints, except tuberculosis
32. Lumbago, myalgia, myositis, stiff neck, and other muscular pains
33. Other disease of the organs of locomotion
34. Congenital malformations and other diseases of early infancy
35. Other and ill-defined causes, including senility
36. Psoriasis

Even a casual inspection of this long and imposing list will convince one of the vastness of the problem of chronic disease in the United States and of the large number of people who might conceivably be classified as "chronically ill." The important factors to be considered, before a person can be considered to have a long-term illness from a nursing standpoint, are the amount of change the illness will make in the person's life *and* the ability of the person to withstand and adjust to that change.

Long-term illness inevitably introduces physical changes. Some of these changes are the result of the disease itself. Although almost all of the diseases listed by the Joint Commission have a primary focus in one organ or set of tissues within the body, they also induce malfunction, disproportion, or dysequilibrium within other organs and tissues. Some of this malfunction is undoubtedly pathological, some may be the result of what Hans Selye has termed the "general adaptation syndrome," and some of these reactions may be actual compensatory efforts made by the body to replace the work of its diseased member or to allow it to rest.

More specifically, under conditions of prolonged inactivity, as bed rest, the actual basal metabolic requirements of the body for oxygen and nutrition are reduced. It has been observed that people who are hospitalized for long periods of time frequently develop severe respiratory, gastrointestinal, urinary, and skin infections. Some of these may be due to the increased exposure to bacteria, but more probably these patients no longer have the physiological ability to resist pathogenic invasions.

Other organs and systems are generally and specifically affected by the physical and social inactivity which are natural sequelae of long-term illness. The efficiency of venous circulation is dependent, in part, upon muscular activity. Respiratory volume and alveolar expansion increase with physical exercise. Bowel elimination is facilitated by regular physical activity and also by the action of gravity when the individual is in a standing or sitting position. A person's appetite is undeniably influenced by the smell of good food, cheerful surroundings, congenial friends, and attractive service. In addition, the peristaltic activity, which is a part of the mechanical process of digestion, is increased with regular exercise. When a person is confined to bed, or to a room, or even the narrow geographic limits of hospital or home, many of the simple factors which promote optimum physiological functioning may be inaccessible to him, leading to wasting and atrophy of skin, muscles, and other organs and tissues. The more severely disabled persons with greater mobility limitations often present increasingly complex overt nursing problems of physiological dysfunction which may be traced to or profoundly influenced by their inactivity.

What effect does long-term illness have upon the psychosocial functioning of the individual? To some extent, the answers to this question depend upon the ethnic, cultural, and socioeconomic groups from which the person comes. Of equal importance in the attempt to determine how psychosocial function is affected in any given person is an understanding of the patient's role and position within the family members who may be available to help and to support him. What cannot be denied is that just as there are inevitable physiological changes during the course of a long-term illness, so are there inevitable psychological changes. However, at this time, there is no documented evidence to prove any relationship between the kind of disability a patient may have and the kind of behavior he may exhibit in his attempts to adjust to his disability.

More specifically, there are some psychosocial responses which are commonly observed. The very physical conditions of his illness usually force any patient (whether he has a short- or a long-term illness) into a dependency relationship with those who are caring for him. Institutional policies and procedures often reinforce this kind of regression which may be most therapeutic during the *acute* phase of any illness. With fuller realization and understanding of his prognosis, the patient who cannot be cured or who faces months or years of treatment may understandably experience feelings of disbelief (denial) or hopelessness and helplessness which can perpetuate this regressive stage. If his cultural and social group put value on the "sick role" or if his past experiences lead him to enjoy this dependence, he may never be able to consider, let alone actively participate in, any form of rehabilitation.

Another mental mechanism which effectively inhibits the rehabilitative process is that of denial. Obviously, if there is nothing wrong with a person, there is no need to try to rehabilitate him!

Not all of the mental mechanisms are obstructive. Most successful rehabilitation occurs when people with long-term illnesses learn to use such mechanisms as compensation, substitution, and sublimation. What must be emphasized here is that people do not usually choose on a conscious voluntary basis the mental mechanisms they will use when confronted with a given stress or crisis.

Long-term illness in one of its members must also cause changes in the family structure, relationships, and roles. Consider what might happen to the family of a young construction worker with two preschool children who falls from a scaffolding and becomes a paraplegic. His self-image will change radically as he watches the physical changes of his own body. He can no longer support his family. If his wife goes to work, who will take care of the children? This is only a tiny glimpse of the impact a long-term illness can have upon a family and upon its individual members.

An additional factor which needs to be considered when one is thinking about the ways in which long-term illness affects the psychosocial functioning of a person is the limitations placed upon social interaction with friends and peers. If the patient is institutionalized, his "peer group" may consist only of those patients who happen to occupy beds in the same room or on the same hospital ward. If he is confined to his home, then this group may consist of the few people who can and will spare the time and make the effort to come and see him. Thus, if the person with a long-term illness becomes increasingly self-centered, it is easy to understand, since he often has no one else to divert him and to occupy his thoughts and time.

BIBLIOGRAPHY

1. Bier, Ruth Irwin: Rehabilitation on a shoe string, American Journal of Nursing **61**:98-100, Aug. 1961.
2. Brown, Esther Lucille: Newer dimensions of patient care. Part I. The use of the physical and social environment of the general hospital for therapeutic purposes, New York, 1961, Russell Sage Foundation.
3. Cantril, Hadley: A study of aspirations, Scientific American **208**:41-45, Feb. 1963.
4. Dericks, Virginia C.: Rehabilitation of patients with ileostomy, American Journal of Nursing **61**:48-51, May 1961.
5. Drake, Melba F.: Rehabilitation: an added dimension in nursing care, American Journal of Nursing **61**:1105-1106, Aug. 1960.
6. Eysenck, H. J.: The Measurement of Motivation, Scientific American **208**:130-140, May 1963.
7. Gilmore, Stuart I.: Rehabilitation after laryngectomy, American Journal of Nursing **61**:87-89, Jan. 1961.
8. Greene, Georgina, and Robbins, Lavina: A rehabilitation nursing record, American Journal of Nursing **61**:82-88, March 1961.
9. Henley, Barbara M.: Helping the elderly find community services, American Journal of Nursing **63**:89-92, April 1963.
10. Kaufman, Margaret A., and Brown, Dorothy E.: Pain wears many faces, American Journal of Nursing **61**:48-51, Jan. 1961.
11. Larsen, Virginia L.: What hospitalization means to patients, American Journal of Nursing **61**:44-47, May 1961.
12. Madden, Barbara Williams, and Affeldt, John E.: To prevent helplessness and deformities, American Journal of Nursing **62**:59-61, Dec. 1962.

13. McCabe, Gracia S.: Cultural influences on patient behavior, American Journal of Nursing **60:**1101-1104, Aug. 1960.
14. Morrissey, Alice B.: Rehabilitation nursing, New York, 1951, G. P. Putnam's Sons, Inc., pp. 67-207.
15. Moser, Doris: An understanding approach to the aphasic patient, American Journal of Nursing **61:**52-55, April 1961.
16. Nursing Outlook: Nursing in rehabilitation services **10:**564-626, Sept. 1962 (entire issue).
17. Paulser, Dorothy: Patients give tests, too, American Journal of Nursing **62:**58-59, Aug. 1962.
18. Peszczynski, Mieczyslaw: The rehabilitation potential of the late adult hemiplegic, American Journal of Nursing **63:**111-114, April 1962.
19. Rusk, Howard A., et al.: Rehabilitation medicine, St. Louis, 1958, The C. V. Mosby Co., pp. 25-82, 136-164.
20. Schwartz, Doris: Medication errors made by aged patients, American Journal of Nursing **62:**51-53, Aug. 1963.
21. Schwartz, Doris: Nursing needs of chronically ill ambulatory patients, Nursing Research **9:**185-189, Fall 1960.
22. Shapiro, Edith: The social worker—a member of the team, Nursing Outlook **9:**98-99, Feb. 1961.
23. Simon, J. Richard, and Chastain, Sally S.: Take a systematic look at your patients, Nursing Outlook **8:**509-512, Sept. 1960.
24. Terry, Florence Jones, et al.: Principles and technics of rehabilitation nursing, St. Louis, 1957, The C. V. Mosby Co., pp. 44-55, 88-116.
25. Wolff, Ilse S.: Referral—a process and a skill, Nursing Outlook **10:**253-256, April 1962.

Chapter 23

Nursing care of patients with long-term illness

The process of rehabilitation nursing begins whenever any patient is admitted to the hospital for any reason. Even though we are particularly concerned, in this unit, with the patient who has long-term nursing problems, the immediate and acute problems of any patient must always receive priority in direct nursing care.

Actually it is in the attention the nurse gives to the patient's immediate nursing problems that she begins to establish the climate and the relationship for later rehabilitative efforts. In addition, all of the prophylactic measures undertaken during the acute phase of illness to prevent cross infection by hypostatic pneumonia and to avoid the development of decubitus ulcers, contractures, deformities, and thrombi are essentially rehabilitative in nature. They ensure the maintenance of as much potential ability as is possible. This is as important to the patient with a short-term illness as it is to the patient with a long-term illness. For the registered nurse, rehabilitation is a philosophy of patient care rather than any given series of techniques and procedures. Rehabilitation presupposes a desire to help restore the patient to the highest possible level of physical, mental, emotional, social, and economic adjustment and function after he has sustained an injury or acute illness. Most often it is a teaching process for the nurse and a learning process for the patient.

How do people learn? Or, a more pertinent question might be, why do people learn? The simplest answer is because they want to! Many of us have sat through a lecture in which a learned teacher spoke for two hours and were unable to remember a single thing he said half an hour after the class was over. We were not motivated intrinsically (i.e., we felt no inner need to know) or extrinsically (we felt that there would be no reward or punishment for not paying attention) to listen and to learn. This is the key to all successful teaching. A nurse can spend 100 hours teaching a patient to irrigate his colostomy, but if the patient does not feel that it is important for him to know how to do this procedure, he will not learn it.

Learning is an activity, sometimes passive (as when you read) and sometimes active (as when you practiced making an occupied bed). It occurs as a response to an identified need, a gap which must be filled before a desired goal can be reached. The goal must be understandable to the learner, and it must be important to him, or he will never expend the necessary physical and mental energy required in the process of attaining it, which is learning.

Now, how do people learn? Many physical skills are learned through imitation, repetition, and trial and error. Thus, a patient begins to learn to irrigate his colostomy the very first time the nurse irrigates it for him, as he observes what is being done, what equipment is being used, and how. Each time the nurse does the irrigation, the patient learns a little bit more. This underscores the importance of consistency in performing such procedures. The patient will usually learn more quickly if the irrigation is done in a place where there are no distractions and at a time when he is not hungry or tired or worried so that he can devote full attention to this business of learning.

People also learn by association; i.e., they associate, or connect, a new fact with an old familiar one. Thus many people know that diabetic patients cannot eat sugar. Slowly, the patient with diabetes can learn that sugar is a carbohydrate food, that other carbohydrate foods are bread, potatoes, etc., that he cannot eat too much of these foods because insulin is necessary to metabolize them and his own body no longer produces insulin, etc., etc.

What methods can a nurse use to help patients learn? Perhaps the best is personal example. How can you expect a patient to be interested in learning to give himself his own insulin injection if the nurse herself is all thumbs? A second method which should be familiar to all students of nursing is to allow the patient plenty of time for practice and to have patience. Assembling a syringe and drawing up insulin and injecting it requires a series of intricate fine motor skills which are not developed in one attempt. In conjunction with this, it is wise to utilize some of the forms of extrinsic motivation: point out how much progress he has made, praise him for his efforts, even when they fail. It often takes more courage for a patient to attempt to learn than we are aware of.

Additional methods which are often helpful are the use of such visual aids as pamphlets, wall charts, and models. Patients usually need an opportunity to ask questions and to discuss the material they have seen or read. Time must be planned for this if the optimum value of such material is to be realized. This also provides an opportunity for the nurse to evaluate how much the patient has learned and to correct any erroneous information he may have obtained.

Although the learner is identified as a patient in all of our previous discussion, the learner can also be, and often is, a member of the patient's family. This is usually the case when the patient is a young child or a person who is severely handicapped either mentally or physically.

Probably much of what a patient learns is "picked up" in an incidental fashion, just as much of what anyone learns comes to us through our ordinary daily experiences in living. However, the knowledge and skills that we retain and that become a part of us are usually those which we consciously sought to attain. This points out the need for the nurse to plan what will be taught and how and to strive to create an environment in which the patient realizes that he is learning.

As we emphasized before, people learn what they want to learn; they are rehabilitated to the degree which seems most desirable to them and also to the degree which they are capable of attaining. The patient with paraplegia may want to walk again. Many paraplegics can ambulate with the aid of crutches and braces, but not independent of these appliances.

How are realistic optimal goals for patients with long-term illnesses determined? Since rehabilitation focuses on a person, not a disease, or a social condition, or an economic problem, many different disciplines contribute to the evaluation process. The nurse contributes an interpretation of the nursing problems the patient presents and frequently acts as a coordinator and referring agent for the different members of the rehabilitation team. Thus the doctor, physical therapist, nurse, and dietitian are all concerned with the physical abilities and disabilities of the patient. The psychiatrist, psychologist, social worker, recreational therapist, occupational therapist, vocational counselor, clergyman, and nurse are concerned with his mental, psychosocial, and economic abilities. The people who are most concerned with his abilities and disabilities are the patient and his family, who can frequently become important, effective working members of the rehabilitation team if given the opportunity. Once it is agreed that the goals set must be understood by and desirable to the patient and his family, the value of the patient and his family as team members is easily seen.

The process of evaluating the long-range nursing problems of the patient and of determining optimal goals consists of assessing the patient's assets and liabilities in terms of his physical, emotional, and intellectual capacities. This involves not only the identification of the overt and covert problems which the patient currently presents, but also the prediction of problems which might occur. Most nurses do some of this automatically when they do such things as using a footboard or bed cradle for patients who will be confined to bed for a long period. They are aware that patients who are in bed for prolonged periods often develop footdrop, so they take measures to prevent it.

If you agree that the major emphasis in rehabilitative effort is on learning, then it is important to assess the intellectual capacity of the patient, since most (although not all) learning is an intellectual activity. When we say that the patient with a long-term illness must understand the optimal goals which he is striving for, some mental activity is implied, since understanding is essentially an intellectual function.

Some of the clues which help in assessing a patient's intellectual capacity include the following:

1. How much formal education has he had?

2. Does he read?
   (a) How much does he read (time)?
   (b) What kinds of printed material does he read?
3. What kinds of radio and television programs does he express an interest in and does he watch?
4. Listen to his conversation. What topics does he choose to discuss? What words does he use when he is talking?
5. What kind of a job did he have before he became ill?
6. What kinds of community activities did he participate in?

The composite picture provided by the answers to these questions will present a fairly accurate evaluation of the patient's intellectual abilities. It supplies the nurse with enough information to teach the patient on a level which he can comprehend. The hypertensive patient who is a lawyer or a Ph.D. will often learn more about his low-fat, low-salt diet when he understands the reasons for it, whereas detailed explanations of respiratory physiology might actually inhibit the learning of respiratory exercises by the patient with emphysema who has never gone past the third grade.

The desire to learn is of equal importance. Even the most intelligent person cannot learn to use a prosthesis if he is afraid to try or if he is not given emotional support during his attempts.

Helpful clues which give some indication of a patient's emotional functioning are found in the answers to the following questions:

1. How does he express anger, frustration, happiness? Can he express these feelings?
   (a) Does he ever cry?
   (b) Does he ever complain? To whom?
   (c) Does he try to be "helpful," or is he really helpful on the ward?
2. Does he talk about his illness, limitations, or handicap?
3. Is he always "sweet," "cooperative," and compliant?
4. Who visits him? When? For how long? What do they talk about or do?
   (a) Who does he seek out on the ward? Or must he be sought out?
   (b) Does he ever "disappear"?
5. How does he indicate his dependence and/or independence? What does he want done for him? What does he want most for himself?

Many of these questions can also be applied to the family members. This will give a valuable indication of their emotional strengths and ability to help support the patient.

A word of caution needs to be included whenever discussing the evaluation of another person's emotional status. There are no precise instruments to be used in this measurement; most of our information is drawn from our own inferences, which are strongly influenced by our own values, beliefs, and cultural background. The nurse with an Anglo-Saxon background may erroneously infer that a weeping patient from another background is "weak." Thus it is essential that the nurse be aware of her own value system and learn as much possible about the behavioral expectations and values of other kinds of people.

With this precaution in mind, it is important to evaluate, at least tentatively, the emotional abilities and disabilities of the patient with a long-term illness. It is normal for such people to feel anger, frustration, disappointment, helplessness, fear, and depression. It is normal for them to want recognition, approval, attention, and acceptance. Knowing this, and recognizing it, the nurse can frequently provide socially acceptable ways of meeting these needs and allowing for tension release without retaliating in kind. Much has been written about the therapeutic environment or milieu, particularly as it applies to the treatment of the mentally ill in a psychiatric setting. Most of these same principles apply equally to the patient with a physical illness. Most of our institutions are established to meet the physical needs of patients; with imagination and care, the thoughtful nurse can also help to meet many of the psychosocial needs of people with long-term illness as well.

The third phase of determining the optimal goals of the patient is to assess his physical abilities and disabilities. The physician determines the amount and extent of damage done and the degree to which this can be medically repaired, corrected, or compensated. The nurse determines the number and amount of overt nursing problems and plans for their solution. Many of these fall into the area of the Activities of Daily Living (ADL) and are concerned with the simple maintenance chores of feeding, bathing, toilet activities, and other areas of self-care. They also usually include assessment of the patient's mobility—is he able to get out of bed, walk, or get into a wheelchair, climb stairs, etc? Many extremely useful checklists which evaluate the patient's ability to perform these Activities of Daily Living have been formulated and are in general use in most hospitals today. Samples may be found in almost any textbook on rehabilitation nursing.

In addition to these checklists, the nurse can further evaluate the patient's physical abilities by answering the following questions:

1. What is the condition of his skin? Is it reddened, irritated, excoriated?
   (a) Are there many caries in his teeth?
2. What kind of position does he assume in bed, in a chair?
   (a) Does he have any contractures? Are any likely to develop?
   (b) Are there any irregularities in his gait?
   (c) What body areas are subject to pressure from bedding, chairs, braces, splints, or bandages?
3. How much active exercise can he tolerate? How quickly does he become fatigued or lose interest?
   (a) How is fatigue manifested?
   (b) Must he take frequent rest periods?
4. How well can he see, hear? How accurately can he judge depth and distance?
5. Does he have any infections? Where? How long has he had them?
6. What foods does he eat? How much protein, carbohydrate, and fat

does he consume in a twenty-four hour period? Is his diet deficient in any of the essential vitamins or minerals?

7. Does he have a regular elimination pattern? Do his intake and output balance?
8. What medications is he taking? What effect do these drugs have if they are taken over a long period of time?

As you have probably recognized, this evaluation of the patient's physical problems is merely a repetition of the earlier chapters of this book which dealt with the overt nursing problems of physiological dysfunction. Its only expansion is the concept of predicting what *might* happen, with the implication that the nurse will take positive action to prevent or to minimize as many of these problems as possible.

The results of these three evaluations are used in formulating the nursing care plan in which the patient's immediate and long-term nursing problems are identified and the nursing care for each is specified. Usually the solution to individual problems is the result of the joint efforts of the nurse and another member of the rehabilitation team, or the solution of the nursing problem may be the recognition by the nurse that this particular problem should be referred to the social worker, occupational therapist, clergyman, or whomever else is best equipped to deal with it. Successful rehabilitation demands that each member of the team respects and understands the contributions each discipline makes toward the well-being of the person who has a long-term illness.

BIBLIOGRAPHY

1. Apple, Dorrian (editor): Sociological studies of health and sickness, New York, 1960, McGraw-Hill Book Co., Inc.
2. Cherkasky, Martin: Patient services in chronic disease, Public Health Reports **73:**978-981, Nov. 1958.
3. Ford, Loretta C.: The 5 elements of progressive patient care, Nursing Outlook **8:**436-439, Aug. 1960.
4. Health Education and Welfare Indicators, Washington, D. C., Dec. 1961, United States Department of Health, Education, and Welfare, Superintendent of Documents, U. S. Government Printing Office.
5. Martin, Harry W., and Prange, Arthur J.: The stages of illness—psychosocial approach, Nursing Outlook **10:**168-171, March 1962.
6. Morrissey, Alice B.: Rehabilitation nursing, New York, 1951, G. P. Putnam's Sons, Inc., pp. 3-62.
7. Rienow, Robert, and Rienow, Leona Train: The desperate world of the senior citizen, Saturday Review **44:**11-13, 55-56, Jan. 28, 1961.
8. Rusk, Howard A., et al.: Rehabilitation medicine, St. Louis, 1958, The C. V. Mosby Co., pp. 1-77.
9. Selye, Hans: The stress of life, New York, 1956, McGraw-Hill Book Co., Inc.
10. Shafer, Kathleen Newton, et al.: Medical-surgical nursing, ed. 2, St. Louis, 1961, The C. V. Mosby Co., pp. 10-45.
11. Shock, Nathan W.: The physiology of aging, Scientific American **206:**100-110, Jan. 1962.
12. Smith, Louise C.: Factors influencing continuity of nursing service. A study sponsored by National League for Nursing, Inc. Directed by Institute of Research and Service in Nursing Education, Teachers College, Columbia University, 1962.
13. Terry, Florence Jones, et al.: Principles and technics of rehabilitation nursing, St. Louis, 1957, The C. V. Mosby Co., pp. 13-41.

14. Thompson, Prescott W.: Let's take a good look at the aging, American Journal of Nursing **61**:76-79, March 1961.
15. Waterman, Theda L., and Lang, Valorus F.: Chronic illness, St. Louis, 1955, The C. V. Mosby Co.
16. Williams, Griffith W.: Illness and personality, American Journal of Nursing **63**:85-87, June 1963.

Appendix

STERILIZATION (HEAT) AND DISINFECTION (CHEMICALS)
Heat

Type of heat	*Length of time (average)*	*Article**
Steam under pressure (autoclave)	15–30 min.	Instruments, packs, gloves, glassware, syringes, sutures
Dry heat	1–2 hr.	Sharp or cutting instruments, needles, ground glassware
Boiling water	10–30 min.	Nonrusting, noncutting instruments

*Must be cleaned before exposed to heat.

Disinfection

Commonly used disinfectants include the following:
Phenol (creosote preparations)
Hexachlorophine, 1:100
Zephiran chloride, 1:1000
Alcohol, 70%
Bichloride of mercury, 1:1000
ST 37 hexylresorcinol
Iodine, 0.5-2.0%

1. Anything to be disinfected must be thoroughly cleaned first.
2. The article should be completely covered by solution.
3. The article should remain in solution for the specified length of time.
4. The length of time desired will vary with the strength of the solution.
5. The disinfectant should be removed before the article is reused.

PARACENTESIS (SURGICAL PUNCTURE OF A BODY CAVITY)
Common elements

1. Causes
   (a) Local inflammation
   (b) Obstructions from new growths
   (c) Interference in normal circulation
   (d) Fluid and electrolyte imbalance
2. Purposes
   (a) For diagnosis
   (b) Relief of pressure, discomfort, or pain
3. Anesthesia is used for all procedures: local (Novocain) for all except myringotomy, which is done under general anesthesia
4. Procedures all done by doctor
5. Surgical asepsis required

Types

1. Abdominal paracentesis (abdomen tap)
2. Thoracentesis (chest tap)
3. Rachicentesis (spinal tap-lumbar puncture)
4. Pericardial aspiration
5. Myringotomy (eardrum)
6. Paracentesis, anterior chamber of eye

Types of paracentesis

Abdominal paracentesis	Thoracentesis	Rachicentesis	Pericardial aspiration	Myringotomy	Anterior chamber of eye
Collection of fluid in peritoneal cavity	Collection of fluid in pleural space	Fluid in subarachnoid space	Fluid in pericardial sac	Used in treatment of acute purulent otitis media to provide drainage and relieve pressure in middle ear	Collection of fluid in anterior chamber
Causes: Tumors Cysts Cardiac disease Nephritis Severe anemia Cirrhosis of liver	*Causes:* Tumors following pneumonia Accompanying inflammation of adjacent organs Trauma	Usually done for diagnostic reasons to make diagnosis of tumor, isolate specific organism, or to introduce medication	*Causes:* Pericarditis Rheumatic fever Trauma		*Causes:* Tension due to glaucoma Corneal ulceration Trauma
Position of patient: Sitting up, facing doctor (provide footrest, armrest backrest)	*Position of patient:* Sitting up, back to doctor (provide footrest, table for patient to lean on)	*Position of patient:* Lying on side near edge of bed, Knees drawn up, head down (curve spine)	*Position of patient:* Dependent upon condition of patient	*Position of patient:* Done in operating room	*Position of patient:* Done in operating room under local anesthesia
Site of puncture: Midline of abdomen between umbilicus and symphysis	*Site of puncture:* Between 5th and 6th intercostal spaces in axillary line *or* between 7th and 8th intercostal spaces in scapular line	*Site of puncture:* Between 2nd and 3rd *or* 3rd and 4th lumbar vertebrae	*Site of puncture:* 5th left intercostal space	*Site of puncture:* Eardrum	*Site of puncture:* At joining of sclera and cornea
Cautions: Patient must void! May puncture urinary bladder	*Cautions:* Watch for signs of air (pneumothorax), respiratory distress, color change	*Cautions:* Patient to remain flat (no pillow) after treatment completed			

Equipment common to all types of paracentesis

Sterile:
Novocain
2 c.c. syringe: #25 needle, #22 needle
Gauze dressings, 4 × 4
Fenestrated sheet for drape
Gloves for doctor
Specimen tubes

Unsterile:
Solution for skin "prep"
Basin for refuse
Adhesive tape

Equipment special for each procedure

Abdominal paracentesis	*Thoracentesis*	*Rachicentesis*	*Pericardial aspiration*	*Myringotomy*	*Anterior chamber of eye*
Sterile:	*Sterile:*	*Sterile:*	*Sterile:*	Done in operating room	Done in operating room
Trocars and cannulae	Three-way stop cock	Three-way stop cock	20 or 50 c.c. syringe with long needles		
Scalpel with blade	Aspirating bottle with stopper and tubing	Ayer water manometer			
Scissors		Drugs if to be given			
Needle holder					
Suture needles with silk					
Tissue forceps					
Unsterile:					
Abdominal binder					
Pins					

Charting of paracentesis procedures

Name of procedure:
Doctor doing it:
Amount of fluid obtained:
Specimens to laboratory:
Condition of patient:

COMPARISON OF DIABETIC COMA AND INSULIN SHOCK

	Diabetic coma	*Insulin shock*
History		
Food	Excessive	Insufficient
Insulin	Insufficient	Excessive
Onset	Gradual: hours or days	Sudden, except with protamine zinc insulin, 24-48 hr.
Physical examination		
Appearance	Extremely ill and drowsy	Very weak and anxious
Skin	Dry and flushed	Pale, cold, clammy
Infection	Usually present	Absent
Fever	Frequent	Absent
Gastrointestinal symptoms		
Mouth	Dry	Drooling
Thirst	Intense	Absent
Hunger	Absent	Intense
Vomiting	Common	Rare (nausea)
Pain: abdominal	Frequent	Absent
Respiration	Exaggerated, air hunger (Kussmaul breathing)	Normal or shallow
Breath	Acetone odor, usual	Acetone odor may be present
Blood pressure	Low	Normal or elevated
Pulse	Weak and rapid	Full and rapid
Eyeballs	Soft	Normal
Vision	Dim	Diplopia (dilated pupils)
Tremor	Absent	Frequent
Convulsions	None	In late stages
Laboratory findings		
Urine sugar	High	Absent in 2nd specimen
Diacetic acid	High	Absent in 2nd specimen
Blood sugar	Normal or high	Below 60 mg./100 ml.
CO_2 combining power	Below 20 vol./100 ml.	Above 50 vol./100 ml.
Course		
Improvement	Gradual, within 6 to 12 hr. following use of insulin	Rapid following carbohydrate administration (1) Candy (2) Orange juice (3) Glucose or substitute

COMMONLY USED BODY POSITIONS

Name	Essence of position	Indication
Fowler's—high	Sitting upright in bed with support	Severe dyspnea from almost any cause
Semi-Fowler	Head elevated at 45°-60° angle	Upper respiratory infection, postoperative peritonitis, respiratory difficulty
Lateral prone	Patient lying on side with	Rectal examination, rectal
Sims' right or left	upper leg flexed	irrigations, patient comfort
Lithotomy	Patient lying on back, thighs flexed, lower extremities supported in stirrups	Delivery, vaginal examination and treatment, rectal examinations and treatments
Trendelenberg	Body on inclined plane with head lower than trunk and extremities	Shock Vaginal bleeding
Genupectoral (knee-chest)	Kneeling, arms and head resting on same surface as knees	Rectal examinations, proctoscopies, postpartum exercise
Dorsal recumbent	Lying on back, hips and legs flexed	Vaginal examinations and treatments, catheterization, rectal examination
Supine or dorsal	Flat in bed, lying on back	Physical examination
Prone	Lying on abdomen	Intramuscular injection, changes of position
Jackknife	Lying on side, acute flexion of head and shoulders downward and knees and thighs upward, spine curved	Lumbar puncture

COMMON IRRIGATIONS OF BODY CAVITIES
Common elements

1. Purposes
    (a) Remove contents
    (b) Relieve inflammation
    (c) Relieve discomfort or pain
    (d) Introduce medication
2. Solution inserted slowly
3. Solution temperature, 100°-105° F.
4. Tubes commonly lubricated with water-soluble surgical jelly
5. Equipment
    (a) Container for solution
    (b) Solution
    (c) Receptacle for return flow
    (d) Clean-up materials—before and after
    (e) Protection for patient from inflow or outflow

Common areas

1. Stomach
2. Bladder
3. Rectum and colon (enema and colonic)
4. Colostomy

Areas commonly irrigated

| | Stomach (lavage) | Bladder | Colon and rectum | | Colostomy |
			Enema	Colonic	
Cause	Retention, poison ingestion, preparation for surgery	Retention, infection, surgical preparation	Retention, constipation, surgical preparation	Constipation, surgical preparation	Remove contents, establish habit patterns
Tubing	Levin	Catheter	Rectal tube	Two rectal tubes, one smaller	Catheter
Insertion	To appropriate mark on tube	1½"-2"	4"-6"	6" inflow 3"-4" outflow	3"-6"
Height inflow	10"-12" above stomach	6"-8" above meatus	12"-18" above rectum	12"-18" above rectum	12"-18" above stoma
Solutions	Tap water, soda bicarbonate, normal saline, poison antidote	Normal saline, sterile water; medication may be added	Tap water, normal saline, mild soap solution	Tap water, normal saline, soda bicarbonate (1-2%)	Tap water, normal saline
Amount	500 ml. at one time until clear or up to amount ordered	150-400 ml. at one time until clear or up to amount ordered	1000-1500 ml.; maybe until clear	½ gal. up to 2 or 3 gal.	200-500 ml., increasing up to 100 ml.; patient comfort may indicate more
Technique	Clean	Sterile	Clean	Clean	Clean
Return due to	Gravity	Gravity	Peristalsis	Peristalsis	Peristalsis

Glossary

abscess A localized collection of pus, the fluid product of inflammation.

acidosis A disease characterized by reduced alkali reserve (lowered bicarbonate) of blood and body fluids.

acromegaly A disorder associated with excessive secretion of the anterior pituitary gland and characterized by enlargement of bones and soft parts, the head, hands and feet, and thorax.

alkalosis A condition in which the alkali reserve (bicarbonate) of body fluids is high.

allergy A condition in which the body cells are hypersensitive to a specific substance or substances that are usually harmless.

analgesic A pain-relieving remedy.

anaphylactic Exaggerated sensitivity to foreign protein.

anemia A condition characterized by a deficiency in the number of red blood cells and/or the amount of hemoglobin.

anesthesia Loss of sensation or feeling.

aneurysm A sac formed by dilatation of an artery.

angina pectoris Severe constricting thoracic pain, usually radiating to the left shoulder and arm; due to reduced blood supply to the heart muscle.

anion An ion with a charge of negative electricity.

ankylosis Immobility or consolidation of a joint.

anorexia Loss of appetite for food.

anoxia Decreased amount of oxygen; oxygen deficiency.

antacids Agents that counteract or neutralize acidity.

antibiotic A substance produced by living microorganisms that inhibits the growth of other microorganisms.

antibody A substance in body fluids formed in response to an antigen.

anticholinergics Antagonistic to passage of impulses through parasympathetic nerve fibers.

antigen Any material that stimulates the production of antibodies.

antipyretic A remedy that reduces fever or temperature.

anuria Suppression of urine due to failure in renal function.

apathy Indifference or no emotional response.

aphasia A weakening or loss of language facility (reading, writing, or speaking).

apnea Absence of breath or respiration.

appendicitis Inflammation of the vermiform appendix.

arrhythmia Variation or loss of rhythm in the heartbeat.

arteriogram An x-ray photograph of blood vessels.

arteriosclerosis obliterans Hardening of the arteries leading to narrowing and occlusion of the lumen of the artery.

ascites An abnormal accumulation of fluid in the peritoneal cavity.

asepsis The absence of living pathogenic organisms.

asphyxia Suffocation as a result of interference with oxygenation of the blood.

aspiration Removal by suction from a body cavity.

asthma A disorder characterized by paroxysmal attacks of dyspnea.

astringent Causing contraction of soft tissues and arresting discharges.

atelectasis Lack of air in a portion of the lungs, due either to failure to expand at birth or to the collapse of an adult lung.

atherosclerosis A form of arteriosclerosis due to the deposit of lipids in the intima and reduction of the size of the lumen of the vessel.

atrophy A wasting away or diminution in size of tissues, organs, or the entire body due to lack of nutrition.

auricular fibrillation A condition in which the normal heart rhythm is replaced by rapid irregular contractions of the auricles, working independently of the ventricles.

autistic Self-centered.

biopsy Gross and microscopic examination of tissues or cells taken from a living body.

bronchiectasis Chronic dilatation of the bronchi.

bronchogram An x-ray film of the tracheobronchial tree.

bronchoscopy Instrumental inspection of the interior of a bronchus.

cachexia A state of profound ill health marked by a general lack of nutrition and wasting.

calculus A hard inorganic body formed in a body cavity or tissue; a stone.

carcinoma Malignant neoplasm derived from epithelial tissue.

cathartic A drug causing active intestinal peristalsis.

cation An ion with a charge of positive electricity.

chemotaxis The reaction of living protoplasm with attraction or repulsion to a chemical stimulus.

chemotherapy Prevention and treatment of disease by chemical substances or drugs.

cholera An acute epidemic infectious disease characterized by profuse watery diarrhea, muscular cramps, vomiting, dehydration, and collapse.

chorea A condition characterized by irregular, spasmodic, involuntary jerking movements.

cirrhosis A chronic interstitial inflammation with hardening, degeneration, and atrophy of any organ, especially the liver.

colitis Inflammation of the colon.

colostomy The surgical establishment of an artificial opening into the colon.

coma A state of deep stupor from which the patient cannot be aroused.

concussion A violent shaking or jarring or the injury to a soft structure that results.

congestion Hyperemia in the vessels of an organ or a part.

constipation Sluggishness or inaction of the bowels.

conversion Change from one state to another; the expression of an emotion as a physical manifestation.

convulsion A violent, involuntary contraction of voluntary muscles.

covert Covered over, private, hidden, secret.

crisis A turning point in the course of an acute disease.

cyanosis A bluish color of the skin due to insufficient oxygenation of the blood.

cystitis Inflammation of the bladder.

cystoscopy Visual examination of the interior of the bladder by means of a cystoscope.

decompression The removal of pressure.

decubitus ulcer A bed sore due to prolonged pressure from lying in bed.

degeneration Deterioration; a change in cells or tissues to a lower or less active form.

dehydration Removal or loss of water, or the resulting condition.

delirium State of mental confusion and motor restlessness, characterized by disorientation, illusions, and hallucinations.

delusion A fixed, false belief that cannot be corrected.

dementia Mental deterioration.

depression A feeling of dejection and an absence of cheerfulness.

dermatitis Inflammation of the skin.

detergent An agent which cleanses.

diabetes insipidus A metabolic condition characterized by the excretion of large amounts of urine and extreme thirst.

SOUTHERN MISSIONARY COLLEGE
Division of Nursing Library

diabetes mellitus A chronic metabolic condition in which sugar is elevated in the bloodstream and excreted in abnormal amounts in the urine, usually attributed to disease of the pancreas.

diaphoresis Perspiration, sweating.

diarrhea Frequent discharge of more or less fluid fecal matter.

diplopia Double vision.

disinfection The destruction of pathogenic microorganisms and their disease-producing products.

disorientation Loss of the ability to place one's self in time and space.

distention State of being distended, or stretched out, enlarged, or swollen.

diuretic An agent that increases the secretion of urine.

diverticulosis The presence of a number of diverticula (a pouch or sac opening from a tubular or round organ) in the intestine.

dysphagia Difficulty in swallowing.

dyspnea Difficulty in breathing.

dysuria Difficulty or pain in urination.

ecchymosis An extravasation of blood into the skin; black and blue spot.

eczema An acute or chronic skin inflammation with multiform lesions.

edema An accumulation of excessive fluid in the intercellular tissue spaces of the body.

electroencephalogram A record of the electrical waves in the brain.

embolus A plug or clot occluding a blood vessel.

emesis Vomiting.

emollient A softening or soothing agent.

empathy Feeling with another person or object.

encephalitis Inflammation of the brain.

enema The injection of fluid into the rectum for therapeutic purposes.

enterostomy The surgical establishment of an artificial opening into the intestine through the abdominal wall.

erythema Redness of the skin due to congestion.

esophagoscopy Instrumental inspection of the interior of the esophagus.

exophthalmus Abnormal protrusion of the eyeballs.

extravasation An escape of fluid such as blood from a vessel into the tissues.

fibroma A benign neoplasm composed of fibrous connective tissue.

fistula An abnormal passage leading from a cavity or hollow organ to the surface or from one abscess cavity or hollow organ to another.

flatulence The presence of an abnormal amount of gas in the stomach or bowel.

flatus Gas in the digestive tract.

fluoroscopy Examination of an object by means of a fluoroscope.

gangrene Massive death or necrosis of tissue combined with putrefaction.

gastritis Inflammation of the stomach.

gastroscopy Instrumental examination of the stomach.

gastrostomy The surgical establishment of an artificial opening into the stomach.

geriatric Relating to old age.

glomerulonephritis A renal disease characterized by inflammatory changes in the glomerulus.

glycosuria The excretion of abnormal amounts of sugar in the urine.

goiter An enlargement of the thyroid gland.

hallucination A sense perception not founded on reality.

hematemesis Vomiting of blood.

hematinic Improving the hemoglobin or red blood count of the blood.

hematuria The discharge of blood or blood cells in the urine.

hemiparesis Muscle weakness affecting one side of the body only.

hemiplegia Paralysis of one side of the body.

hemophilia A hereditary disorder characterized by impaired clotting time of the blood, transmitted by females to males.

hemoptysis The spitting of blood.

hepatitis Inflammation of the liver.

hernia The projection of a loop or part of an organ or tissue from its natural cavity.

homeostasis Equilibrium in the living body with respect to chemical reaction, fluid content, and temperature.

hydronephrosis Dilatation of the kidney pelvis with urine.

hyperemia Congestion; an increased amount of blood in a part.

hyperesthesia Exaggerated sensibility to a sensory stimulus.

hyperglycemia An increased concentration of sugar in the blood.

hyperplasia An increase in the size of a tissue or an organ.

hypertension High arterial blood pressure.

hyperthyroidism A condition produced by excessive secretion of the thyroid gland.

hypertrophy A general increase in size of a tissue or organ.

hypnosis An induced condition of artificial sleep during which the subject responds to suggestion.

hypnotic A drug causing sleep.

hypodermoclysis The subcutaneous injection of a solution.

hypostatic pneumonia Pneumonia resulting from lack of activity.

hypothermia A subnormal body temperature.

hypothyroidism A clinical state resulting from decreased secretion of the thyroid gland.

hypoxia See *anoxia*.

icterus index The relative level of bilirubin in blood serum or plasma.

idiosyncrasy An individual mental or physical characteristic or peculiarity.

ileitis Inflammation of the ileum.

ileostomy The surgical establishment of an artificial opening into the ilium.

immunization The process of rendering a subject immune.

impaction State of being firmly lodged or wedged.

incontinence Inability to retain a discharge.

infarct Necrosis of tissue due to loss of blood circulation.

infestation Invasion by animal parasites.

influenza Acute infectious epidemic disease with fever, catarrhal inflammation of the respiratory or gastrointestinal tract, or nervous disturbances including headache, insomnia, convulsions, delirium, or depression.

infusion The therapeutic introduction of fluid into a vein.

insecticide An agent that destroys insects.

interstitial Situated in spaces or interstices within a structure.

intracellular Within a cell.

intramuscular Within a muscle.

intravascular Within the blood vessels or lymphatics.

intussusception Telescoping of one segment of the intestine into another.

jaundice A yellow color of the skin and deeper tissues due to bile pigment.

ketonuria Acetone bodies in the urine.

lavage The irrigation or washing out of a hollow organ.

laxative A mild cathartic.

lethargy A state of inaction or indifference; torpor or sluggishness.

lysis The gradual decline of the symptoms of an acute disease.

malaise A vague feeling of discomfort and uneasiness.

malignancy Virulency; referring to a cancerous growth as distinguished from a benign neoplasm.

meningitis Inflammation of the membranes of the brain or spinal cord.

micturition Urination.

myelogram X-ray picture of the spinal cord.

myoma A benign neoplasm composed of muscular tissue.

myringotomy Incision of the tympanic membrane.

narcosis Unconscious state produced by a narcotic drug.

narcotic A drug that produces stupor or sleep and allays pain.

nausea Sickness of the stomach; tendency to vomit.

necrosis The death of one or more cells.

negativism A tendency to do the opposite of what most people would do or of what one is requested to do.

nephrosclerosis Sclerosis or hardening of the kidney.

obstipation Intractable constipation.

oliguria Scanty urination.

orthopnea Discomfort on breathing in any but the erect position.

osteoma A benign neoplasm composed of osteoblastic connective tissue.

palliative Alleviating symptoms without cure.

pallor Paleness.

palpation Examination by means of the hand.

pancreatitis Inflammation of the pancreas.

paracentesis Surgical puncture of a cavity for the purpose of removing fluid.

paralgesia Abnormal or painful sensation.

paralysis Loss or impairment of motor and/or sensory function in a muscle through injury or disease of its nerve supply.

paraplegia Paralysis of both lower extremities and the lower part of the body.

paresis Partial or incomplete paralysis.

paresthesia An abnormal sensation such as burning, pricking, or numbness.

pathogen Any virus, microorganism, or other substance capable of producing disease.

pellagra A clinical deficiency due to lack of vitamin B characterized by gastrointestinal disturbances, erythema followed by desquamation, and nervous disorders.

peritonitis Inflammation of the peritoneum.

pneumothorax The presence of air or gas in the pleural cavity.

polydipsia Excessive thirst.

polyuria Excessive excretion of urine.

prolapse A falling down or sinking of an organ or part through an external orifice.

prophylaxis The prevention of disease.

proctoscopy Instrumental examination of the rectum and anus.

psoriasis A chronic inflammatory skin disease characterized by scaly red patches.

psychoneurosis An emotional disorder of mild or moderate intensity.

psychosis A severe emotional disorder.

psychosomatic Pertaining to the relationship of the mind and the body.

ptosis A drooping of an organ or part.

pyelonephritis Inflammation of the kidney and the renal pelvis.

pyemia The presence of pus in the blood.

pyrexia Fever.

quadriparesis Weakness of the muscles of the four extremities.

quadriplegia Paralysis of the four extremities and the body trunk.

radiopaque A substance that does not permit the passage of x-rays or any other form of radiation.

rationalization The use of a plausible justification for some act really performed for an unworthy reason.

reaction formation The exsessive development of its opposite trait to cover the existence of an unacceptable trait.

regression Return to a former state.

repression The submerging of a conscious thought into the unconscious sphere.

resuscitation To revive; to restore to life after apparent death.

retention Keeping in the body what normally should be discharged, as urine or feces.

rickets A clinical deficiency due to a lack of vitamin D occurring in infants and young children and characterized by softening of the bones and malnutrition.

sarcoma A highly malignant tumor composed of connective tissue neoplasm.

sclerosis An induration or hardening.

sedative An agent that is calming and quieting.

senile Pertaining to old age.

septicemia A systemic disease due to the presence of pathogenic microorganisms or their toxins in the blood.

shock Peripheral circulatory collapse.

sigmoidoscopy Instrumental examination of the interior of the sigmoid colon.

sign Objective evidence of a disease.

somnifacient An agent that produces sleep.

spasm An involuntary convulsive muscular contraction.

stasis Stagnation of the blood or other fluids.

sterile Free from living microorganisms.

sterilization The process of the destruction of all microorganisms in or about an object.

stricture A localized contraction or stenosis of a tubular structure.

suppression Complete failure of secretion of a fluid, as urine or bile.

surrogate Something or someone put in the place of another.

symptom Any perceptible change from the normal in function, appearance, or sensation indicative of disease.

syncope Fainting.

tenesmus Painful straining to evacuate the bowels.

thoracentesis A surgical puncture into the cavity of the chest to remove accumulated fluid.

thromboangiitis Inflammation of the inner lining of a blood vessel with thrombosis.

thrombophlebitis Inflammation of a vein—accompanied by thrombus formation.

thrombus A blood clot occluding a blood vessel.

toxoid A toxin treated to destroy its toxic property but still capable of inducing the production of antibodies.

tracheotomy The surgical establishment of an opening into the trachea.

tranquilizer A drug that promotes tranquility by calming without depressing patients.

tremor Quivering; shaking.

tumor Neoplasm; an enlargement due to a mass of cells multiplying independently of the normal rate of growth and serving no useful purpose.

turgor Normal cell tension; swelling.

ulcer An open lesion on the surface of the skin or mucous membrane.

uremia A toxic condition resulting from an excess of urea and other nitrogenous wastes in the blood.

urticaria Hives; an eruption of pale wheals accompanied by severe itching.

vaccine A preparation of dead or attenuated organisms that stimulate defense mechanisms and are used to prevent disease.

varices Enlarged and twisted veins.

vasoconstrictor An agent that constricts blood vessels.

vasopressor An agent that raises blood pressure.

vector Any living carrier that transfers pathogenic microorganism from the sick to the well.

ventriculogram An x-ray of the ventricles of the brain.

vertigo Sensation of dizziness; a feeling of an irregular or whirling motion.

virus An ultramicroscopic group of pathogens.

volvulus A twisting of the bowel upon itself causing obstruction.

vomitus Matter ejected from the stomach.

Index

Date	DUE		
9/13/64	Res Neu I		
8/1/65	"		

Library Bureau Cat. No. 1138

SOUTHERN MISSIONARY COLLEGE
Division of Nursing Library